The World of Surgery
1945–1985

JAMES D. HARDY, M.D.
The World of Surgery
1945–1985
Memoirs of One Participant

upp
UNIVERSITY OF PENNSYLVANIA PRESS
Philadelphia

Copyright © 1986 by the University of Pennsylvania Press
All rights reserved

Library of Congress Cataloging-in-Publication Data

Hardy, James D., 1918–
   The world of surgery, 1945–1985.

   Includes index.
   1. Hardy, James D., 1918–   2. Surgeons—United
States—Biography.   3. Surgery—History—20th century.
I. Title. [DNLM: 1. Surgery—personal narratives.
WZ 100 H2694]
   RD27.35.H38A38   1986   617'.092'4 [B]   85-26340
ISBN 0-8122-8000-8 (alk. paper)

Printed in the United States of America

TO MY WIFE

O happy eyes
How much you have seen
For better, for worse;
How fair it has been!
—Goethe, *Faust II*

CONTENTS

Preface ix

PART I. *Alabama 1918–1938*

CHAPTER 1 *Growing Up in Alabama* 5
CHAPTER 2 *College at the University of Alabama* 19

PART II. *Philadelphia 1938–1951*

CHAPTER 3 *Medical School at the University of Pennsylvania* 31
CHAPTER 4 *Internship at University of Pennsylvania Hospital* 58
CHAPTER 5 *Medical Resident at Penn* 70
CHAPTER 6 *With the U.S. Army in England, France, and Germany (From a Medical Officer's Journal)* 78
CHAPTER 7 *The 1940s: The Rise of Physiologic Surgery* 120
CHAPTER 8 *Isidor Schwaner Ravdin* 124
CHAPTER 9 *Resident in General Surgery at Penn* 132
CHAPTER 10 *Resident in Thoracic Surgery and Surgical Staff at Penn* 144
CHAPTER 11 *The 1950s: Cardiovascular Surgery Comes of Age* 159

PART III. *Memphis 1951–1955*

CHAPTER 12 *The Medical College of the University of Tennessee: Surgery Staff Member and Director of Surgical Research* 167

PART IV. *Jackson 1955–*

CHAPTER 13 *A New Medical School Is Established in Jackson* 183

CHAPTER 14 Human Organ Transplantation   240
CHAPTER 15 The First Lung Transplant in Man   264
CHAPTER 16 The First Heart Transplant in Man   269
CHAPTER 17 The Developing Department of Surgery: Further Progress   289
CHAPTER 18 Called Urgently to Peru   313
CHAPTER 19 National and International Participation and Awards   320
CHAPTER 20 The 1970s: The Practice of Surgery Is Changing   339
CHAPTER 21 The Surgeon Becomes the Patient: My Own Operations   343
CHAPTER 22 Family   351
CHAPTER 23 A Look Backward and a Summing Up   362

Index   373

PREFACE

I am well aware that a certain degree of presumption is inevitably associated with the writing of one's memoirs. This tacit sacrifice of humility has in fact been the only major constraint in the writing of this book. Nonetheless, the manuscript, intellectually discarded in the permanent files many times, has now been published. For unless a manuscript is actually rendered into print and published, it is rarely preserved.

The Civil War diary of my paternal grandfather, for whom I was named, surfaced and was printed and circulated privately a great many years after his death. It gave insights into his early years and character that could not have been known in any other way. In contrast, my own father spoke rarely of his childhood and almost never about his father, although I knew from a man who had worked for both of them that there had been an easy relationship between the two. When I had reached the age when one becomes interested in knowing more about one's parents' earlier lives, it was too late. Hence, if nothing else, this book may serve to impart to my children something of their father's orientation and life experiences. However, I hope that it may also reflect the world of surgery in the United States from 1945 to 1985. Surely this period will be looked upon as one in which great advances in surgical physiology and anesthesiology were made, when many new surgical specialties developed and flowered, and when arterial surgery, open-heart surgery, organ transplantation, and the artificial heart and other medical prostheses came into clinical surgical practice.

The most difficult decision in writing an autobiography, other than whether or not to write it in the first place, is that of what and how much to reveal. Some biographies offer virtually no insight into what genetic and environmental forces shaped their subjects' early and most formative years, as if the individuals had sprung full-grown upon the scene. This represents only half a life. Furthermore, if the early years are not presented with at least some degree of candor and objectivity, the space consumed would be better used elsewhere in the volume. This forthrightness applies with special poignancy to my childhood in Alabama, for by the time I went to Philadelphia to medical school at the age of twenty, my codes and principles were pretty well set, though they were perhaps not fixed permanently until about thirty-five.

Having come from a fairly large and closely knit family, I could have asked each living member to review my remembrances of those days long ago. In the end I did not do this, for inevitably their memories would vary and, in that case, whose would I adopt?

The book presents my recollections about many persons, issues, and events. However, being a collector—some would say a pack rat—I have had available annual notebooks dating back to internship days, a journal kept during military service in World War II, and, in addition, large files of correspondence, diaries kept over various years, and the complete files of the Department of Surgery since the opening of the University of Mississippi Medical Center in 1955. Even so, my conversations or statements imparted to others were rarely written down verbatim at the time; thus, my recollections of them must naturally be imperfect. In this respect, therefore, I ask a certain indulgence from the reader. Moreover, I should emphasize that this volume is in fact a memoir, not a formal history of United States and world surgery during the period covered. The particular value of a memoir, however, as opposed to a history by a removed and thus detached historian, is that the special perceptions of the author, at the time, are thus recorded.

Finally, some words of appreciation. First, my deep gratitude to my parents, wife, and children is reflected throughout the volume. They have illuminated the eternal dimensions of family life. Beyond this, it is not possible to acknowledge individually the host of people who have contributed to my life and career, including those who to a degree may have disputed the way but who in so doing contributed to my inner growth and perceptivity.

Teachers at all levels—high school, college, medical school, and hospital residencies—served as role models and brought me slowly to realize that I would be honored to teach. Relationships with students at all levels have been the single most rewarding and continuously challenging activity of my professional life. A close second has been the privilege of knowing the innate nobility of countless sick patients in all stations of life.

Virtually my entire professional career has been spent at the University of Mississippi Medical Center; for affording me this opportunity, I tender particular appreciation and respect to the memories of Chancellor J. D. Williams and Dean David S. Pankratz.

To assist the completion of the manuscript itself, I asked several people to read the material for gross errors of fact and to make critical suggestions. For this, keen appreciation is expressed particularly to Mrs. Jean Bunge and Dr. Thomas M. Blake. Last, but most important, Mrs. Evelyn G. Gardiner's outstanding word processor activity throughout numerous drafts of the manuscript, and Mrs. Virginia W. Keith's always superb proofreading, are gratefully acknowledged. The efficiency, editing, and accuracy of the University of Pennsylvania Press have been exemplary.

The World of Surgery
1945–1985

PART I

*Alabama
1918–1938*

CHAPTER 1

Growing Up in Alabama

Hamburg, Germany, September 7, 1983

The meeting of the general assembly of the International Society of Surgery. The president: "I am pleased to announce that the new president-elect is Dr. James D. Hardy of Jackson, Mississippi, U.S.A. He will serve as president of the next congress in Paris in 1985 and thereafter preside as international president through our congress in Sydney, Australia, in 1987."

It's a long way to Hamburg from the small hamlet of Newala, Alabama, in 1918.

Julia Ann Poynor married Fred Henry Hardy in 1917, when they were thirty-five and fifty, respectively. She was a very attractive brunette with brown eyes and hair, and he was a handsome man with early gray hair and bright blue eyes. In 1918, my mother was sent to the hospital in Birmingham by our family doctor because she seemed too big for normal pregnancy. A baby boy, Julian Patterson Hardy, weighing five and a half pounds, was born uneventfully on May 14. However, things did not look quite right with the mother. Suddenly the nurse exclaimed, "I think there's another one, Mrs. Hardy." And, indeed, James Daniel Hardy, weighing four and a half pounds, followed Julian at an interval of sixteen minutes, allowing Julian always to claim that he was the oldest. A twin is special, and Julian was a special twin. There were to be few cross words between us and never animosity.

Mother returned home to Newala, Alabama, thirty-five miles south of Birmingham, which was a long way then. This hamlet, located about two miles from an old cemetery atop a hill said to be the geographical center of Alabama, was virtually "Hardyville." Father's lime plant, which manufactured calcium oxide from natural limestone, was the principal, indeed the only, industrial enterprise in

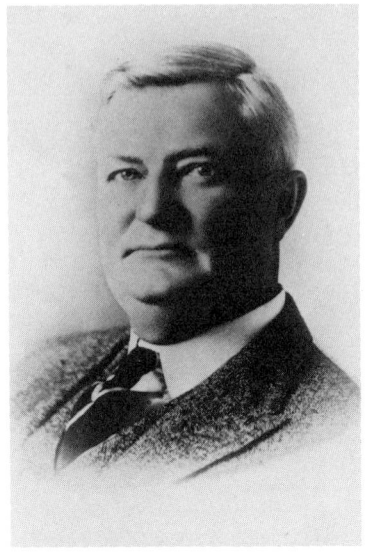
Fred Henry Hardy

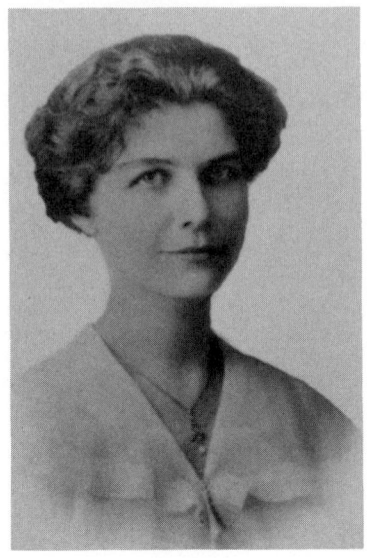
Julia Poynor Hardy

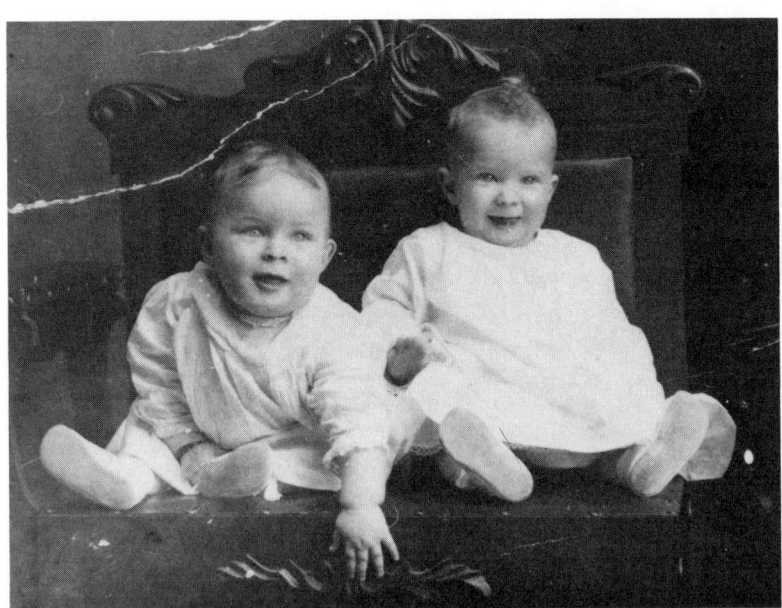
Julian Patterson Hardy (left) *and James Daniel Hardy*

that farming community. Native limestone was hauled from the deep quarry about a half mile away; the tramcar was then hoisted up an incline and the rock was dumped into one of the forty- to sixty-foot-tall open furnaces (kilns). The calcium carbonate limestone then settled through the intense heat, over a period of about forty-eight hours, and was harvested below as white calcium oxide, lime. It was sold in bulk or reduced to a white powder and bagged. We also farmed and ran the small post office. The name Newala, from "New" for New York and "Ala" for Alabama, was coined by my father, who had been born in New York state, his wife, in Alabama. Father had grown up in nearby Calera where his father, James Daniel Hardy, also had manufactured lime. A deep, virtually pure limestone deposit ran through Shelby County.

Father had attended the University of Tennessee and Maryville College, both in Knoxville. His ancestors were of Scottish extraction and Presbyterian.

Mother, whose family was of English ancestry and Episcopalian, was from Mt. Hebron near Eutaw, Alabama. Her father, Captain Diggs Poynor, had graduated from Virginia Military Institute and had taught military science and tactics at the University of Alabama

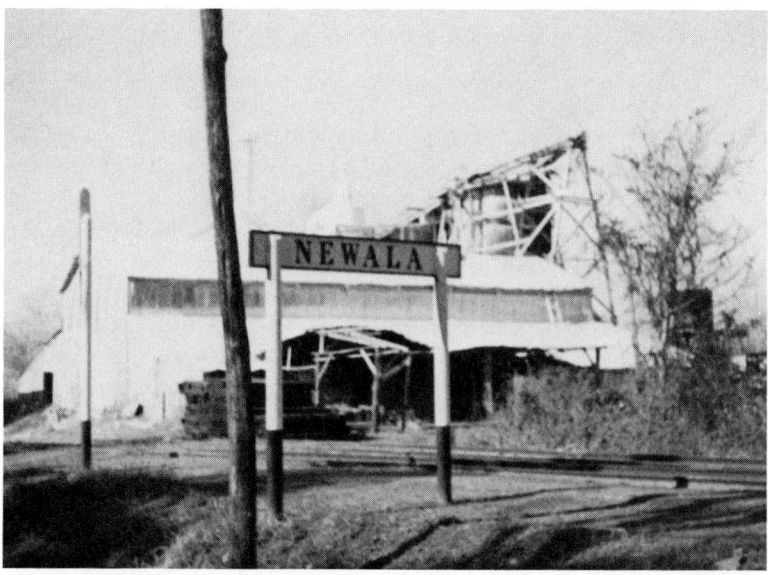

Newala Lime Works, Newala, Alabama

at Tuscaloosa from 1861 to 1865. After the Civil War he bought a plantation at Mt. Hebron, about fifty miles away, and founded a private one-room school which emphasized Latin, Greek, mathematics, and English. Mother and her sisters were expected to learn to sew, play the piano, and cook—though there were always black cooks in the kitchen. My mother went from her father's school to the University of Alabama, where she graduated summa cum laude and Phi Beta Kappa, and subsequently received an advanced degree in Latin from Columbia University, an unusual accomplishment for a woman in those days. In due course she taught Latin at Alabama College for Women at Montevallo.

Marriage and family came late, but then rapidly. Mother had the new fraternal twins, James with curly blond hair and blue eyes, and Julian with darker straight hair and grey-blue eyes; in addition, she had four stepchildren, aged seven to fifteen, whose mother had died some years earlier. Eighteen months later Taylor, my youngest brother, was added to this household of six children. Mother usually fed Julian, Taylor, and me our supper on the back steps, before the rest of the family. We would always look west and say, "Goodnight, Mr. Sun."

The oldest of the four stepchildren, Agnes ("Sister"), was to go to Alabama College for Women, four miles distant in Montevallo, and John to the University of Alabama soon after that. Later, Emily ("Dolly") also went to Montevallo College, and Fred, the youngest, to Auburn.

We were a happy family and remained close as we grew up, I think in part because of Mother's absolute dedication to winning the love and respect of her four stepchildren, who reciprocated warmly. We were all treated the same, share and share alike.

Our house was not ornate, but it was home and a solid refuge. We had running water, a rarity in that community, by virtue of the lime plant's needs. Heating was by open fireplace, or wood and coal stove. We used kerosene (coal oil) lamps, later a Delco generator to make our own electricity, and eventually power from the Alabama Power Company. The frame house was often cold and drafty, and respiratory infections played a prominent part in our lives. There was no effective treatment for the sinister lobar pneumonia, long before sulfonamides and antibiotics, but mustard plasters were applied to the chest for counter-irritation, and sponge baths and aspirin were given to control the fever. The doctor's most important contribution was to sit up with the patient and wait for the fever to break (the "crisis"), a good prognostic sign.

say the Presbyterian "forgive us our *debts*, as we forgive our *debtors*" instead of the Episcopalian "forgive us our *trespasses*, as we forgive those who *trespass* against us."

Julian and I abruptly came face to face with the reality of school at the age of six. Actually, since Mother had been a schoolteacher, first teaching Latin and mathematics in high school and then at Alabama College for Women before she married, we had been taught since earliest childhood. In fact, Mother continued to correct our spelling and grammar in our college letters and for the rest of her life. Not satisfied with the Newala public grade school, for which Father had given the land, Mother bought two standard school desks and chairs, and Julian and I "went to school" from eight to twelve in the front room, or parlor as it was called. Taylor, a year and a half younger and with no one to play with, was apt to lie on the floor and listen, and he often chirped up with an answer before we could. Julian once fumed, "I wish the baby was here; he'd know the answer." Classes were interrupted one day when it was found that the Negro who dumped the limerock into the kilns had been overcome by fumes and had fallen in. He had been slowly cooked, and had to be hoisted out by his strong leather belt. His wife was given one hundred dollars, even though there was no such thing as workmen's compensation then and no payment of any sort was required. Although the modern workmen's compensation system is often abused, I often think back to John Grady and realize its necessity.

Another episode at about this time concerned Jimmie Lee Johnson, who was shot by an irate husband as he fled the man's home. The .30–.30 rifle bullet blew a two-inch hole in his tibia, and the inevitable infection set in. He went back and forth to the hospital in Selma for months on end but steadfastly refused amputation. And he proved to be right, for the wound finally healed. He walked on an elevated shoe, but he got back his prestigious job of firing the steam boiler that ran the lime-manufacturing machinery. Far into the future, this experience was to render me very conservative in amputating legs as a surgeon.

Julian and I enrolled in the fourth grade in the local school when we were eight. After three years at Newala grade school, learning nothing that I remember, though I recall our young schoolteacher had trouble keeping order, we rode the school bus to the consolidated high school at Montevallo.

The seventh-grade homeroom teacher was Miss Rispah ("Ripsaw") Dudley, from "right down on the Rappahannock River in Virginia." She was probably in her mid-forties at the time, and was rather short and plump. Her dark hair was beginning to show faint streaks of gray, and her cavernous bosom became the seemingly bottomless repository for such varied items confiscated from misbehaving boys as marbles, spinning tops, and even, some hinted, frogs. She was a firm disciplinarian but jolly, and we liked and respected her.

Miss Dudley's specialty was geography, which she loved, and I recall that one class project was to construct a large-scale map of the United States, each student being responsible for one state. My assigned state was Colorado, on which I pasted a sheep and a cow and various other products of Colorado (but not skiing). The completed map hung on her homeroom wall for years. I have always had a special feeling for Colorado since then.

During this year, however, I got pneumonia and was a long time shaking it off. Lobar pneumonia was then a dread disease. A neighboring dairy farmer died of it in just three or four days, and thereafter his dairy and young family soon disintegrated. Father, John, Fred, and Taylor each almost died of pneumonia. As soon as a diagnosis of pneumonia was made, the car would be sent for Mrs. Sarah Crim who lived near Calera, about three miles away. "Miz Sarah," as she was called, would put on her white uniform, pack her suitcase, and move into our home for the duration of the illness. A rather short and roly-poly brunette of perhaps forty-five, she was a tower of strength in our midst. She saw to it that the doctor's orders for mustard plasters to the chest, cool sponge baths, and aspirin were carried out. She relieved Mother at the bedside, and she was unfailingly optimistic. Few people in hospitals can appreciate the respect and authority accorded the trained nurse in a rural community.

Dr. C. O. Lawrence, the local physician, would come out from Calera as often as he could, and as the crisis approached he would sit by the bedside all night drinking coffee, leaving at daylight to begin his daily office and house calls. Later on, he was accused of using a controlled substance and he moved away, but no accusation could have altered what he meant to us.

For my illness this time, my parents had chosen Dr. Lawrence, who believed in "feeding a fever," rather than another one who believed in "starving a fever." Among doctors the treatment for fevers other than malaria (which was treated with quinine) was otherwise much the same; only such symptomatic treatments as those mentioned above were available, since there were no antibacterial drugs then. Once I was out of bed, our doctor recommended that I be taken to a specialist in Montgomery. The pediatrician ordered that I stay out of school for three months. My parents took his advice, since I was clearly "doing porely," but I tried to keep up with the schoolwork and, at the end of the term, was given special examinations. I passed (without distinction) and was allowed to go on to the eighth grade with Julian the next fall. Meanwhile, I had formed a life-long habit of reading.

I had no more serious illnesses in high school, but I did develop one pesky problem that taught me early the difference between a good bedside manner and a secure laboratory diagnosis. I had contracted an intestinal parasite which we later learned was the result of inadequately cooked pork. Over a period of about a year, I was taken to two different local doctors who prescribed numerous treatments of one sort or another to no avail. One day Father saw me looking thoroughly dejected and asked, "Son, what's the matter?" I replied that I was still passing the parasite and was terribly discouraged. He told me to jump in the car and drive about twelve miles to where our former doctor had moved. Dr. Lawrence said at once that the only way to be sure was to send a stool specimen to the state laboratory in Montgomery. The correct diagnosis was returned in days, I took a single dose of the appropriate medicine, and I was completely cured.

When I was in high school, Miss Zelinski arrived from Chicago to be the music teacher. Can you imagine the name Zelinski in Montevallo, Alabama? Virtually every soul had an Anglo-Saxon name, for the blacks usually bore the family names of people who had once owned slaves. Everybody was Protestant, with the exception of a Jewish family and a family suspiciously whispered to be *Catholics* who disappeared to Birmingham occasionally and were said to have gone to something called mass. The Jewish family, the Klotzmans, were in the dry goods business. We always dropped by their store to visit, and I had my eye on a pair of hunting boots that were on sale for $2.75. "Joe," I said, "I haven't saved quite enough money yet. How much will the boots be after the sale?" Shielding his mouth with his hand, he replied, "Same thing," and I knew he meant the same for me.

Miss Zelinski, a petite, dark brunette presumably of Polish extraction, was a dynamo. She taught both choral singing and band, and she could play a variety of the school's venerable instruments.

Miss Lillian ("Big Lil") Barksdale had homeroom for the eighth grade, and she taught civics and history. Tall, rarely smiling, not quite gaunt, with her brown hair drawn severely in a bun at the nape of her neck, she projected a stern visage. And yet, she was not nearly as sinister as she looked, and she certainly taught well. I remember one day when the august county superintendent of education, and parents, were to visit our civics class. Miss Barksdale had named me President Hoover, and I was to conduct a meeting of my cabinet consisting of specified classmates. Well, we were conducting the nation's business quite smoothly until I turned to Postmaster General Reid and asked him if he thought the letter stamp could be reduced from two cents to one. Unfortunately, Mr. Postmaster General panicked, turned red, and finally blurted out that he did not think the American people would stand for this reduction. At this the audience began to giggle, and from then on the cabinet meeting lost momentum.

Meanwhile, I was suffering some of the things that boys often have to suffer. I had very curly hair, the only one in the family except Mother who did, and my brothers teased me mercilessly. I apparently had got over a slight lisp, which I don't remember, but I had to wear braces on my teeth. And the pimples of approaching puberty were endless, no matter how many cakes of Fleischmann's yeast I choked down on the advice of our family doctor.

At home at Newala (note that I did not say *in* Newala, for the place was hardly big enough to be *in*) my father believed in hard work and in chores and routine tasks for boys. He also made it possible for us to work and get paid for it. Since he was the only employer within walking distance, he alone could hire us. Although children were not allowed to work around the lime kilns, the manufacturing plant, or down in the limestone quarry—this was because of exposed machinery and other hazards, though injuries were remarkably few—one could first be water boy to the workmen, then later hoe corn from sunup to sundown for fifty cents a day. Grown men with families got $1.00 a day or sometimes $1.25. This looks like a pathetic amount, but the depression was at hand and a large loaf of bread cost only five cents. Most people had gardens. Finally, a boy could graduate to having his own horse or mule to plough, or to scrape dirt off the limerock. Also, each year I farmed my own plot of an acre or so and in addition raised chickens. I sold the produce in the commissary and bought a case of wonderful-smelling shotgun shells in the fall.

Extended families and close ties with relatives were still the norm in Alabama. My only living grandparent was our maternal grandmother, and she would tell us about how the Federal troops had burned everything when they came through during the Civil War. The South still smarted from defeat and Reconstruction, and "the Nawth" and (damn) Yankees were still viewed with considerable suspicion and circumspection. About this time Uncle Dudley Poynor, one of Mother's brothers who, after graduating from the University of Alabama, had returned home to run the family plantation, gave me a lifelong interest. "James," he asked, "do you hunt?" I did hunt. "What do you hunt?" Squirrels and rabbits. "Son," he gravely intoned, wearing a pained expression, "*gentlemen* hunt birds [quail]." He then gave me a superb German short-haired liver-and-white pointer bitch, Belle, and thereafter I was to have a pointer wherever possible, and to enjoy this sport with my comrade in arms, the dog.

One day Father bought a load of cattle that included a young Jersey heifer. He said we could have her calves if we learned to milk her, and we named her Little Rose. Sadly, one day a sharp rock thrown by one of us cut her right eye, and all the clear jellylike insides ran down her face, rendering the eye blind. It was my first stark realization of what careless stoning could do to an animal. We also learned about the "let down" reflex long before we studied the posterior pituitary gland in medical school: any farmer knew that a cow, especially if angry, might not "give down" her milk until put with her calf.

During the depression our finances went from bad to worse. Whereas only an order for a box-car load of lime was welcomed during the 1920s, soon an order for a truckload was a time for rejoicing, and finally even a fifty-pound bag was sold with alacrity. It was a time of no building construction, there was less water purification, and farmers bought almost no lime.

Theft became an increasing problem, and cattle were slaughtered in the pasture. Ripe corn ears were ripped off in the field during darkness. The commissary was burglarized, and one night someone tinkered with the car out in the garage, about sixty feet from the house. Hoboes came daily, asking for handouts.

One particular vignette of those depression days stands out in my mind. A little black boy, "Buck" Hawkins, son of one of the neighborhood workmen, came over on a Christmas morning. I asked, "Buck, did you have a good Christmas?"

"Yeah," he said, "I'se had a good Christmas."

"What did Santa Claus bring you, Buck?"

"A orange," he replied.

Finally, one day we saw Mother crying and gradually wormed the truth out of her: Our beloved place, modest as it was, had been advertised for sale in the county newspaper for nonpayment of taxes. What would we do, Father now being over sixty? It was the lowest point of the depression for us.

Blessed be his name, a Mr. Aaron of Meridian, Mississippi, took a five-thousand-dollar mortgage on the house, the lime plant, and the approximately twelve-hundred acres of land. The taxes were paid and the equipment repaired. This enabled us to get some lime business as President Roosevelt got public works building under way. We finally dug out of the pit, but not before a prolonged and bitter strike precipitated by the firing of a union member chronically drunk on the job—his was the crucial one of running the hoisting engine that pulled the loaded tramcars out of the deep limestone quarry. This irresponsible strike—at times violent (electrical transformers were dynamited and strategic points were manned with rifles) and militantly prolonged by strikers from regional coal mines—was to color permanently my attitude toward unions. Many years later, as soon as possible, I paid off the mortgage on our home. I took my wife and the girls out to dinner, in full party dress, and had a "mortgage burning ceremony."

As the depression deepened, spending money was truly scarce. Our allowance was thirty-five cents a week. Since movie admission was twenty-five cents, one had to let the girl go in first on her own finances, after which the boy would go in, happen to see her there, and slip in beside her in the conveniently empty seat. Afterward, we would either have two five-cent sodas at Wilson's Drug Store or, more often, a Coke at her home. We also played a lot of bridge. Though we had little money, one thing we did have was gasoline from the Newala pump—as much as Father could spare—and having the car to drive around in was a lot.

Happily, my financial situation was improved by the launching of a dance orchestra by three Mahaffeys, the three youngest Hardys, and three others. Actually, I was not invited to play at the beginning. They did not need my clarinet, which I had bought second hand by selling vegetables, but they did need a trombone, so I bought one for twenty dollars at a pawn shop in Birmingham. I gradually taught myself to play by matching on the trombone notes that Mother struck on the piano. (Mother played the instrument, too, at first.) The "Bama Skippers" played successfully until the Hardys scattered to college.

I went out for varsity football my junior year in high school. I weighed only about 120 pounds and, as I was not an adept ball handler, my only hope was to make it in the line. Unfortunately, I was only able to make the second team or "scrubs" that year, while Julian played quarterback. Mother, who took the car and a load of players to the away games each Friday afternoon of the season, said, "But, James, you are doing the noble part." I said I didn't want to do the noble part, I wanted to play on the varsity. The next year I weighed over 130 pounds and made the team at right guard. Our team had two and one-half sets of twins. I have always valued the high school football—the anticipation of the relished Friday-afternoon competition, the camaraderie of the team members, the adjustment to "you win some, you lose some," the singleness of purpose, and the realization that while hard physical contact between men may smart considerably, it will not prove fatal. Lastly, one learns that victory may lie just one last thrust ahead, so never quit—not a bad motto for a surgeon.

Even though it was 1934, there was never any question in our family that we were going to college. We had our choice: Alabama or Auburn. It never occurred to us to go anywhere else, even if our parents could have afforded it.

Like most high school students, I had no very specific career plans. My earliest inclination had been to be a farmer, for I enjoyed seeing crops and livestock grow, still do. But with the years, it had become obvious that farming was a very uncertain business: it either did *not* rain, and the crop was "burned up," or it *did* rain, so much and so long that the weeds took over the crop because one could not get in to cultivate or harvest it. Moreover, there really did not seem to be enough intellectual content in farming. Perhaps not surprisingly, of the five boys in the family, none wanted to continue the lime business after what we had seen during the depression. Next, the idea of being a teacher, perhaps of English, intrigued me, for languages ran strong in Mother's family. However, as college became more imminent, I fell under the influence of two of my peers. My two best nonfamily cronies were Alan Gresky and Glen Elliott. They were perhaps two years older than I, played tennis well, and I admired them. Both had entered premed at Alabama the year before, and they urged me to try it. Julian simply joined me. These friends later dropped out of premed: Glen was called up as an officer and was a full colonel when I last heard early in World War II, and Alan became a physicist at Oak Ridge Institute of Nuclear Studies.

When a representative of the University of Alabama visited our high school to talk with prospective students, Julian and I told him we were thinking of premed, though there had been no doctors in our family. He promptly discouraged us, saying that a medical education was too long and that our father could not afford the cost, especially with Taylor coming to college soon. But the college interviewer did not know my parents. Father said that if he couldn't sell lime he could always sell a load of cattle to pay for board and tuition, and Mother successfully reapplied to teach Latin at "the college."

Thus, my senior year went along with a rush, with football, a lead in the senior play, playing in the dance band, fun, and of course classes. One omission in my education was to prove a hardship later: the school taught virtually no science, and mathematics ended with plane geometry and perhaps a smattering of algebra. Just before the last six weeks of school, a good friend of mine and I were told that our grades were tied and that the final six weeks would decide who would lead the senior class. Well, John made an A in French and I made a B; as a result he gave the valedictorian address and I the salutatorian address.

And so, on to *college*. As we departed the home environment, I announced that I had milked my last cow and taken my last dose of castor oil. That has stood.

CHAPTER 2

College at the University of Alabama

Julian and I went to college one day in early September, 1935, in a Chevrolet sedan which sported a spare tire on each side of the hood. We had learned to drive several years earlier, simply by trial and error in the middle of a large, flat hayfield where we could hit nothing. However, I think Father drove us over to Tuscaloosa. It was only sixty miles away, but the trip over dirt roads and shallow creeks that had to be forded was arduous. Mother was rather silent, but Father gave us a serious talk on the perils and pitfalls of misspent time and activities at college. At seventeen, we were just as impatient with, and impervious to, such advice as my own children were to be in the years to come. ("Daddy is going to give us one of his heavy talks, Girls.")

Mother had arranged through friends for us to room in a private home in town, about a mile from the university campus. She reasoned that we would be looked after and would have a quiet place to study, away from the distractions and frivolities of campus dormitory life. As it turned out, however, we wasted a large amount of time walking back and forth, and there were temptations right there in the home. Since we had all three of our meals there, we made the twenty- to thirty-minute walk to classes in the morning, then two ways again for dinner (as the noon meal was called in the South), and then back for supper. And, if we had to go back to school later for some reason, another forty to sixty minutes were lost. Moreover, at night we were hungry and unable to begin studying hard until we had had something to eat. As often as not, the landlady's son was late, and the usually good supper was always held up until Sonny arrived. Afterward, Sonny and his father would urge Julian and me to play "just two or three hands" of bridge before we settled down for the evening—and you know how that stretched on and on. When we finally started studying, it was often late and we were tired. We wasted a great deal of time that year.

Another problem with living off campus was that we did not have the benefit of information and advice from classmates and upperclassmen in premed. I had a nagging uneasiness that all was not well with my classwork, but in high school I had taken everything in stride and I had no serious doubt that, if necessary, I could do well on the midterm examinations by cramming. Also, I had made the football band with my fine new golden trombone, which I had bought with my dance-band money the previous summer, and each weekend we went to Birmingham or elsewhere with the football team. Bear Bryant was playing end at the time. Later I began to travel around the state with the glee club (Schumann's "Träumerei" was my sentimental favorite). Pi Kappa Alpha fraternity activities also took time. Hell week was memorable for much hazing, including paddling: one midnight I was sent out to find thirteen one-gallon syrup buckets by six the next morning; another midnight I was sent on a (successful) search for a white rat (I did not know at the time that such a thing existed); and on the last night we stripped and were doused with thick syrup from scalp to toe, overlaid with corn flakes and then clothing, and then dumped blindfolded on a deserted road about fifteen miles out in the country. And, at the end, there was a gripping and almost mystical secret initiation ceremony, read by the president by the light of a single, flickering candle in the otherwise dark attic chapter room: "I shall hold myself worthy of opprobrium and scorn if. . . ."

Clearly, I was heeding the advice of some fraternity men that I should not let my studies interfere with my college education. It was a great time in many ways but, still, we were teenagers trying to find ourselves, and I felt a vague unhappiness at being pulled in so many directions. My mid-year grades were generally acceptable, good in English and German but with a D in algebra. This flirtation with disaster in math was a warning that I noted but did not heed.

The decision to accept the opportunity to exchange my rifle in the ROTC for my trombone in the military band was one of the best decisions of my life, for it led to playing in the concert orchestra and acquiring a lasting appreciation for classical music. As a land grant college, Alabama required two years of ROTC for all able-bodied male students, the others being required to take physical education. "Colonel" Carleton Butler, a mustachioed brunette whose long, straight black hair flopped forward over his eyes and then backward with movements of his head, was director of all three instrumental groups—the football and military bands and the concert orchestra. A recent arrival from a school in Birmingham, he was a musician to his toes. The bands, of course, concentrated on standard Sousa marches and school songs, the concert orchestra on classical overtures (*Oberon, Die Meistersinger,* etc.) and waltzes.

In the spring I wrote my parents a status report. I felt quite secure in German and in English composition, somewhat less so in chemistry and zoology, and least of all in trigonometry. Freshman inorganic chemistry was essentially a lecture course to a large class, with little individual or laboratory instruction. In zoology, however, the teachers did know each student by name. C. G. Breckinridge was a demanding but master instructor. Father wrote back, "Son, here's where I get in the game. When I have a problem, I hire an expert. Go hire a math tutor, whatever it costs." Several of us did so, but the woman had ten such students in difficulty, and no one got special attention. Julian and I remained deeply apprehensive. With a weak high school background in math to start with, we had let too many months pass without really understanding how to derive the formulas and then work the problems.

The day of reckoning came. When the trigonometry questions were handed out on the final exam, I saw at a glance that I would fail. A good friend, a French horn player from Pittsburgh and an excellent math student, looked back and saw my face and whispered, "Hardy, do you want some help?" I saw I needed the answer to only one question to pass, and I was sorely tempted. I admit it. But I knew in my heart that I deserved just what I was getting. And I knew that neither I nor my parents could countenance cheating. I shook my head ruefully, no, and proceeded to do the best I could. It did not help that we had sat up all night studying, a stupid act that I never repeated. We were so dazed from lack of sleep that we weren't able to use what we did know, which was not enough.

I failed trigonometry.

And it had probably cost me Phi Beta Kappa. What a collapse. I had netted an A in English composition and German, and B's and C's on the rest. But I had failed a course. It was a colossal humiliation. When she heard, Mother wept quietly, and I well knew how terribly disappointed she was, after all her efforts.

My first real failure in life.

The next two weeks were a miserable time, while I reexamined myself and my future. Bad as the situation was, though, I was still glad I had not cheated.

This event was clearly a major turning point in my life. I had not been fully "sold" on medicine, but now I determined to show myself and my PiKA fraternity brothers that I could master premed, even if I dropped out later. I could hardly wait to begin at Alabama College for Women, which accepted boys for summer school. The two courses I took were excellent and indeed memorable. The psychology course was taught by Dr. Helen Vickery, one of the best teachers I ever had. The other course was sociology, conducted by a Dr. Alice Keliher who came from the University of Chicago just for the summer sessions. She was a fine teacher, but she clearly considered herself on safari there in Alabama. She was surprised when we assured her that we had never seen a lynching and knew of none that had occurred in Shelby County—though of course, sadly, lynchings had occasionally occurred elsewhere in the state.

That summer, with hard work, I got straight A's, fully transferable to the university. This helped my grade point average at Alabama considerably, giving me a solid B average. More important, it did much for my self-respect. I took trigonometry over, put in time on it, worked all the problems correctly, and made an A. And from there on nothing was left to chance.

Our second year, Julian and I lived in a dormitory right on campus and only about twenty yards from the PiKA house (though he had pledged SAE). I ate at the "Bullpen," the dining hall of one of the largest dormitories on campus, along with the freshman football players. Three meals a day, seven days a week, cost forty-five dollars for three months.

My priorities had changed drastically. Now the extracurricular college "education," while not abandoned, was kept firmly in place and my studies came first. I sharply limited my bridge playing, but continued glee club, football band, military band (required), and concert orchestra. The talk was of classes and professors, and the atmosphere was purposeful. A medical student came into our room one night, bringing a book which he said we should read. It was Lloyd C. Douglas's *Magnificent Obsession*. René Vallery-Radot's *Life of Pasteur* and Eve Curie's biography of her mother, Madame Curie, also inspired me.

About this time the Sunday section of the *Birmingham News* published a photograph of Nobel Prize winner Alexis Carrel and

Charles A. Lindberg, who had collaborated on developing a perfusion pump that allowed tissues to be kept alive for months. Almost fifty years later, I was to be invited to write a companion article at the time of republication of Carrel's 1908 organ transplantation paper in the *Journal of the American Medical Association*, some of his work for which the prize was awarded in 1912.

Organic chemistry was taught by "Dr. Jack" Montgomery. It was a good course, consisting of well-developed lectures and solid supervision in the laboratory. Near the end of the first semester he commented, not once but twice, that if a student could correctly advance through all the chemical steps required to convert an aldehyde to a ketone, the student would make a hundred on the final examination. Gary Cumbie (now practicing medicine in Andalusia, Alabama) called me the night before the exam and suggested that, if I had finished studying (he knew I always studied alone), we go over to the education building, which had blackboards on three walls, and write out in sequence all the chemical reactions involved in the conversion of an aldehyde to a ketone. The next day, the only question on the exam was the aldehyde-to-ketone conversion, and I made the one hundred. As a result, "Dr. Jack," chairman of premedical advisers, became my very strong advocate as medical school applications loomed. That summer we "lived" physics, a very clean and precise science.

And so the second year ended, and it should be noted that by this time the ranks of premedical students who had begun the freshman year had thinned considerably. Now things were vastly different. My self-confidence and standing as an able premedical student were solid. In addition to other recognition, I had been appointed by the faculty to arrange speakers and programs for the premedical students during my upcoming third (senior) year.

On one somewhat amusing occasion, the professor of English literature asked me if I would tutor a football player who was also in the class. Having eaten with the freshman players the previous year, I was sympathetic, for I knew well the huge physical effort extracted from them from early afternoon until dark. However, I cautiously explained to the professor that all I did was to feed him back his own lecture material. To this he replied, "If he can feed back anywhere near the same thing, he'll pass, and he's got a coaching job already if he can just get out of college." (He did.)

The senior year was fun. As a paid teaching assistant I covered mammalian (cat) anatomy, general biology, and botany. Actually, I'd had almost no botany before and was just one jump ahead of the students. The nicest thing about being a teaching fellow was the intimate daily contact with members of the zoology faculty.

An intriguing assignment popped up during the fall. Dr. Henry Walker, chairman of zoology, wanted me to take the snake exhibit to the Alabama State Fair in Birmingham. I was a bit taken aback by this assignment, but the man who was to have taken the exhibit was sick. The professor said that I must at least know the common snakes, coming from a farm, but he gave me a book anyway. I was introduced to an imposing collection of rattlers, moccasins, coral snakes, and various nonpoisonous snakes, virtually all of which I was thoroughly familiar with. A deeply sunburned and weather-beaten woman first asked to see a joint snake (said to fly into pieces when struck but then to reconstitute itself after dark), and then wanted to see a hoop snake (said to catch its own tail and roll down a hill like a wheel). "Madam," I replied, "science recognizes no such reptiles." Late in the day I got some heckling from two premed classmates who happened by.

The senior year afforded the opportunity for more electives than had been possible before. Astronomy, genetics, and atomic structure were of special interest to me. Atomic structure was taught by Dr. George Palmer. Ahead of his time, he was goodnaturedly ridiculed by many students as an ancient, visionary alchemist trying to convert lead to gold. He was later to become the first president of the Alabama Atomic Power Association. In 1965 I wrote to him on learning of an operation:

Dear Doctor Palmer:

You will not remember me, but I was in your atomic structure class in 1937. Little did I realize at the time how important isotopes would one day be in my clinical research work. However, the groundwork I got in your class was a delight when the proper time came for its exploitation.

I learned recently from Doctor Gordon King, who was a classmate of mine at Alabama, that he had operated upon you some time ago. Actually, I had asked how you were doing these days, which prompted his information.

I send my very best wishes and hope I shall see you one of these times in Tuscaloosa.

He replied:

Dear Dr. Hardy:

I appreciate your letter very much indeed!

It is so seldom we ever get a letter like the one you sent me. Students usually wish recommendations and you never hear about them otherwise. Now and then someone thanks you.

Teaching is its own reward—satisfaction. You do many things as a teacher which you get little credit for but the satisfaction. For example, a speech I made started the Southern Research Institute (Birmingham). It would not have happened if I had not spoken to thousands of Birminghamians. I organized the Southern Association of Science and Industry which helped to bring science and its applications to the south sooner.

Genetics was taught by Dr. Berwind P. Kaufmann. He ran a very tough course and the students considered him "very scientific," i.e., "you get only what [the grade] you make." He was to become head of the Carnegie Institute of Genetics on Long Island. These courses prepared me to welcome space exploration, isotope research, and organ transplantation, years later.

The major problem of my senior year was to find a medical school. Alabama's medical school at Tuscaloosa offered only the first two years; I wanted to take all four years at the same place, preferably in the East. On the advice of James Donald, a brilliant second-year medical student from a medical family in Alabama, I applied to the University of Pennsylvania. The Donald clan of physicians believed that the University of Pennsylvania offered an ideal blend of science and practical treatment. It was also the oldest medical school in the United States. Penn replied that no decision would be made until March, but when, under pressure to enroll at Alabama, I urged an earlier decision, I was accepted by telegram in late October. My keen pleasure was tempered somewhat by the sober realization that now Julian and I would be apart for the first time—but we were always to remain close throughout our lives. Julian enrolled at Alabama in Tuscaloosa to be near his future wife, Marion Doughty, who was still in college.

Near the end of the year I was invited to join the Department of German and pursue a doctorate in that discipline, perhaps in part because of my thesis, "The Life of Goethe as Reflected in *Faust*." I had also become a favorite of Herr Doktor Foster, my professor and chairman of the department. "Herr Hardy," he would telephone some evenings, "would you like to walk around the quadrangle?"

"Jawohl, Herr Doktor!"

We would later have a bowl of ice cream at the "Supe" Store, and then use in sentences the ten difficult words presented in the afternoon *Birmingham News*. Dr. Foster was a gentleman of the old school and a veritable "Mr. Chips"—his wife had died and he was lonely.

Though I was honored by the department's invitation, my parents agreed with me that I should go on to medical school, and the offer was respectfully declined.

Julian and I graduated from Alabama in the very hot concrete football stadium late on the afternoon of Tuesday, May 24, 1938. We both had majored in chemistry and taken minors in zoology and German. Even back then, though premedical students were urged to get a broad liberal education, they loaded up on science courses. At least one, and sometimes two, foreign languages, often German

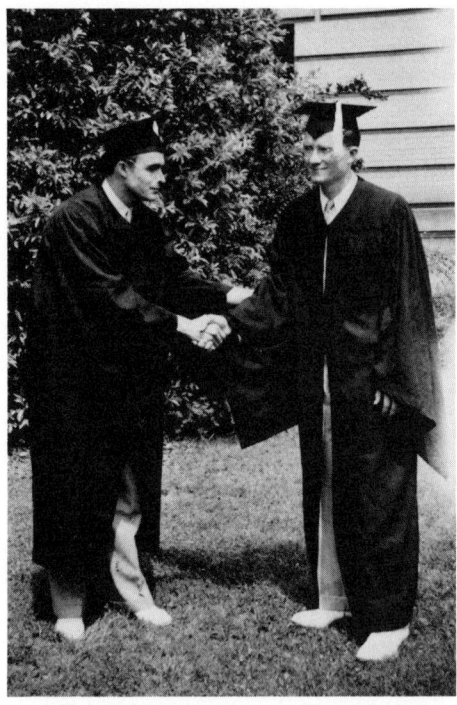

Gary Cumbie (left) *and JDH, graduating from the University of Alabama.*

and French, were required for admission to some medical schools.

That summer I worked for my father and played with the Bama Skippers dance orchestra. It was again a time to read nonrequired books, and the librarians at Montevallo College spoiled me shamelessly—as have the members of this most generous profession throughout my life, including Miss Frances Houston at the University of Pennsylvania Medical Library, Miss Irene Jones at the University of Tennessee Medical Library in Memphis, and Miss Irene Graham at the University of Mississippi Medical Center. I also set up my own telescope, above the horizon atop the tallest lime kiln, and studied Jupiter's moons, Saturn's rings, constellations, and other phenomena of the nocturnal sky.

PART II
Philadelphia 1938–1951

CHAPTER 3

Medical School at the University of Pennsylvania

Arrival for medical school

September came, my suitcase and new trunk were packed, and Mother and Father drove me up to Birmingham to take the train to Philadelphia. The coaches in those days were not air conditioned—what was? The stifling heat in the car during the night forced me to raise the window, and cinders from the locomotive peppered my clothes and white shirt. The train left Birmingham in the evening, went through Atlanta, and arrived in Philadelphia the next afternoon. I was never one to sleep sitting up, despite the many night drives with the Bama Skippers dance band, and so was awake at daylight when the train passed through Virginia. The apple trees just outside the window were loaded down with beautiful green or red apples in receding orchards.

Tired but full of anticipation, I got off the train in 30th Street Station in Philadelphia. I found two Alabama transfers, James Donald and Henry Hodo, there to meet me. We all piled into a taxi and rode out to the Penn dormitories. My room, in the graduate dormitory Morris Hall, was up steep stairs on the fourth floor, just under the roof, with an attic window and a sloping ceiling. It would be isolated, private, and ideal for studying, if the steam heat made it up that far. Immediately across the hall was Tom Magruder, a medical student whose father was a surgeon in Birmingham. Just next door was a veterinary student, and I came to be impressed that he had to know the anatomy not only of mammals, such as dogs and cows, but also of chickens and other creatures as well. He worked very hard.

Going to the dormitory mail office to rent a box, I found a long letter from Mother in which she imagined she'd been at Penn for several days, had looked around, and was describing what it was like. It was a very moving message, and my fond memory of it is painful only in that I always wanted to do that for my own children when they went away to college and later to graduate schools, but I usually didn't get around to it, to my persisting regret.

The next day, by way of rushing me, Phi Chi medical fraternity upperclassmen took me over to on-campus University Hospital, the medical students' mecca, to watch an operation. Professor I. S. Ravdin, a Phi Chi and a short chubby man, stood back from the operating table where removal of a gallbladder was in progress, his sterile gloved hands folded across his rotund abdomen to avoid contamination. He told us a bit about the patient's history, and then introduced his first assistant, Dr. Jonathan Rhoads, who he said had come up from Johns Hopkins. Little did I dream then what a large role these two men would one day play in my career.

Medical fraternities were then still important social and dining centers, since only a handful of the students were married. I joined Phi Chi, a lodge traditionally popular with Southerners and only two short blocks from the University Hospital and the medical school.

That first Sunday afternoon I saw a notice that led me to Irvine Auditorium on the Penn campus. There, a WPA orchestra accompanied a child prodigy of twelve or fourteen who played Tchaikovsky's Violin Concerto splendidly.

Seeing black men with authority over white people was a new experience for me. The chef at the Christian Association Building, where we often waited on tables for our meal and a dollar, was black. He was in charge at night, and he always treated us with jovial courtesy, though some of us had a heavy Southern accent. Everyone called him Mister. (One incidental note: Since we could not leave to begin studying until all the tables had been cleared, we had a vested interest in the speed with which various dinner groups ate. The anthropologists were slower than the archeologists, but just barely.)

On one occasion, seated at one of the tables for four in the Phi Chi house at dinner, I was complaining stridently of having to eat fish on Friday because the Catholics required it when one of my best new friends said quietly, "Jim, before you say any more, I should tell you I'm Catholic." However, there was no way you could've told it; he looked just like anybody else.

Still another surprise was the subtle, and sometimes not so subtle, anti-Semitism. Montevallo had had only the one Jewish family, which was thoroughly a part of the community, and to me there had been little visible anti-Semitism at college. But the situation was decidedly different in Philadelphia. I have found, all over the world, that the larger the minority, the greater the prejudice.

It was probably about this time that I began to drink coffee, at least regularly, always permitting myself the morning cup or so and a glance at the *Philadelphia Inquirer,* for our fellow Philadelphian Benjamin Franklin was said to have extolled the cumulative importance of such small repetitive daily pleasures, in contrast with the few great events that occur but seldom in a lifetime.

The first day of medical school

On the first day of medical school, 120 freshmen met in a high-rise classroom with long circular benches. We represented many states, though the largest single segment came from Pennsylvania and New England. The number of Phi Beta Kappa keys in evidence, back then when vests and watch chains were popular, was indeed impressive, and the quality of the students was generally very good. However, as time passed, a few students proved to be marginal: some did not apply themselves adequately, others worked desperately hard but simply could not do better. One student, who was chronically at risk in some course or other, never seemed disturbed. In fact, he once stated casually that the bottom half of the class was what made the upper half possible.

Dean William Pepper welcomed us. Tall, mustached as I recall, he looked the very picture of a dean. He said that each one of us represented ten applications. (After the six-week exams he assembled us again and reminded us that we were the chosen ones—but said they were afraid they might have chosen the wrong ones.) He told us that we would wear a necktie and jacket at all times and advised that we begin studying at once. This advice was quite unnecessary in my case, after my early experience in college. The discipline (and success) of consistent study had been learned well. I had come to medical school embracing fully Thomas Carlyle's dictum, as I recall it, that the problem is not to *see* what lies in the distance, but to *do* what lies clearly at hand. I combined unabashed idealism with a deep respect for professors that was not all that far from reverence. I studied five or six hours a night.

The chairman of the Department of Anatomy was Eliot Clark. The instructor of our section in gross anatomy was Henry Lee Spangler, a young physician of recent vintage. He had a habit of giving pop quizzes, and he became increasingly impressed that I usu-

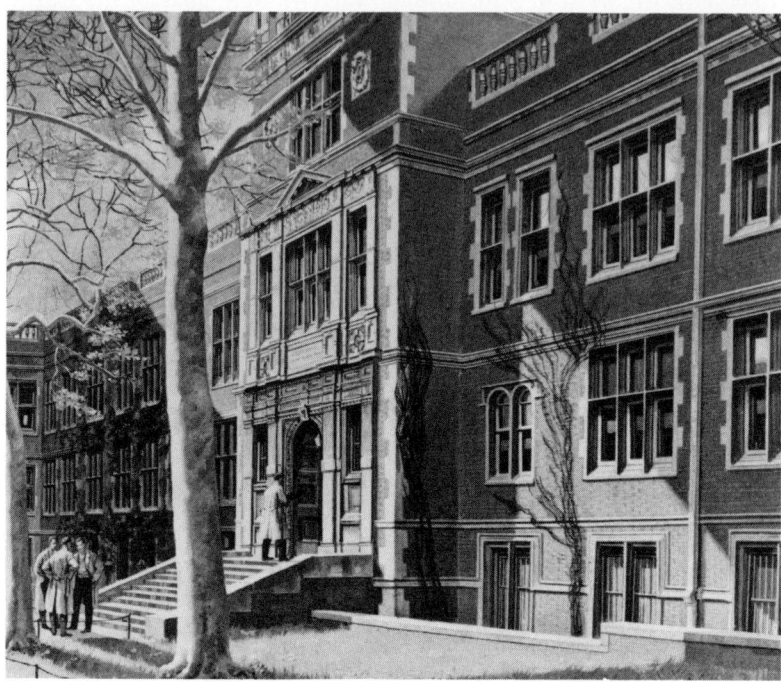

University of Pennsylvania School of Medicine by Frank Reilly, presented to the school as part of the "Collegia Medica Squibb" program by E. R. Squibb & Sons

ally did well. One day he abruptly announced to the four of us at our dissection table that he would predict right then that Hardy would intern at the University Hospital, the pinnacle of achievement in his mind and in ours. I did not tell him I had taught mammalian anatomy the year before: he did not ask me.

Our cadaver was an elderly male whom we named Caleb the Cadaver. I wondered, from time to time, who he had been, but generally we did not dwell on such thoughts. We respected the bodies, but sepulchral formality was not observed. The smell of the gross anatomy lab and the preserved cadavers permeated our hair and clothing. We freshmen were always discernible to experienced nostrils. Also, the grease seeped into the covers of the dissection manuals. Noting this, Jack Lafferty wrote the publisher and suggested that impermeable covers be substituted. To everyone's surprise, the publisher did just that and made Lafferty a present of a handsome, brand-new set of the dissection guide.

The first afternoon in histology, after the formal lecture (I think by Professor George de Renyi), Dr. Mary Hogue, the section teacher, came along as we were getting out our microscopes and opening the large box of slides which we would be studying for the semester. She asked the man on my right, Lincoln Godfrey, where he had gone to college. "Harvard, madam," he replied. She expressed much admiration for Harvard and then moved to me. When I answered, "The University of Alabama," she asked where the school was located. She then moved on to the man on my left, Malcolm Hayward. He too was from Harvard, and thus received warm congratulations. My two neighbors, who of course knew each other well, began to tease me about my college and the backward South in general. They said the teacher should not be blamed for not knowing where the University of Alabama was, since few people even knew where the state of Alabama was. They joked that Southerners were all so anemic from hookworm disease that when they became amorously aroused they fainted from blood loss. I listened to all this, as I looked through the slides in the box. Then I said, "I'll make you fellows a bet," as I placed two fifty-cent pieces on the table. "I'll bet you both that I will identify correctly seven out of any ten you select from these slides that we'll be studying." They promptly placed their bets, and I identified eight of the ten. After that they subsided. I did, however, acknowledge to them the obvious, that I'd had histology the previous year.

The point was, Alabama gave a tough and effective premed course. To be sure, it was heavily weighted toward zoology, with general biology the freshman year, then comparative anatomy, embryology, and histology. In contrast, some of my freshman classmates at Penn had had only general biology in college. And since in 1938–39 gross anatomy was still a massive course, extending over almost two-thirds of the freshman year, with histology prominent also, I obviously had a head start, which gave me more time to study biochemistry and physiology when they began in the second half of the year.

Dr. George de Renyi gave superb lectures in embryology, folding his jacket over his head to depict progressive stages of the embryo.

Physiological chemistry began after Christmas and it was rugged, with early quizzes on our knowledge of inorganic, then organic, and next physical chemistry. I could hardly believe the speed and efficiency with which Robert Fisher, across from me, set up his equipment, finished the experiment, and left for the afternoon. (I determined to become ever more organized.) Bob later became chairman of neurosurgery at the University of Oklahoma and still later at his college alma mater, Rutgers. Nor could I understand how Ferdinand Weisbrod could make 96 on quizzes, while I struggled to break 80. Dr. David L. Drabkin told us that students like Weisbrod were wine to the faculty's blood, and I could certainly believe him. The best chemistry course I'd had in college was quantitative analysis, and with its support I finally got a B in biochemistry. However, part of the grade was derived from a bonus given for identifying and then quantifying an elective unknown. My result was so close to the standard distributed that our section instructor, Dr. Henry F. Smythe, Jr., came over to my lab desk and asked, "Hardy, where was it you said you went to college?" When I answered, "The University of Alabama," he wanted to know who had taught the course in quantitative analysis. I would have written Dr. James L. Kassner back at Alabama but, though my grade in his course had been most gratifying, he had been so stern and reserved that we students were afraid of him and I doubted he would appreciate my letter.

It was not until years later, after considerable research and a master's degree in the subject, that I really felt comfortable in biochemistry. Nevertheless, when in biochemistry we examined racemic levo- and dextrorotary crystals described by Pasteur, I felt a great appreciation that I was afforded the opportunity to see great things discovered by great men.

But physiology was different. I liked it from the start, for physiology is the science of bodily function, of how the body works. If one knows how it works normally, one can usually figure out when it is working abnormally. Having done that, one can hope to make an accurate diagnosis, which must precede and point to appropriate treatment. This was the first freshman-year subject to which I'd had no formal exposure in college, and it offered considerable challenge. Near the middle of the course, we were offered electives in research and four of us, including Robert Mayock and Robert Helm, took up work with Joseph Doupe, a laboratory instructor who was down from Canada that year. We studied the suspected inhibiting role of fat introduced into the duodenum by stomach tube upon the quantitative and qualitative secretion of gastric acid and digestive enzymes. Using ourselves as the experimental subjects, we proved the point well. At the end of the year we were called upon to present our work to the assembled class and faculty in one of the large lecture halls, and my group insisted that I give the report, my first research presentation. Later, Dr. Henry C. Bassett, the chairman of the department, called me in. He asked my future plans and, regarding research, remarked that to make a discovery one must have either a new idea or a better method, and that, above all, one should not use a method inferior to the best currently available.

On Saturday mornings, from time to time, we had a clinical correlation hour in the medical auditorium of the University Hospital; it was intended to show us the relationship of the basic science courses we were taking to the treatment of patients. After a number of poor speakers, resulting in a massive dwindling of student attendance, Dr. Bernard Comroe, an arthritis specialist, was assigned to restore interest. This charismatic physician brought in things to see and feel—patients with knobby hands, swollen knees, and twisted feet, who came right along between the rows of students. Student attendance rose meteorically. This experience taught me the value of showing patients, and of laying on hands. We were told that the physician should always touch the patient, but should be careful with women lest the gesture be misinterpreted. Incidentally, one might consider the foot safe enough but no, some people cannot bear to have their feet touched. When in doubt, one is wise simply to shake hands.

In May I received my birthday check from my father. He had promised Julian, Taylor, and me one hundred dollars if we did not smoke before we were twenty-one. The check was for only twenty-one cents, but with Julian also in medical school and Taylor in law school back at Alabama, I understood and still have it. The important motivation had been the challenge, not the money.

The first year: looking back

The courses in my first year, consisting mainly of lectures and laboratory work with a considerable amount of one-on-one instruction, were generally good. However, the work seemed to be largely an extension of college, and a general cohesiveness and focus appeared lacking. Perhaps this was unavoidable due to the inexperience of the students being taught.

While studies were ninety to ninety-five percent of our focus, there *was* life outside the classroom and laboratories. We either played tennis on the university courts down by the Schuylkill River or went downtown to look and shop, or took in a movie or, sometimes, the risqué Faye's Burlesque on Market Street. We occasionally visited the Philadelphia Museum of Art; if memory serves, the large painting *Prometheus Bound*, in which vultures ate away Prometheus's liver as fast as it regenerated, was hung at the first landing of the stairs. Later on, when Dr. Ravdin talked about "the irresistible urge of the liver to regenerate," I wondered if the ancients had been aware of the remarkable biological phenomenon that, when a portion of the liver is removed, the organ will regenerate to a size approximately equal to its previous volume.

We also had Friday evening upper-balcony student tickets to the Philadelphia Orchestra. Leopold Stokowski was initially the conductor. With his snow-white mane, he made a striking appearance. Highly volatile, he once halted the concert when someone was allowed to enter late, noisily. Eugene Ormandy followed, and I recall he once had emergency treatment at University Hospital for subdeltoid bursitis, before the afternoon concert—a painful affliction for a great orchestra conductor. The Philadelphia Music Appreciation Committee distributed classical music albums at a cost of only $1.50. Numerous friends and I began our libraries in this way. If memory serves, the performers were not divulged, but the music sounded very much like that of the Philadelphia Orchestra. I always felt that Philadelphia liked students.

Saturday evening was sometimes passed at the Phi Chi house or around the corner at Smokey Joe's, a poorly lit beer joint. Two Saturdays a month, however, I worked from noon until midnight at an NYA (National Youth Administration) job in the bacteriology preparation room in the basement of the medical school (wonderful solitude!). Sunday morning was devoted to the *Philadelphia Inquirer* and to the *New York Times* with its section "The Week in Review," plus church irregularly. But Sunday afternoon was often a time of loneliness. It was hard to meet congenial girls as a stranger in Philadelphia.

Very rarely, we treated ourselves to a seafood dinner at the old original Bookbinders way down on Walnut Street near the Front Street wharves. One night we found that the check was more than we had calculated, and we had to leave a really minimal tip for the waiter. Disgusted, he held the coin between his thumb and forefinger and asked us loudly and repeatedly if we could spare it. We were mortified.

More often we went to a spaghetti place, Victor di Stephano's on Broad Street, where selections were played on request from a huge collection of classical recordings as the patrons sipped Chianti over red checkered tablecloths by candlelight.

My one sortie out of Philadelphia during the freshman year, other than home at Christmas, was to visit classmate Jim Kitchen's home in the Pocono Mountains over the Thanksgiving holidays. Driving up into the mountains, we saw the wind gusts swirling the dry snow along the road ahead. The next day we went out into the snow, and I tried skiing, snowshoeing, and ice skating on a small pond. That night in bed I became terribly warm and began to sweat. I was deeply concerned, for the next round of exams was to start the following week. I stayed under all the covers and sweated the night through. When I got out of bed next morning, however, I was surprised to feel quite normal. Going down to breakfast with the family, I sheepishly related to Dr. Kitchen that I'd had pneumonia during the night but had recovered by morning. Mrs. Kitchen laughed and said she had never dreamed I would use all the covers on the bed; since I was from the deep South she had just wanted me to have all the warmth I could possibly need!

Finally the freshman year was over. My grades were 97 in microscopic anatomy, 90 in gross anatomy, 88 in physiology, and 85 in biochemistry. Obviously, the best grades were in the two anatomy courses, both of which I had already had in college. I didn't know where I'd ranked in the class, but all things considered, I was satisfied.

That summer I got a job as "doctor," teacher, and director of athletics in an NYA camp in rural Alabama, where two groups of unemployed teenage boys were rotated on a two-week basis building a schoolhouse. We were housed in old Civilian Conservation Corps barracks. The staff consisted of a Mr. Smith, whose chief claim to fame was that he had been (then) Senator Claude Pepper's campaign manager for president of the student body at the University of Alabama, a male cook, and myself. Mr. Smith was in charge. Fortunately, my medical expertise was never required. We got a small music group going; our theme song was "The Wabash Cannonball." As for teaching, I decided that the most useful subjects I could offer were current events, which were moving all of us toward war, and English grammar. In the former regard, I was rewarded when some of the boys charged over one morning in early September to tell me that Great Britain had indeed just declared war on Germany over the invasion of Poland.

The Sophomore Year

The second year began smoothly, as we were all seasoned veterans. A few classmates were no longer to be seen, but Pennsylvania actually flunked out few students. With the sophomore year came the realization that we were now really studying medicine.

That year and thereafter I lived in the Phi Chi fraternity house. Bacteriology and pathology, the two fall disciplines, were both solid courses that required a great deal of laboratory time. In the former, we noted that bacteria did not grow immediately adjacent to some molds on old culture plates, but unlike Sir Alexander Fleming, we did not perceive the significance of this phenomenon, which led him to discover penicillin. "To see the world in a grain of sand. . . ." Virtually no virology or genetics was presented, and rather little immunology.

Pathology, on the other hand, was not so different from what it is today, with lectures, microscopic pathology, gross pathology, and the autopsy service. Brief research electives were offered. Pathophysiology was stressed less then than it is now. From pathology I developed a lasting pedagogical conviction that the entire grade for a major course should not rest on a single examination. A midterm examination was given and, for students who had done poorly, a final examination. The rest were exempted from the final. Having had flu and considerable fever when taking the midterm, however, I felt I knew more pathology than I had displayed, for microscopic pathology was but an extension of normal histology. Though exempted, my request to take the final was denied. The grade was decent but, in any future teaching by me, students would have multiple grade sources to reduce the role of chance.

During the fall, Julian had applied to Penn as a transfer from the two-year medical school at Alabama. When he did not get a positive reply, I made an appointment with Dean Pepper, who sent for my own medical school record for the freshman year. He looked it over while puffing on his pipe. He then spun back to face me and said, "If Dean Graves at Alabama backs your twin brother, we'll take him." Julian was accepted for the junior class the following fall.

Pharmacology, physical diagnosis, and neurology occupied the second semester of the sophomore year. Physical diagnosis included what is now called introduction to clinical medicine, with examinations performed on ourselves and on an occasional patient, under supervision. Neurology was a weak and poorly organized course. It had been announced that it was going to be completely reorganized, I think by Dr. Detlev Bronk. However, he was called to war work in Washington so often that we rarely saw him.

Pharmacology was perhaps the best course we had in medical school, taught by six very able physician-scientists. Emphatically, each week revolved around the Friday afternoon quiz in pharmacology. After the final weekly test, I was called in by one of the instructors, Dr. Robert Dripps. He showed me that I had misread one of the three questions and had gone in the wrong direction—but accurately. I was stunned. *Anybody* knew better than that! He went on to say, however, that since my overall average had been the best in the class, the faculty had met. He then smiled and showed me the front of the bluebook. The grade was 100.

During the spring a five-man "ethics committee," consisting of one representative from each class plus a faculty chairman, was appointed through the dean's office to look into medical school cheating. I found the way of the reformer an uncomfortable one. Two students in my class were caught and expelled, but I had not reported them personally. Actually, cheating was not widespread, but the cleverest one was never caught. We were under the Honor Code, but it was no more effective then than it is now insofar as student reporting of cheating was concerned. (The University of Mississippi School of Medicine formally abolished the honor system some years ago in favor of effective proctoring of examinations.)

I casually elected to take ROTC in medical school, for no better reason than that I could go to camp at Carlisle Barracks in the summer after the sophomore year and would be commissioned a first lieutenant on graduation from medical school. This fateful decision was ultimately to determine my marriage and my medical career.

But we did have a good time at Carlisle. The four of us in my tent were all classmates at Penn. Just after reveille one morning, I had been commanding the company at close order drill when someone from the rear rank yelled, "Come on, Hardy, dismiss us. We'll be late for breakfast."

"I'm fixin' to," I answered—a Southern colloquialism that convulsed those Northern "troops" with laughter. From this I got the nickname "Fixin' to" Hardy.

One incident that accentuated my personal perception that the neurology course was uninspired, and mine was the general one in the class, occurred while we were at Carlisle. I received a letter from Assistant Dean Edward Thorpe asking me to state honestly whether or not I had answered all four of the questions on the final examination; he said I had done well on the other three questions and would pass, but that my grade would have been much higher if the other question had been turned in. I had indeed answered all four questions. With the commandant's permission, I took the train down to Philadelphia and went straight to neurophysiologist McCooch's office. He was away, but there I saw a profusion of examination bluebooks piled in disorder on his desk. I soon found my missing question and took it to Dean Thorpe's office to be graded.

Then one day, when we were drilling on the parade ground, there came over the campwide loudspeaker system the order for everyone in the command to assemble in the grandstand for an announcement. I shall never forget that moment, for here again fate intervened in my future. The commandant said, very simply, "Gentlemen, France fell this morning."

How could that be? There was Marshal Gamelin, who *Life* magazine said was the greatest general of his time. And the impregnable Maginot line. And the vaunted French army, supposedly the best in the world. But France had fallen in almost a matter of days after the German onslaught.

The commandant went on to say that, inevitably, we would all be in the war very soon. It was still 1940, a year before the bombing of Pearl Harbor, but I knew in my bones the colonel was right.

MEDICAL SCHOOL THEN AND NOW

Before going on to the junior year, it is useful to contrast medical school in the 1940s with that in the 1980s. In large part, medical education today bears a strong resemblance to that of forty years ago, especially with regard to the third and fourth years. After all, what the student needs is a critical mass of factual information, exposure to patients, hands-on experience, and the incredibly capable human mind which integrates all these to provide a clinically competent physician. But certainly changes in the components have come about, especially in the freshman and sophomore years.

The student body

The number of freshman medical students admitted to medical schools in the United States in 1938 was approximately five thousand, whereas it is over sixteen thousand today. Currently, however, the number is beginning to decline, due to the perception that there will be a significant surplus of physicians by 1990. Of course the population has increased, but the number of medical students has increased disproportionately as a result of federal subsidies to medical schools for admitting more students and the establishment of more schools. One has the general impression that the overall quality of the students now being admitted has declined slightly, and certainly the perceived attractiveness of medicine as a career has diminished somewhat in recent years in the view of many of the most able college students. This may be due, in part, to the expense of a medical education and to the long years of training required. The wife of a surgeon said to me recently that she did not want her very bright daughter to enter medicine. "It takes their youth!"

Another major difference in the student body is in its composition. In my class there were only three women and one black man (who left after the freshman year). Now, in some schools, one-third to even one-half the class may be female, and other minorities are also well represented. This in itself has changed the image and the social and sociological environment of medical school classes. The fact that many of the female students become married, often to classmates, and then have babies—this, too, exerts a subtle humanizing and maturing influence on the male classmates. Indeed, at least half the members of each class have married, either in college or before finishing medical school, and they may have several children. Most students have an apartment, a car, and multiple other expenses, for which they borrow substantial sums of money to get through medical school. Already in debt at graduation, they seem far more oriented toward getting out and making money than was the case with my own class: we lived in a single room, we did not marry, we had no car—but then we had little debt. Medical fraternities were very important as social centers. They are now virtually gone, but single students thus often have no supportive base of operations.

Financial pressures plus (and perhaps because of) family pressures and at times divorce appear to cause more scholastic difficulties and psychiatric stress than was the case forty years ago. Federal and other grants-in-aid are far less readily available. To the best of my memory, not one student dropped out of our class because of emotional difficulties. Moreover, the scourge of psychedelic drugs, marijuana, and cocaine was unheard of.

Modern students are more openly critical of teaching at all levels and are much more ready to speak out about true or imagined grievances. This is true of the population in general. However, none of this is completely new: recall the ancient professor who replied that his job was to cast artificial pearls before genuine swine. Students today still complain of scut work, night call, poor teaching rounds, not getting to present their cases at rounds, and so forth.

But even with having to contend with all the above pressure, most medical students today are fine, solid entrants into the profession. In passing, it should be noted that if outside financial aid becomes too restricted, some minorities may be denied and medical school thus restricted to the well-to-do, with all the associated sociological repercussions.

The curriculum

A major organizational change in the curriculum has consisted of a vast reduction in the number of formal lectures and classes. Another remarkable change has been the drastic reduction, almost the elimination, of laboratory time in physiology, pharmacology, and microbiology. Anatomy hours have also been pared very sharply.

The reason given for the reduction in laboratory hours is that the modern students have already covered the material in college. Having recently had two daughters go through college and medical school, I would have to agree that college science courses today cut at least as deeply, in many instances, as did our similar courses in medical school. But I, for one, have wondered aloud whether something subtle but very valuable may not have been lost along with the laboratories. In my day, the relaxed hours in the laboratory afforded the chance for relaxed philosophical chats with the instructors, during which we came to know them better—time that I remember so favorably from my own labs in medical school. For example, while waiting for some progressing chemical reaction to finish in biochemistry, several of us would gather around Dr. David L. Drabkin or Dr. Samuel Guerin. I recall the former's comparing Penn, Cornell, Columbia Physicians and Surgeons, and Harvard medical schools one day. He said that comparative standings would vary, from time to time, and that Cornell was especially strong just then. But, he went on to say, a *great* school rarely fell very far because its overall depth in good faculty would sustain it. A school that was prominent through the reputation of just a few especially able faculty members, however, was highly vulnerable and, once fallen, was likely to be many years regaining its former prestige. Drabkin was an internationally known authority on the biochemistry of hemoglobin. A mathematician, he imparted to us the faculty of mathematical precision. He said that some scientists had made their reputations by recalculating the data published by others, providing new insights.

In Dr. Guerin, who was just getting into isotopic research, I found an ally some years later when I began using isotopes in my own research. He eventually became dean of the medical school.

Furthermore, will we produce as many capable clinical investigators when the students have so little bench laboratory experience in medical school? Of course, the phasing out of student laboratory time may afford the faculty more time for their own research, but after all, many basic science faculties had students only four or five months of the year, even in the old days. I once heard a major professor say that medical school would be a great place if there were no medical students (i.e., he could do his research full time, the year round). A jest, of course, but with a kernel of truthful admission. What one remembers best, when all is over, is not courses but individual able professors who serve as role models for the rest of one's life. Our pharmacology course was great in 1940 because the superb instructors gave it their complete attention. When an experiment was put on, *it worked*.

Today, since medical students are as busy as ever, what has replaced the time given up by anatomy, for example? Statistics, genetics, human behavior, psychiatry, and family medicine have been significantly expanded. Obsolete material has been continuously weeded out to keep the body of information offered as fresh and current as possible.

The content of the junior and senior years varies from year to year and from school to school, but basically the clinical clerkships remain as they were forty years ago. The students do get to do more routine procedures, like those interns perform, than we did, but otherwise there is little difference, only new diseases and new treatments for old diseases. ("The questions don't change, only the answers.") The pure block system has essentially replaced the old block system, which allowed daily cross-block lectures to the whole class. With the pure block system, the student is assigned solely to a given specialty (e.g., surgery) and during those three months he receives no lectures from any other specialties, such as pediatrics. Again, the number of lectures has been sharply reduced throughout the whole curriculum, especially in the clinical third and fourth years. Personally, I enjoy a well-organized lecture on a topic. For example, some years ago in London I happened to drop by the Royal College of Surgeons and heard a magnificent lecture dealing with catechol amines by one John Vane. (In 1982, Vane shared the Nobel Prize.) I thought to myself, *the lecture lives!*

There is, of course, a cleanness and simplicity about the pure block system, but it does have its drawbacks, it seems to me. For one thing, many students learn better by having the same mass of material presented over a longer period of time and by a degree of repetition (reinforcement). For another, the prolonged, if less concentrated, exposure of faculty to students, and of students to faculty, can lead to better "bonding" between the two. With the pure block system, a student might have the surgery rotation the first three months of the junior year, and then never again meaningfully encounter the discipline unless entering a surgical specialty. Finally, in the pure block system the sections of the class actually see little of each other after the sophomore year. In contrast, much class solidarity was achieved our senior year by attending (enthusiastically) Dr. O. H. Perry Pepper's seminar each Friday afternoon from four to five o'clock. For example, the very last Friday afternoon of our senior year, Dr. Pepper, chairman of the Department of Medicine and a marvelously charismatic teacher and clinician, walked into the medical amphitheater and said to our class, already seated and fully attentive, "I looked up my log of the first patient I ever showed this class four years ago. I have another patient with that same disease waiting outside. I wonder if anyone remembers what the disease was?" With one voice, the class thundered, "*Herpes zoster ophthalmicus!*"

The modern extensive senior electives taken at other medical centers and, indeed, in foreign countries were nonexistent in my medical school days.

The Junior Year

For the medical student, the first and third years are the worst. Survival is the first-year objective, for few students are dropped after that. But the third year is a key one, for an enormous volume of information must be asssimilated in internal medicine with its numerous subdivisions, pediatrics, obstetrics and gynecology, psychiatry, general surgery, ophthalmology, neurosurgery, orthopedics, urology, otolaryngology, and public health. This book learning must be achieved at the same time the student is learning how to work with sick patients. Some students do not blossom until they reach the third year, while others who were outstanding in the basic science courses tend to lose ground during the clinical years. Each specialty had its own textbook which supplemented its lectures, small conferences, clinics, and individual patient workups. We did not go on the hospital floors until our senior year. My personal error during the third year was that I tried to learn too much detail, sometimes not perceiving the major points.

Julian and I arrived in Philadelphia a day or so early, this September of 1940. We had agreed to serve as student helpers with the bicentennial celebration of the University of Pennsylvania. My specific assignment was to stand on the stage beside the public address electrical cord as the dignitaries from all over the world came up to take their seats, saying, "Watch your step, please. Please watch your step." I had an excellent vantage point.

It was a lastingly memorable occasion: President Franklin Delano Roosevelt was the keynote speaker. I had long heard how great he was, or conversely what a Lucifer he was, and I was certainly interested in what he would look like. Great was my surprise to see how crippled he was, unable to walk without strong support.

After Roosevelt had been helped to the lectern, he was stable and needed no further assistance during the standing address which lasted perhaps thirty minutes. And he was superb. It was easy to see why he won elections, carried the country with his fireside chats, and was very likely to be reelected in November.

He began slowly, saying complimentary things suitable to the occasion with great presence, assurance, and a bell-like voice. Next he reviewed in general terms the war in Europe and some of the problems facing the country. Then he moved smoothly into political waters, though never mentioning the Republicans or anyone else.by name. I can tell you that just about everybody in that large audience in Convention Hall was with the president. Even so, each succeeding day I realized he had inserted into his address powerful political time bombs. He was magnificent.

Then classes began. We rotated through the various clinics during the third year, with a lecture each afternoon to the whole class by a faculty member in one of the clinical specialties. The quality of the lecturers varied considerably but was generally good.

Julian and I were on medicine clinic first. And here we first, also, became familiar with the patient stratum that is more likely to address the physician as "Doc" than the more dignified "Doctor." I remember particularly a large, considerably obese lady whose chart was inches thick, signifying many, many visits to the University Hospital in the past. There was really no major scientific problem, though she did have mild-to-moderate degenerative arthritis in her knees, not uncommon in seriously overweight patients. But she wanted some medicine. Having been taught in pharmacology not to prescribe drugs except for specific purposes, Julian and I refused. We then sought out Dr. Arthur Phillips, our chief, who had to review our case and see the patient with us. He listened to us and then said, "Boys, this happens again every year. You're not in pure science now, you are treating a patient. The lady is going to get herself some medicine somehow, perhaps by coming back tomorrow with the chance she'll be seen by someone else, or by going to the emergency room or even to another hospital. The psychological effect of taking medicine is very important to her. Let's give her a prescription that has a bright color, tastes good, won't harm, and doesn't cost much. She'll be satisfied and, believe it or not, she'll feel better, too." She got the medicine and we got the message.

With experience, it became increasingly clear that to make a correct diagnosis one could readily discard numerous possibilities and then concentrate, with tests as indicated, on the remaining and most likely choices.

Easily the most spectacular professor we had the third year was Dr. John Stokes, who taught dermatology and syphilology. He was a world authority on syphilis and his textbook *Dermatology and Syphilology* was a veritable bible in the field. Dr. Stokes kept us all nervous at the two-hour session in the amphitheater each Thursday morning from nine to eleven. He would come in with all his staff and about six patients who were placed behind blinds. Two students would be assigned to each patient to take the history, do a physical examination, and come up with a diagnosis to be presented to the class about thirty minutes later. The students had never seen the patient before and were sorely under the gun.

Meanwhile, Stokes had the seating arrangement of the class before him on the lectern, and he fired questions on the reading assignment. (When he called "Hardy," I would always ask which one and he would usually name Julian.) And he would say the most shocking things, for sex, venereal disease, and such intimate relationships were simply not discussed openly in those days. He asked a student what people did after intercourse. When the student made some lame reply, Stokes said, "I can tell you're a virgin. *They sleep.*" Or,

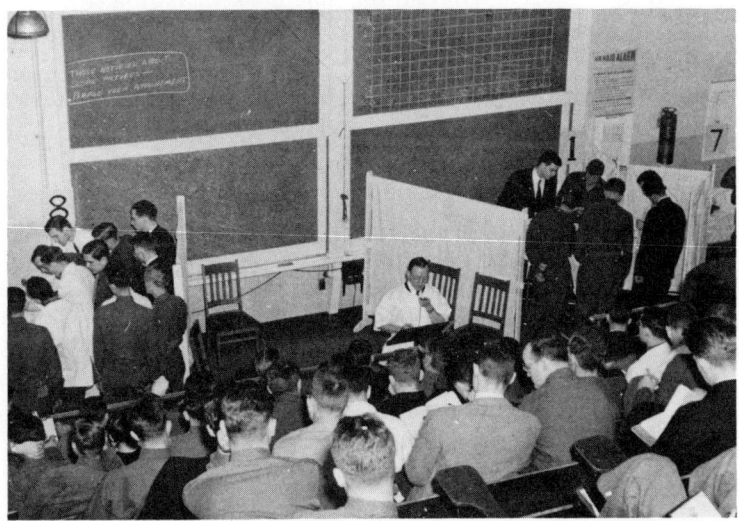

Professor John Stokes' class, medical amphitheater

"Don't ask the man if he's had gonorrhea. Ask him *how often* he's had gonorrhea. Asked in this way, he'll usually admit to at least one dose." On another occasion he told us, "One positive test for syphilis will convict a day laborer. Two positives will convict a white-collar worker. Three positives will convict a bank president. But, gentlemen, sometimes four positive Wassermanns will not convict a clergyman!" We were commanded to remain forever vigilant, always with a "high index of suspicion." I don't know how much dermatology I learned in that course, but I came out suspecting almost anyone of harboring syphilis.

Dr. Richard Kern was another very effective lecturer, in infectious diseases and allergy. He was later to be editor of the *American Journal of Medical Sciences* for many years. Tall and imposing, he had a dramatic way of waggling his long index finger at the class and making his points emphatically. For example, he stressed that not all that wheezes is asthma—meaning that partial obstruction of a bronchus by a tumor might be responsible, a point that led me to diagnose lung malignancy in my mother. To control rabies, *muzzle the dog;* this became a byword with the students. Regarding a severe and dangerous upper respiratory tract infection, he demanded bed rest ("When you have a fire in the attic, put it out before it spreads below [to the lungs]"). He said that any doctor could make at least enough money to get along, that the commodity most important in life was *time*.

Surgery lectures were given by Drs. Isidor Ravdin and Eldridge Eliason, and they presented stark contrast. Ravdin always gave a very orderly, well-prepared exposition of the assigned subject, usually reading the presentation and showing a patient at the close of the hour. Eliason, on the other hand, virtually never seemed to have prepared anything formally. He almost invariably brought in patients and gave a clinic, as it were, but driving home the selected points he wished to make. Thus, the two teaching styles were so different that it would be hard to decide which was the more effective. Actually, both methods were effective, but one had to appreciate that Ravdin took his teaching responsibility as more demanding than did Eliason.

Obstetrics and gynecology afforded me an opportunity, indeed, a necessity, for the best cramming effort of all my educational experience. The lectures, by Dr. Carl Bachman in obstetrics and Dr. Franklin Payne in gynecology, were well organized and very good, and there was also a textbook. However, since there was only one examination, the final at the end of the year, I had done little related studying owing to pressure from all the other courses that had given multiple tests along the way. We had a free day between each two major final examinations. Obstetrics and gynecology came in its turn: it received forty-eight hours of intense attention—and modesty forbids divulging my grade in that course.

Clinical pharmacology was a small course conducted by Dr. Isaac Starr. It is cited particularly to note my first introduction to the existence of a physiologist with the identical name James Daniel Hardy, whose work with the dolorimeter at Cornell was presented (one aspirin gave almost as much pain relief as two, codeine was of course more effective than aspirin, and morphine better than either). The dolorimeter was one of the four questions on the final examination (I remembered the answer only because of the name). In due course we began to receive mistakenly addressed requests for each other's reprints. This confusion was accentuated after I had left Philadelphia and he had taken a position at the University of Pennsylvania. I was even offered an honorary degree from his college alma mater, to the keen embarrassment of the president. We eventually met and found that we might be distant relatives.

As steward of the Phi Chi house that year, I planned all the meals and ran the dining activities, this for free room and board. All went well until a student from Maine, Paul Burke, drew up and circulated a petition. He complained of a nutritional deficiency, to wit, potatoes. I had substituted rice too often, and potatoes were returned prominently to the menus.

In October Julian and I were called home urgently. Father was critically and probably terminally ill. Always substantially obese, he had had diabetes for some years, requiring insulin daily; he hated to inject himself but did so stoically, except for brief periods when he would feel so well that he would skip the injection and promptly get into trouble. After my freshman year, a "cardiologist" in Birmingham had told Father in my presence he would be dead in six months from heart failure, but that it might be a little longer if he would lose one hundred pounds, which Father promptly proceeded to do. I thought then, and I think now, that it was a brutal thing for a doctor to say; he might or might not know the heart, but he certainly did not know human sensitivities.

Father, at seventy-four, died from heart failure secondary to the atherosclerotic complications of obesity, diabetes, hypertension, and advanced age. In addition to the sadness of losing a parent, I regretted not having been closer to him after I was grown. After I'd gone to college, we'd rarely had the long talks on the side porch during the summer evenings that we'd had when I was a boy.

One particular problem, especially from Mother's immediate standpoint, was that no will could be found, though I had been present some years before when Father had made a will as he faced emergency gallbladder surgery. The probate court moved at a snail's pace, and the importance of a current will was all too apparent.

Then, on Sunday, December 7, 1941, came the attack on Pearl Harbor. I remember exactly where I was, as does almost every other adult American of that time. I was upstairs at the Phi Chi house studying when someone yelled the news up the stairway.

In the spring I received a letter from Genevra ("Gene") Ziegler, secretary of Alpha Omega Alpha (AOA), the medical school scholarship honor society, telling me that I had been elected to membership. It meant I ranked among the first five of my junior class. At the subsequent business meeting Franklin Murphy, the current president, abruptly nominated me for president and the nomination carried into election, since no one else was proposed. I felt embarrassed, for I wondered whether the four other new junior members might not have preferred some one of themselves but were reluctant to nominate a second person. I wrote Mother later that night that I hoped Father would have felt I'd done my part, for my education had indeed been a joint venture with my parents as major participants.

After exams, I was to work for room and board at the Alabama State (Bryce) Mental Hospital at Tuscaloosa as a summer extern. I was assigned to Dr. Peabody B. Mayfield, one of the staff psychiatrists.

It was a pleasure to work under the wing of "Dr. Peabody." He had a very practical approach to his work and a constantly cheerful attitude in circumstances that could have been very depressing, with the heavy load of patients. He permitted himself small liberties in writing to the patients' relatives. For instance, he wrote one family that, no, their son could not be discharged because "he is still possessed of the same philandering proclivities for which he was originally incarcerated." It was a long time before he got a reply: "Dear Dr. Mayfield, the reason we ain't writ back was the creek was up and we couldn't git across to the schoolteacher to git her to read your letter."

Dr. Peabody instructed me in the basics of taking a psychiatric history. First you ask the patient if he hears voices that nobody else hears. If he says yes, he is definitely psychotic. Next you ask him if the voices say good things or bad things. If good things, he is a schizophrenic, hebephrenic type; if bad things, he is schizophrenic, paranoid type. The only major modality for treatment was shock therapy, consisting of electroshock or induction with insulin or Metrazole. None of the modern drugs had been developed. It was instructive (and embarrassing) to see how bold the long sex-starved women became. Invitations to a visit after dark were commonplace. Later on, I became more knowledgeable regarding the problems generated by long-term separation of mature men and women in mental hospitals, prisons, and the military.

Although I sat in on psychiatry conferences, my specific responsibility, along with the other summer extern, was to give the inmates physical examinations, two thousand of which were scheduled for the summer. To keep us honest, they told us that one patient was known to have dextrocardia. It was August before the other student appeared at the communal dinner table one noon with a broad grin on his face: He had found the "right" heart.

We were able to play tennis late most afternoons, and as the years passed, the time I was willing to devote to sports went to tennis in the hope of becoming proficient in at least one direction.

That summer Hitler invaded Russia.

The Senior Year

The senior year was the best of any school year ever. The pressure was off, for outside the dean's office on the bulletin board had been posted the ranking of the entire class at the end of the junior year, the only ranking that counted because the senior grades were irrelevant. From these rankings would come our internships, the next step in front of us.

We rotated to other hospitals for a part of the clinical experience. I was assigned to a very good medicine service down at venerable Pennsylvania Hospital, founded by Benjamin Franklin (as we were reminded from time to time), and to weak teaching of surgery at Presbyterian Hospital. Fortunately my obstetrics was at the University Hospital. We also had conferences at ancient Philadelphia General (Old Blockley) Hospital, where the massive volume and severity of the pathology were remarkable.

The relaxed freedom of the senior year gave me the opportunity to read widely as I'd not done for years, other than to study the textbooks. Each weekend I took home a load of current medical periodicals.

Another pleasure was that of working with our AOA faculty sponsor, Dr. Francis C. Wood, cardiologist and later chairman of the Department of Medicine. This increased my interest in the heart and the circulation. Further, five of us took on a Department of Surgery research project dealing with the effect of sulfanilamide powder on wound healing, supervised by Harold Zintel, a surgery resident. Dr. Ravdin had suggested the project after being flown to Honolulu immediately after the attack on Pearl Harbor to inspect the wounded and to report on the medical support system. The British Army was recommending the local application of the sulfanilamide powder by the wounded man himself, and it had been used at Pearl Harbor. However, did it impair wound healing? We found by studies in dogs that it did not.

Still another project was the competition for the History of Medicine Prize. The title I selected was "The History and Importance of

Military Field Hygiene." This led to trips to the Philadelphia College of Physicians Library and down to the Surgeon General's Library in Washington for original source material. I devoted a lot of time to the manuscript, and several weeks after its submission Miss Lillian ("Dean") Gallagher, the dean's assistant, informed me, very confidentially, that I would win the prize. I "very confidentially" told Julian but no one else. But to my sharp disappointment, someone else's name appeared in the printed program at graduation. He had submitted his paper at the last possible moment. Julian had seen the announcement first and, characteristically, touched my elbow and said, "James, don't let it bother you." But there was a sequel. A week or so later we took the Alabama State Medical Board examinations, and four of the ten discussion questions, now in wartime, had to do with topics discussed in my medical history manuscript. I had to sympathize with whoever had to read my voluminous answers to those four questions.

Yet another interest was that of trying to determine, from microscopic slides at Philadelphia General Hospital, just when the condition of sarcoidosis had been clearly separated from routine tuberculosis. Some of these lymph node slides were in the museum of Sir William Osler, probably the best-known physician of his time. I did not settle the question but I learned a lot about sarcoidosis, which was to prove useful on several future occasions. Moreover, I also became interested in Osler, and he and his Pulitzer Prize–winning biographer, Harvey Cushing, are prominently represented in my collection of medical history books.

Internship was the major consideration the senior year. The national internship matching system was still far in the future. I knew I wanted to intern at the Hospital of the University of Pennsylvania. HUP then took fifteen students from Penn, selected from the top twenty-five percent of the class, and five from other universities. All internships at Penn were of the rotating type. My first interview appointment was with Dr. T. Grier Miller, head of the Division of Gastroenterology and co-developer of the Miller-Abbott intestinal tube. He greeted me pleasantly and then handed me a sheet of paper. He directed that I write down the fifteen men in my class I would most like to intern with. This was not an easy task, for I liked practically everyone in the class, but I focused on intelligence, integrity, industry, dependability, compatibility with others, and stamina. He looked over my list and remarked that my own name had appeared on every list handed in so far by others. And that was about all there was to the interview.

Next I went to see Dr. Eldridge Eliason, chairman of the Department of Surgery. Everyone knew that being appropriately dressed in a suit and tie, with a recent haircut and clean fingernails, was important to him, for he was the embodiment of the suave, wavy gray-haired, well-dressed, and immaculately clean bachelor. Having looked me over, he asked where I was applying. I answered, "Just this hospital, Dr. Eliason."

To this he raised an eyebrow, looked at me narrowly, and said, "What if you didn't get it?"

I replied that I'd rush over and see the dean, at which he broke out laughing and said, "That's an honest answer if I ever heard one. Well, that's all."

What I did not tell him was that I had already been over to ask the dean to write me a letter for an internship at the University of Michigan, as a backup. He had said, "Hardy, do you really want to go to Michigan?"

"No, sir, I'd rather intern here."

"Then I'm not going to waste my time writing to Michigan."

Thus I felt reasonably secure. And so it came to pass. Julian was to return to Alabama for internship and residency in obstetrics and gynecology, and private practice in Birmingham.

In mid-April, on Undergraduate Medical Association Day, our group gave our research paper, "The Effect of Sulfonamides on Wound Healing." We won a prize, and with our money Donald Freshwater (later an outstanding neurosurgeon), Charles Neer (later an orthopaedist and world authority on the shoulder), William Harris (later a prominent general surgeon in Birmingham), and I presented Harold Zintel, our surgery resident supervisor, with a briefcase. But even more exciting, Dr. Ravdin called us into his research office over in the medical school and said, "Boys, where do you want to publish it?" We were astonished and elated, having had no idea it could be published. It appeared in the journal *Surgery*, and was my first publication.

About that time, as president of AOA, I went to the dean's office to get the names of the top five students in the junior class, who were eligible for AOA. Miss Gallagher said, "Being from Alabama, Mr. Hardy, you're not going to like this. Number three is the Negro student, Barnes."

"That doesn't bother me in the slightest, Miss Gallagher," I replied. "He probably had to work twice as hard to get there."

Another responsibility was that of inviting the annual AOA lecturer. On Dr. Perry Pepper's advice, Dr. Alfred Blalock, who had recently come from Vanderbilt to be chairman of surgery at Johns Hopkins, was invited to present his highly interesting recent research in which he had shown that removal of a thymoma improved in some instances the condition of the patient with myasthenia gravis. He declined because of war work in Washington, and Walter Bauer of Harvard spoke on changes in the synovial fluid of the knee joint in arthritis.

The most prestigious senior prize awarded to a medical student at Pennsylvania was the Spencer Morris Prize of approximately nine hundred dollars. It consisted of a preliminary written session, following which the survivors met a faculty member for an oral examination. One afternoon twenty-five or so members of our class assembled in the pathology-bacteriology laboratory for the written examination. To our surprise it consisted of only one question: "Write a paper on any medical subject of your choice." On the face of it, like a timed open-book exam, this should have been a welcome

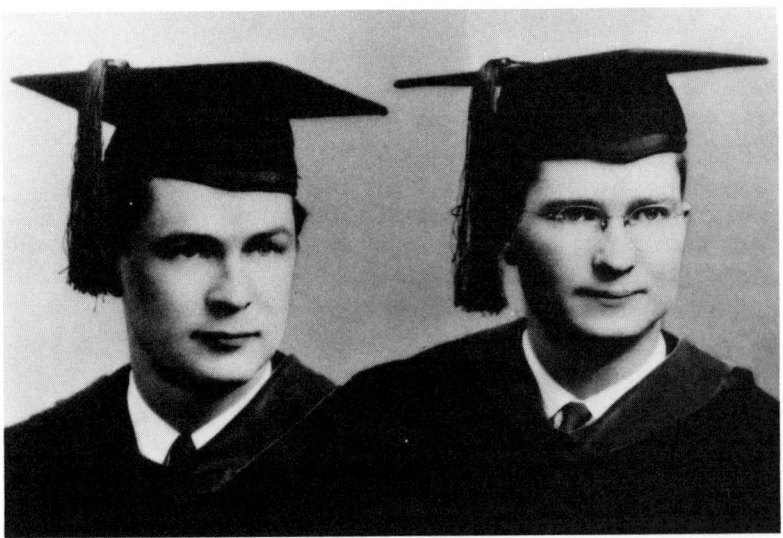

Julian Patterson Hardy (left) *and JDH, graduating from medical school at the University of Pennsylvania.*

challenge. However, one had to choose a topic quickly and get started. I chose hyper- and hypoinsulinism. It would be possible to embellish the piece with a bit of medical history since Seale Harris, possibly the first to predict that insulinomas would be discovered, had practiced in Birmingham. Five of us advanced to the oral exam, and James M. Walker, appropriately in my opinion, was the eventual winner. Certainly I well knew that I was not. It had been the first oral examination of my experience—I was very nervous and had done poorly, even on very fair questions. I made up my mind then that if I was ever involved in teaching, I would see to it that students experienced enough oral quizzes to become accustomed to taking them.

Mother had come up to Philadelphia for our graduation. The night before she arrived, some of us who had been together for four years began downtown and tried to drink one beer in every bar all the way back to the university. I had had to drop out even before we reached the bridge over the Schuylkill River, but apparently this was not soon enough. Mother said, "James, you look so pale. You must have been working terribly hard."

At graduation I was commissioned 1st Lieutenant 0-448702 and Julian 0-448703.

CHAPTER 4

Internship at University of Pennsylvania Hospital

No doctor will *ever* forget his internship.

For one thing, it represents, once again, elevation to a still higher echelon. The competition stiffens noticeably when the student moves from high school to college (in premed at least), and then from college to medical school. But up to the internship one is protected, as it were, in a cocoon of prescribed studies, where adequate grades constitute status and emotional safety. With the internship, however, the importance of grades recedes abruptly, and the preeminence of clinical performance moves front and center.

The good intern is now able to select and use, in the complex setting of the hospital, the immediately pertinent information learned in medical school. This must be achieved despite frequently stressful, often eighteen-hour days. He has to carry out the innumerable details of good patient care while maintaining a positive attitude and pleasant relationships with staff, his residents, nurses, patients, and medical students. Above all, the intern, no matter how brilliant in medical school, must quickly establish a reputation for *dependability*. This requires continuous entry, in one's pocket notebook, of all the countless details of each patient's status, studies and procedures to be scheduled immediately to avoid wasting hospitalization time, and suggestions and instructions of the staff physician, as well as the maintenance of accurate, current, and complete hospital chart records. The intern must also exhibit *availability*, always alert for his signal and never leaving the hospital without properly signing out to his covering physician. Finally, all work must be finished as soon as possible, before some new, perhaps emergency, admission comes in.

The internship can be a richly rewarding and even fun experience if approached correctly; otherwise, it can represent one of the most disagreeable periods of the physician's life.

Owing to a massive loss of doctors and nurses to the war effort, the University Hospital had asked for volunteers from our incoming intern group to begin early. I had volunteered and began my internship unofficially in April on the laboratory service. In those days there were no technicians at night, and Lincoln Godfrey, the other intern, and I did urinalyses and blood counts, plated out pus for bacterial growth or sputum for possible tuberculosis, typed pneumococci to permit selection of appropriate antiserum, and ran chemistries for blood sugar levels in diabetes and blood urea nitrogen levels to exclude uremia. It was frequently an all-night job, and I was uneasy over the responsibility for cross matching blood during the night lest an error result in the transfusion of mismatched blood, causing major illness or death of the patient. In fact, I was aware of an instance in which two hospitalized patients had had identical names, and one had received the other's blood, though not fatally. (Later, all hospitals used consecutive *numbers* for hospital admissions instead of depending solely on names.) After Godfrey and I had mutually supported each other for a few nights, each of us covered the laboratory service every other night. During the day we worked in the lab along with the technicians.

My first clinical service was neurosurgery. Before July 1 the service had been covered by two interns, at least one of them in his second year, but the two-year internship was now shortened to one year. Thus the service, accustomed to having the assistance of second-year men, now had only one intern, a first-year man on his first clinical rotation. The war was already changing things drastically in the University Hospital.

Neurosurgery was a murderous service. Despite every economy of time, I got only three to four hours sleep a night, did not go out of the hospital for the entire six weeks, and rarely saw my roommate, John Gislason (later a nationally prominent urologist). He was in bed when I finally got to the room in the early morning hours; before he got up, I left to draw the blood specimens on the patients, check on the X-rays and the blood for transfusion, see all the patients on the service, start the IVs, and be in the operating room on time to scrub for the first case.

It was a time when neurosurgery was exploring the feasibility of ever more radical surgery for removal of brain tumors, but anesthesia still often consisted largely of heavy preoperative morphine dosage and local anesthesia. The brain itself is insensitive to pain. The routine use of general anesthesia with endotracheal intubation and mechanical ventilation was yet to come. The morphine dosage had to approach, but not exceed, overdose levels. The operative mortality rate was substantial by current standards, and it seemed to me that on the ward I was commonly occupied either in trying to stave off disaster from respiratory arrest or, if unsuccessful, in getting permission for the autopsy. It was worth your own life if you failed to get permission for autopsy on that service, for autopsies permitted learning and led to progress.

Despite all this, things were going fairly well until a certain day, one of the worst of my life. The chief was away on vacation and the service was being run by the chief resident, George Markley, a confident and competent man who of course had staff backup available by telephone. The assistant residents were Henry Schenkin and Roger Cheney. Henry was nice to me, within the constraints of being nervous on a service where a minor error could suddenly become a federal offense, but Cheney was a real terror. I virtually despised him.

We were operating on the first patient that morning, with the brain exposed, when the chief of anesthesiology, Robert Dripps, poked his head through the door of the operating room to say that there was a youngster in a crib in the hall who was cyanotic and scarcely breathing, our next case. George turned quickly to me and asked, "How much morphine did you give that kid?"

"Well," I answered, "when I got around to writing the preoperative orders about three o'clock this morning, and not knowing just what the dosage should be, I woke up the intern on pediatrics and asked him the dosage. He said that $1/12$ grain, followed in three hours by another $1/12$, should be adequate, and safe."

"You mean, then, that he got $1/6$ grain. That's a good bit for his size. Drop out and see about him."

When I saw the little boy I was appalled, for I first thought he was dead. I stirred him up, to make him breathe, and sent a nurse urgently for anesthesia staff support. They arrived immediately with a tank of oxygen and a face mask, and for hours on end took turns ventilating the totally narcotized child, while the ultimate issue of brain damage and even survival from too little oxygen to the brain remained in doubt. Remember, in those days intratracheal tubes, mechanical ventilators, and effective antidotes to morphine were in their infancy and simply were not available. Today it would not have caused the least concern.

Meanwhile, I suffered the tortures of the damned. Here I was, on my first clinical service, and I may have killed a patient. Doctors may forgive mistakes but they don't forget them. I'd never felt lower in my life. Not only was the patient himself at risk, but also my reputation and career, not to mention the massive abuse I would have to take from Roger Cheney. It was small comfort that the boy's mother, who knew something was wrong but not the abject gravity of the situation, said that an unusual sensitivity to morphine ran in her family.

I was sitting over in a corner of the little patient's room when Cheney came in, having finished the case they had been doing in the operating room. I braced myself for his certain—and this time deserved—abuse and hunkered down. But to my astonishment, Roger put his arm around my shoulders and said quietly, "Jim, we're going to save this kid. We're canceling the rest of the schedule for today so that we can all be here to help. Now remember, we're all with you. We're going to save him. And don't you worry."

I still almost choke up when I recall that poignant moment. For the first time, I saw the real Roger beneath all that burly, bluff demeanor of insecurity, and we became fast friends.

The child recovered completely in eighteen hours or so, but I remain conservative with narcotic dosage to this day.

The neurosurgery rotation finally over, I found that the worst was probably past. On no other rotation during my internship was I subjected to such continuous physical and emotional stress. From then on there was time to enjoy the fellowship of a remarkably able and attractive group of interns which included Robert Fisher, Reid Bahnson, John Gislason, Archibald Fletcher, John Kirklin, Souther Tompkins, and still other equally capable men. In fact, some months later I was able to begin piano lessons. I had found in the dormitory that the trombone was really not a solo instrument and that trombone practice in close quarters did not promote friendships. I already knew how to count time and read notes, the treble clef from the clarinet and the bass clef from the trombone. I called the music department of the university and explained my requirements. I would need to take the lessons at night and might not always get there, but would of course pay whether I got there or not. I don't remember how I paid for the lessons. The internship paid for only room and board and uniforms, but I did sell blood at the Graduate Hospital from time to time.

I was put in touch with Bill Smith, a thin, tense, hyperkinetic brunette about twenty years old, who had a spot on his lung and was 4-F. He was an excellent pianist, especially with regard to technical precision, if not expression. Bill lived with his aunt on Chestnut Street. She was a plump and pleasant middle-aged lady who had psoriasis. She always waylaid me as I came in and as I left, asking for a cure (there was none). From that good lady I learned how to get away from a patient who will not let the doctor go: start moving backward toward the door, conversing pleasantly, then open the door and quickly pop out.

I promised to practice an hour each night on a piano in the intern-residents smoking room (lounge), no matter how late. This got me into a bit of trouble with the hospital administration. Just across a narrow courtyard was the obstetrical wing, and all the windows were open in August because there was no air conditioning. One woman, annoyed by my practicing, called the night superintendent and complained that she didn't come to have her baby in a nightclub. During one lesson, having practiced little, I tried to fake a passage from Beethoven's *Moonlight Sonata*. I thought I'd gotten away with it, but Bill suddenly shouted, "Not bad, but Beethoven was good, too. *Play it his way!*" While I never played the piano very well, a lasting reward was that all four of our children were stimulated to learn.

Pediatrics was a heavy rotation also. Dr. Joseph Stokes, an outstanding authority on and investigator of viral infections and immunological techniques, was chairman of the department. When I looked down those two long rows of benches with mothers holding a legion of squalling kids, I would feel like going back for another cup of coffee before attacking the afternoon multitude. It was winter and many of the children had strep throats, some had pneumonia, and at times one would have meningococcal meningitis. All too often they communicated the streptococcus to *my* throat. Moreover, crucial decisions had to be made: If I took a chance and sent a sick and feverish child home, I might miss a potentially fatal infection; on the other hand, if I admitted the child to the hospital, I would have to do a complete workup that evening. There were intravenous infusions to be given through tiny scalp veins, and lumbar spinal punctures to perform if meningitis was suspected. Each such case was quite time-consuming, and five or six patients, added to the load of the already very active hospital ward service, could tax the time available and perhaps result in skimpy treatment of somebody.

Pediatrics was a rewarding service, though, in that we did a lot of good for a lot of children. The German chemist Gerhard Domagk had discovered prontosil in 1935 (Nobel Prize, 1939), and other sulfonamides were coming along steadily for better treatment of infections. But the pediatric rotation showed me that I did not want to be a pediatrician any more than I wanted to be a neurosurgeon.

Obstetrics and gynecology was a very tidy and orderly service, and generally a happy one. The arrival of a baby is a joyful and exciting event for the family, and most obstetrical patients do well—there are almost no deaths. My principal project on the labor floor was to avoid precipitous delivery, "precips," in the patient's room without getting the mother to the delivery room for anesthesia before the event. With women who'd already had six or eight children, one had to be fast indeed—in fact, sometimes one had to push back the "crowning" head to avoid a humiliating precip. I managed to avoid this with the help of an able corps of OB nurses and the medical students. Each morning I posted on a suspended balloon "The Order of the Day—No Precips!" (as Marshal Joseph Stalin was then issuing an order of the day to the Russian troops confronting the Germans before Moscow).

Most interns then, and perhaps many now, believed that women perversely delivered more babies at night than in the daytime, just to keep the doctor from getting sleep. Well, I kept a record during my rotation: There was no statistically significant difference in the number delivered between 6 A.M. and 6 P.M. and between 6 P.M. and 6 A.M.

I went on the gynecology service before I hit OB. I asked the outgoing intern to tell me what I should expect and do. "Look," he said, "the nurses run the place. Just make friends with the head nurse, Miss Toberowski. If you act right, she'll tell you just what to do, and she knows more gynecology than you'll ever know." I took his advice, threw myself upon her mercies, and did famously.

At the end of obstetrics and gynecology I was offered a residency with them, but at that time there did not seem to be enough scientific and intellectual challenge. Besides, Julian was already going into that specialty, and one in the family was enough. But I liked that happy service.

I enjoyed general surgery with the Ravdin-Rhoads service, which was being covered by Dr. Rhoads while Dr. Ravdin was with the University Hospital army medical unit in India (the 20th General Hospital in Assam). The two residents were Harold Zintel and

C. Everett ("Chick") Koop. I thought the residents and staff worked harder than any doctors I'd met. Night after night I'd see one of the three striding along some hall of the hospital at 2:00 A.M. or so, only to see him back in the hospital by 6:00 the next morning. It eventually cost one of them tuberculosis and another several episodes of hemorrhage from a peptic ulcer.

My memories of orthopedics are of all the children and teenagers who virtually grew up in the University Hospital, wearing body casts of all sorts for bone tuberculosis, congenital deformities, and chronic staphylococcal osteomyelitis. Almost all the acute fractures were cared for by general surgery.

The eye service was nice, neat, and orderly. It had its own floor, apparently given by one of Dr. Francis Adler's wealthy patients, and thus was the private preserve of his men only. There was no clutter, and the hurly-burly of the rest of the hospital might have been on Mars. There was essentially no night work. I liked the eye service and was offered a residency, but it was too narrow for me.

ENT (ear, nose, and throat) was a very light service also. My most vivid memory is that of performing tonsillectomies under open-drop ether anesthesia. When there was considerable bleeding, which there often was, it became a taxing effort to replace the face mask quickly to give more ether, then remove it quickly and suck out the blood, and then continue the technical procedure—before having to repeat this sequence. No patient died, however, and in due course the open-drop ether was replaced with safe and secure endotracheal anesthesia.

The emergency room was fascinating, with its great variety of problems giving invaluable experience in rapid assessment and prompt disposition of patients (triage). Some patients were admitted to the hospital, some to the outpatient clinics, but most were sent home. Since I had begun the internship early, I elected an extra rotation on the ER. Fortunately, to my knowledge I committed no major errors in judgment there. However, the emergency room of a hospital is its Achilles' heel, because extremely serious medical errors may be made there for many reasons. Traditionally covered by the least-experienced physicians, usually interns, most major hospital emergency departments gradually developed round-the-clock professional staff physician coverage.

Medicine was by far the most important service of my internship. Physiology, pharmacology, and medicine had stimulated my interest in the circulation. Then, for much of the senior year, as president of

AOA I had worked with Dr. Francis C. Wood, a cardiologist, and as I mentioned previously, I had taken his senior elective, given to about five students at the Children's Heart Hospital.

On medicine I coped with my first death when I was the only doctor present. A Negro nurse who had stenosis of the mitral valve had had many attacks of acute heart failure, but each time we had been able to save her. This night, at about 2:00 A.M., she had another severe attack and said, "Dr. Hardy, I'm dying."

I said, "Of course not, we'll pull you out of it."

But she said, "No, Doctor, I'm dying." And she promptly fell back dead in my arms. There had been no time to call the family or the clergy. This was only a few years before the development of cardiac resuscitation and of heart surgery which could have readily relieved the valve obstruction.

One hears it said that doctors fear death more than any other group. I question this, but if it be so, then it is because they know so well how easily and quickly life can be snuffed out.

The service where I had the most contact with the medical chiefs was private medicine, and here I had a lot of luck. For example, Dr. Charles Wolferth, head of cardiology, called me one day and said, "Hardy, I've just examined a Ms. Q. in the office and admitted her to the hospital. She runs a 'cat house' up in Scranton, but she's a jolly soul and she pays her bills."

I went to take the history and do a physical on the "lady," who was overweight, wore a lot of expensive-looking rings and other jewelry, and was indeed jolly. I thought she had considerable fluid in her right chest, so I called Dr. Wolferth and told him I thought we ought to tap her chest to remove the fluid and improve her respiration. He said that I was wrong, that he had just examined her in the office. Brashly, I said, "Dr. Wolferth, I'll bet you fifty cents I can remove at least a liter of fluid."

"You're on," he said. "Go ahead." I removed 1200 ml and simply wrote a few words to that effect in the progress notes. Later that afternoon he came to see her, saw my note, and laughed. The next day Ms. Q. complained when he did not come down immediately when she wanted him to during office hours. He sent word to her that Dr. Hardy was his intern and that he would come only if Dr. Hardy summoned him. When I left the service, he told me to let him know if I ever wanted help with a residency.

One Sunday afternoon I had very carefully examined a patient Dr. Edward Rose, head of the Endocrine Clinic, had admitted that morning for observation because of fever and some shortness of breath. Dr. Rose was blind, having become so after he had been in practice for some years, and was a much sought after master of ceremonies and raconteur at medical fraternity affairs. He had the hospital so memorized that he could enter almost any room, on any floor, essentially unaided, and because of his blindness his other senses were particularly acute. I called Dr. Rose at home and told him I thought I could hear a very localized pneumonia in the patient's left lung. He said that, no, he had listened to her chest with his experienced stethoscope that very morning. Even so, I ventured to ask his permission to get a chest X-ray, since it was not permissible to start sulfonamide therapy without first making a diagnosis. He decided to humor me, since it *was* a teaching hospital. The X-ray did show a patch of pneumonia, I began the sulfonamide treatment, and by next day when he visited the patient again she was better. He didn't say much, but he began to treat me somewhat differently.

Dr. T. Grier Miller, chief of gastroenterology and co-developer of the Miller-Abbott tube, had one of the best bedside manners I have ever known. He would always sit down in the patient's room, no matter how briefly. He usually "laid on hands" by palpating the abdomen, taking the pulse, or listening to the heart or lungs. And he always said something encouraging. To one patient in the terminal stages of acute leukemia, with bleeding from mouth, nose, urinary tract and bowel, and face so swollen that his eyes were almost closed, Dr. Miller said, "Bill, I have good news today. Your blood hemoglobin level has risen." It made the patient's day—he was thrilled. Of course, he had been given a blood transfusion during the night, but he wanted to believe the good news.

One thing bothered me, though. Dr. Miller would ask me the laboratory data on a patient and then look at the laboratory sheet on the chart himself. One day I said to him, "Dr. Miller, sometimes I get the feeling you don't trust me." To this he replied, "I found I couldn't trust your predecessor."

One amusing episode occurred about that time. Dr. Joseph Stokes, chairman of the department of pediatrics, was admitted with severe abdominal cramps and it was decided that a long Miller-Abbott tube was to be passed. I thought Dr. Miller would want to pass this tube himself on his august colleague. Everything was ready at the bedside, the tube cooled in ice water, but when Dr. Miller tried to pass the tube he simply couldn't get it down, and the situation became embarrassing. Abruptly Dr. Miller desisted and motioned me to follow him out of the room. Outside he said, "Hardy, go back in there and pass that tube!" Returning, I said, "Dr. Stokes, the passing of a tube is an act of mutual forbearance on the part of both the physician and the patient. Your eyes will water and you will gag, but keep swallowing." It passed. (Confidentially, at times a surgeon would rather do a major operation than try to perform a minor procedure that the housestaff do every day and indeed excel at.) Every medical student should have to swallow a nasogastric tube so that he or she will know how uncomfortable it is and not leave the tube in place one hour longer than the patient needs it.

Not all was efficiency on private medicine, however. I had learned to circumvent many minor irritations and preventable sleep interruptions. First, I did not remove the bladder catheters, stomach tubes, and IVs at bedtime, lest they need to be restarted during the night; rather, I removed them early in the morning so that they could be reinstituted during the day, if necessary. Second, I routinely wrote pain reliever, laxative, and sleep sedative p.r.n. (*pro re nata*, as the situation demands) on the order sheet. But I had learned not to get upset at being awakened "unnecessarily" by a night nurse, for any number of reasons, the most important being that the patient might actually need me and, also, getting upset tended to prevent subsequent sleep.

At the end of the service Dr. Miller called me into his office and asked, "Jim, what are you going to do next year?"

"Well, Dr. Miller, I'm going to apply for the medical residency, but I hold a commission in the Army and I'll probably have to go."

"We'll see," he said.

Usually only one new medical resident was selected each year, and the chief resident in medicine was by far the most prestigious and respected house officer in the hospital, at least according to the medical students. Since I had a reserve commission, I had no real hope that I would get the medical residency, or be allowed to serve even if I did. The war was now in high gear in 1943.

Each teaching hospital was allowed to declare a certain number of residents essential to its teaching functions. They could not be called up so long as they were on that list. However, with the heavy losses of staff to the military, it was necessary to keep as much help as possible, and it was good strategy to take first as many 4-F's as possible, leaving more flexibility for keeping the commissioned men wherever they were badly needed. I knew that numerous members of our intern group were applying for the medical residency.

Selection day for new medical resident appointments finally arrived. We had heard rumors for days. It seemed that, because of the general shortage of staff, two first-year medical residents were to be taken this year. We all conceded one of these places to Godfrey. In the first place, he was a good man—Harvard, AOA, hard worker, good doctor. Second, he was a Pepper, nephew of Dr. O. H. Perry Pepper, chairman of the Department of Medicine. The Peppers had been prominent in the school for generations and, furthermore, they were a very able lot. Therefore, the rest of us felt we were competing for the second position. We had just had breakfast and were sitting in the intern-residents lounge one morning when the phone rang. Don Freshwater, a fellow intern and my colleague on the medical school senior-year wound healing research, answered it and said, "Jim, it's for you." Picking up the receiver, I realized it was Dr. Pepper himself on the other end of the line.

"Hardy," he asked, "did you apply for the medical residency?"

"Yes, sir, Dr. Pepper, I did."

"Well, we seem to have lost your application." My heart sank. "Let me ask you a few questions. How old are you?" Twenty-five. "Are you married?" No, sir, I'm single. "Do you have a commission?" Yes, sir, I have a commission. "Well, that's all." And he hung up.

"Well, Hardy! That fixes you!" exclaimed Freshwater. And I knew he was right. I was more disappointed than I had intended to be but I did not let on. I got up and went down to the emergency room.

About an hour later I got a call from Miss Ruth Rumble, Dr. Pepper's imposing secretary, saying that Dr. Pepper wanted to see me. I knew he always also called up to his office those who had not gotten his residency, to say he was sorry there were not more openings. I was determined not to show the slightest emotion when I got there, but I felt plenty inside.

I was ushered into his inner office. Dr. Pepper said, "Sit down, Hardy. Have a cigarette?"

"No, thank you, sir, I don't smoke," I replied quietly.

"Hardy," he said, "the selection committee has only one concern about you. We wonder if you're going to be able to support all your women on a medical resident's pay?"

"Dr. Pepper," I exulted, "I'll certainly try!"

"Then you've got it," he said, and reached over his desk to shake my hand. We chatted a few minutes and I learned that the second

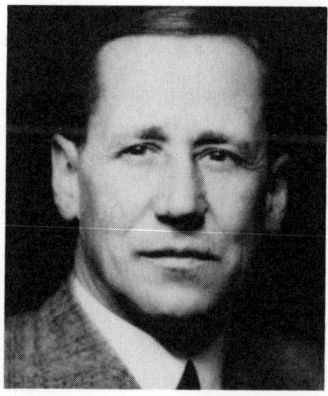

O. H. Perry Pepper

resident was indeed to be his nephew, whom I had liked and admired since our freshman year.

What a triumph. To say I was elated would be the grossest understatement. I would be working in the most prestigious position, in the specialty I liked best, and with a staff that I respected enormously. The world was my oyster.

I began the medical residency in July.

CHAPTER 5

Medical Resident at Penn

The medical residency "year" was a most rewarding nine months, truncated by events to be told. The responsibilities of the resident were not dissimilar to those of the intern, but the resident stayed in one specialty for the year, instead of rotating every four to six weeks as did the interns, and the resident had far more authority, prerogatives, extensive responsibilities, and time to carry on research, interspersed among patient admissions, ward rounds, and conferences. Incidentally, my finances promptly improved: I received seventy dollars per month to serve as hospital Chief Medical Officer (CMO) at night, a stipend as medical resident, and ten dollars for each Addis count on urine specimens.

My daily duties started with rounds on the wards at about 6:00 or 6:30; after breakfast and a glance at the newspaper, I was back on the ward for staff-resident-intern-student rounds at 8:00 A.M. Anyone who has been on a medical service is well aware of how stylized this minuet can be. Moving from bed to bed down the aisle, the intern would give the history and physical examination from memory, the resident would be called upon for his opinion of the situation, and then the "attending" (physician) would elaborate and pontificate. These work rounds usually lasted about two hours.

Small facts assumed major dimensions in the minds of some attendings. A common error was to misstate the patient's age by a year or so, whereupon the patient, if female and if the stated age was too high, would usually issue an embarrassingly firm correction. I introduced the highly effective procedure of placing the age in very small, unobtrusive characters in a corner of the name card on the foot of the patient's bed.

When the attending changed every three months, the whole flavor and aura of the ward changed too. For example, an attending who was a vascular man would tend to see blood vessel problems in many patients, the heart man heart problems, the metabolic man metabolic problems. It was useful to hear different organ systems discussed in depth, but it also taught me that a highly specialized physician can readily miss the overall picture of a patient's disease and personality. In fact, so concerned was Dr. Pepper that a given specialist scheduled to come on the service would tend to pull in too many patients with his type of disease conditions—rendering the ward a poor learning laboratory for the students, interns, and residents—that he would caution me ahead of time not to let this or that ultraspecialist fill the ward with arthritics, or diabetics, or asthmatics, or cardiacs, or still other types. Theoretically I, the resident, had control over which patients were admitted to "my" ward, but obviously common sense suggested that one pay some deference to what the attending wanted to do.

Three days a week one of the ward service chiefs—Dr. Miller, Dr. Wolferth, or Dr. Pepper—would make teaching rounds. Dr. Rose, head of endocrinology, held "unknown case rounds" on the sun porch, where he would listen to each sentence, in fact each word, of the student's history, and then would say what he thought was wrong with the patient—and he would usually be right. All were fine teachers, but Dr. Pepper perhaps had the most charisma. Every so often he would make "look rounds." He would proceed down the aisle, allowing no comment while he looked closely and carefully at each patient in turn. At each bed he would say what he saw and what he thought might be wrong with the patient, and he was astonishingly accurate in many cases.

I vividly remember one patient whom we had diagnosed as having bronchitis and had been treating with sulfonamides (the attending was a specialist in the clinical studies and trials of these drugs). The chief looked at the middle-aged white woman for a few moments, rolled her hair between thumb and forefinger, compressed her ankle, and then said, "This patient has severe myxedema." He pointed to her somewhat puffy face, her dry, brittle hair, and the slight swelling of her ankles. To our dismay and acute embarrassment, tests showed that he was absolutely right: she had profound loss of thyroid function.

Such demonstrations were not lost on me, and I later did the same thing with students myself. Dr. Pepper was very good, but one does not have to be a genius. The answer lies in experience. The value of seeing large numbers of patients (or doing large numbers of operations) cannot be exaggerated. Sir William Osler wrote as follows:

> To study medicine without books, is to sail an uncharted sea;
> But to study medicine without patients, is not to go to sea at all.

Dr. Owen H. Wangensteen, chairman of surgery at the University of Minnesota for many years, once told the story of his visit as a young man to Dr. Harvey Cushing of Harvard, world-famous neurosurgeon and the father of that specialty in this country. "Dr. Cushing," Wangensteen had asked at the end of a brilliant brain operation, "how did you know to go so quickly to the site of the tumor?" This was of course long before the advent of radiologic advances such as arteriograms or CAT scan.

"Experience," answered Cushing, always a severe and precise man in the operating environment, it seems.

When Wangensteen had repeated his question on two more successive mornings, Cushing had replied, "Young man, for the third and last time, *experience.*"

With experience the physician learns to note automatically a host of things as he sees the patient. He notes the general appearance (cancer?—which Leonardo da Vinci could put in the face), the walk (limp? staggering? stiff?—each suggests a different disease), speech, the eyes. Virtually everything about a patient can suggest that a given organic or psychiatric disease is, or is not, a possibility. Poor teeth suggest social and financial status. Tattoos suggest occupation, perhaps periods of intoxication, and potential exposure to venereal disease.

Once morning rounds were over, we set in motion all the decisions made during rounds: tests were ordered, procedures carried out, consultations requested, X-rays scheduled, and so forth. After this, unless I needed to help the intern, check write-ups, or teach students, I was free for the most part to do research between the numerous conferences. Grand Rounds was the major departmental meeting each week, at which instructive patients were presented to the assembled faculty, house staff, and medical students of the department of medicine in the medical amphitheater. My own two major conference responsibilities were to plan grand rounds, and to work with Dr. Pepper on his senior-class seminar. In these two activities I saw a lot of him and I treasured this association. I also took over the job of passing the Miller-Abbott tubes for the whole hospital, using a fluoroscope in the GI Clinic which I'm sure spewed radiation in all directions. When the relationship between radiation exposure and leukemia became well known, I wondered if I might myself not turn up with leukemia, as this was the cause of Dr. Abbott's own death.

Shortly after beginning the year, I went to see Dr. John Lockwood, who was running the Harrison Department of Surgical Research for Dr. Ravdin during the war. I asked him to suggest a jumping-off place for research in the management of surgical infections. (In retrospect it is interesting that, though a resident in medicine, I had turned first to surgery for this guidance.) "Hardy," he said, "infections are a dead issue. Penicillin is going to make surgical infection research irrelevant. I advise you to enter some other field." Looking back at all that has happened since, it is clear that his position was premature, to say the least.

Linc Godfrey and I then asked Dr. Isaac Starr, who developed the ballistocardiograph and later received the Lasker Award (the medical "Nobel Prize" in the United States), to recommend a research project. He suggested that, using his ballisto, with which one could measure (estimate) the output of the heart per minute, we might evaluate the circulatory effects of intravenous fluids given to normal subjects, compared with their effects in dehydrated patients. This was straightforward enough, since we commonly had to give vomiting patients intravenous salt and glucose solutions, often in preparation for surgery to relieve alimentary tract obstruction. Today such a

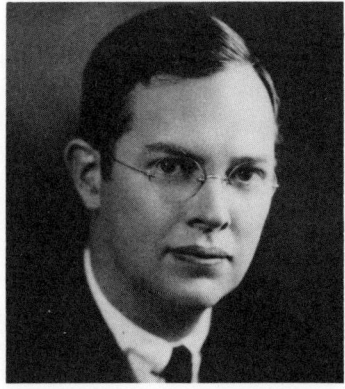

Isaac Starr

study would seem almost too obvious, for all physicians know that such fluid treatment increases cardiac output. In 1943, however, this had not been well documented, since methods for readily measuring cardiac output were crude and in their infancy.

We demonstrated very clearly that intravenous fluids had little effect on normal subjects (ourselves and other interns and residents), but that they substantially increased the previously diminished cardiac output of dehydrated patients. Dr. Starr looked at the data and then said to us, "Boys, you've got a find!" We published our research in the *Journal of the American Medical Association*.

Incidentally, working in Starr's laboratory at the time was Christensen Lambertson, who had won a prize each year at Undergraduate Medical Association Day for still further improvements in equipment he had developed as a teen-ager—college student for walking on the ocean floor at his home on the Jersey shore. One day he disappeared. It seemed he had been whisked to Washington to work on problems related to diving equipment for frogmen.

Another study, one which I worked on alone and published after the war, had to do with whether patients with low serum protein levels absorbed amino acids at a normal rate. First, a tube with four lumens or conduits was constructed, being actually a long Miller-Abbott tube with two small tubes tied along it. Through each of the two small tubes a balloon was inflated to block off a sixty-centimeter segment of the small intestine selected at fluoroscopy. Then, a known concentration of the amino acid solution was instilled at a fixed rate into the intestine just below the first balloon; the solution not absorbed was sucked out when it reached the second balloon. Using a timed interval and rate of infusion, it was possible to calculate how much nitrogen had been absorbed. The normal controls were myself and my fellow interns and residents, but such was the discomfort of swallowing and then tolerating the large (four-lumened) tube for the required eighteen hours on the hard fluoroscopic table, that I never got anyone to volunteer twice. I had no technician and ran every chemical analysis myself in laboratory space provided by Dr. Francis Lukens, a splendid physician, scientist, and gentleman. It was time consuming, yes, but research is never quite the same as when the investigator does every analysis and calculation himself: he knows his data cold, something that is deeply satisfying.

I had learned by now that it is not necessary to be a genius or have some primordial insight in order to do useful research. One simply has to work at it hard and intelligently, as one would otherwise be doing with patients on the floors. Research became a vital part of my professional life during my residency and was to remain so thereafter.

Another project arose from the great need, in 1943, for further studies of the effects of blood loss in wounded soldiers. A massive search was mounted for "plasma expanders" that could be stored on the battlefield and then used to support a patient's blood pressure until blood itself became available for transfusion.

In the blood plasma substitute project, I gave gelatin intravenously to a large number of patient volunteers and residents in order to exclude any reactions or sensitivities to the gelatin itself. Its circulatory effects were studied on the ballistocardiograph table. And from this study I learned something not measurable in grams or centimeters about research policies and politics. One day I was sitting in the corner of Dr. Starr's laboratory, calculating ballisto tracings with a slide rule, when Dr. Starr came in and said, "Jim, I've just come from the research committee that receives reports from different groups doing research in the medical school, and I heard something that disturbed me. The gelatin project was presented, but your name was not mentioned as a participant who would share in publications. What is your arrangement?" I replied that I had been assured my name would appear on any paper in which my data were used. He then said, "Well, I'm concerned about it. I've seen too many young men soured on research by some unhappy early experience. I want you to go over and see John Lockwood, and let me know what you find out."

I first called Dr. Archibald Fletcher, a resident in surgery who had enlisted my very considerable collaboration. He said that my recollection of the publication agreement was of course correct, and he went at once to Dr. C. Everett Koop, resident in surgery and the executive officer for the project. Apparently having been inadequately informed of the informal agreement with me, Dr. Koop took the position that to include my name on publications would require acknowledgement of the fact that I was in another department, thus giving undue credit to the Department of Medicine, as opposed to the Department of Surgery. However, Dr. Lockwood took a different tack and my name was included. The affair led to somewhat bruised feelings, though, and thereafter the interdepartmental collaboration was terminated by mutual agreement.

After the dust had settled, Dr. Starr advised, "Now, Jim, in the future, when you participate with others in a research project, draw up a 'memorandum of understanding' at the outset, before any substantial amount of work has been done. Lay out who is to do what, and list a tentative order for the authors' names to appear on any papers—first author, second author, last author, and so forth. Like a will, it can always be changed later, in the light of subsequent events and personnel changes, but it preserves a written record of the original agreements."

I followed this advice in all significant activities thereafter. It startled colleagues occasionally, appearing to the naive that I did not have complete trust. But with appropriate attention to verbal explanations, it preserved friendships and gave credit where credit was due.

One day in the early spring, Dr. Pepper called me to his office to meet with Dr. Robert Loeb of Columbia-Presbyterian Medical Center in New York, a very influential national figure in the world of internal medicine. He had been charged with the responsibility of assembling in Chicago a research team to find some way to control the ravages of malaria among our troops in the South Pacific, where this disease was often causing more casualties than the Japanese. Dr. Pepper had recommended Franklin Murphy and me, and urged that we take the assignment because it would keep us in touch with the laboratory and with at least some element of clinical medicine while we were in the military service. Certainly there would be few such opportunities in the army ground forces, so I accepted. Dr. Pepper and the University Hospital released me from the essential list immediately. To my dismay, however, while Murphy was approved, the War Department said that I had a commission, had been trained with the army ground forces, and that was where I would be assigned. About a month later I was on my way to Carlisle Barracks.

When I went by to say goodbye to the women in the dean's office, Miss Gallagher, his assistant who had known me since my freshman year, asked, "Dr. Hardy, what have you lined up in the military?"

"Why, nothing, Miss Gallagher," and I recounted my research assignment failure.

"I'll be in touch with you," she said.

My last full day at University Hospital was one of the most memorable. A major military project measuring the effects of blood loss in man was being conducted in Dr. Starr's laboratory. Some large men were bled almost a liter of blood. I volunteered as an experimental subject and was bled almost 1100 ml. As the blood loss approached this point my vision became blurred, and I had to take rapid deep breaths and keep flexing my arms and legs to avoid blacking out. My blood pressure fell to 70 mm Hg and the cardiac output fell by almost 50 percent. When blood loss ceased, however, my vision gradually cleared over the next few minutes and, although I remained very weak and somewhat breathless with a rapid pulse, I did not decompensate again. My blood pressure gradually rose to between 80 and 90 mm Hg, but it did not return to the prebleeding level of 120 throughout the night. For several hours I could not sit up without passing out, but later on I could sit up with my feet on the floor. By morning I could stand weakly, but to observers I "looked and acted like a sick man." This was my last full day in Philadelphia, and I had to go downtown to buy an army footlocker to take to camp at Carlisle Barracks. I made it downtown and got it, but it was just about all I could do to pick up the empty footlocker and get it back to the University Hospital. At this point, I had my stored blood transfused back, and my cardiac output promptly returned to normal. I felt like a new man and departed for vacation in Alabama.

On April 22, Godfrey and I took the train to Harrisburg and thence to Carlisle Barracks. On the way up, Linc, who had celebrated considerably the night before, suddenly said to me very somberly, "Are you nervous?" It was extremely unusual for him to ask any personal question—he was so reserved, so Harvard de rigueur.

"Why, no, Linc, I'm not nervous. After all, we *are* doctors. We won't exactly be in a foxhole, though since we are headed for the infantry we may well be in a battalion aid station."

He said, "Well, whenever I have to change from one place to another, or from one job to another, I get all nervous inside."

I did not think too much about this exchange at the time, though some years later, upon learning of his untimely death, I was to recall with sadness his then apparently trivial question and comment.

CHAPTER 6

With the U.S. Army in England, France, and Germany
(From a Medical Officer's Journal)

Arriving at Harrisburg, we piled into a two-and-one-half-ton truck for the perhaps twenty-mile trip to Carlisle Barracks. After filling out all the army documents, Godfrey and I found ourselves assigned to the second floor of a long barracks, where virtually all the other officers were black dentists who had just graduated from Howard University in Washington. Godfrey was at first incensed, but near the end of our stay he said to me privately, "You know, this is the first time I've ever had social contact with Negroes on an equal level. They're really very nice guys."

And the Negroes were gentlemen. I recorded, then, that "the further I go, the more I am convinced that the chief difference between peoples is that of education. I, for one, hope that the day will come when all races will get even breaks in this world. We all live but once."

It was all business at Carlisle. The next morning, although we had yet to go to the supply building and get our fatigue uniforms, we were first addressed by a colonel in the pouring rain and then drilled by the officers who would command our 53d Officers Training Battalion.

One day I was paged on the parade ground. Miss Gallagher was calling from Philadelphia. She wanted to know if I would like to be assigned to the medical service at McGuire General Hospital, just being completed in Richmond? I would!

In five weeks the staff at Carlisle put on perhaps the best course I'd ever had anywhere—physical conditioning, logistics, the duties of a (medical) train commander, field hygiene, emergency wound management, and much else. It was my first experience with the valuable use of instructional movies, which taught us such things as how to clean a rifle (a dirty rifle misfired as a German closed in for the kill), or how to check for booby traps (the infantryman had checked every last possibility, he thought, but when he pulled the chain on the commode it blew him sky high).

My next orders sent me to the medical officers pool at Stark General Hospital (GH) outside Charleston, South Carolina.

2 JUNE 44: FIRST "PERMANENT" ASSIGNMENT—STARK GENERAL HOSPITAL. Arrived at first station a bit scared. When I snapped a smart salute, the adjutant almost fell out of his chair. (Clearly, military formalities are relaxed considerably "in the field.") Was assigned to the medical services by request—and to cardiology under Cpt. Kaufman (a Penn graduate-school alumnus). Hot as hell here. Roommate in the "Green Mansions," as these torrid barracks which house the MDRP [Medical Department Replacement Pool] are sarcastically termed, is leaving for a GH in Georgia. Hope I get one!

3 JUNE 44: A MARRIAGE CONTACT. Saw Arch Fletcher and he's just received orders to proceed to 6th Sv. Command Headquarters in Chicago. He'd lined up a beach party for the (Saturday) afternoon, but it fell thru when Cpt. Kaufman kept me on duty all afternoon.

Met Weezie Sams, though, and she's a most delightful girl. Brown eyes, brown hair, yellow summer frock, high heels. We went out to dinner, where Arch and I talked Carlisle shop all evening. I'm certain the girls (Weezie and Kay Oates) were bored stiff. [Arch, son of Presbyterian missionaries and ultimately to be a medical missionary himself, had made contact with the girls through the Presbyterian church.]

I quickly found I could share thoughts easily with Weezie, and five years later she became a Hardy. The Sams family, from Atlanta-Decatur, had been transferred to Charleston by the Atlantic Coast Line railroad for the duration of the war. Weezie had recently graduated from Agnes Scott College in Decatur.

4 JUNE 44: REVOLVING ROOMMATES. Went to Folly Beach with Weezie. Grand time. Weather here hottest of experience. Always wet. Rains daily. Terrific humidity. After losing three different roommates in three days, I now have Bill Kirchbaum of NYC—nice chap. This pool is plenty "hot."

7 JUNE 44: HOSPITAL TRAIN MEDICAL OFFICER. Ordered to accompany hospital train of patients to Cushing General Hospital at Framingham, Massachusetts. Can't find Carlisle notes on duties of train commander. Wish I'd listened during those 1400 lectures. I do recall that one must examine toilets and water supply.

First actual experience in commanding men but one of the sgts. is an old hand at this business. The job is his!

8 JUNE 44: AN EFFICIENT OPERATION AT CUSHING GH. Passed through Phila. during night—same old 30th Street Station. Awake to look out upon the beautiful Hudson Valley and River. Passed and glimpsed West Point.

Organization at Cushing GH was astonishing. Backed in, delivered patients, turned over valuables, unloaded baggage, made property exchange, had records signed for, sent telegram advising Stark and War Department of arrival, and backed out again—all in 15 minutes. Framingham was a quaint old New England town. Never saw people who asked so many questions.

[Note: The railroads were invariably most considerate of the needs and comfort of wounded soldiers.]

10 JUNE 44. Returned to Charleston and found four blankets missing. Reported them on survey. "Fault of no one concerned." We're using Carlisle information daily. Very practical course! Also found orders waiting directing me to proceed to McGuire GH. Great luck! Report there 20 June.

21 JUNE 44: ARRIVAL AT McGUIRE GH, RICHMOND. Mamma's birthday and wedding anniversary. Arrived in Richmond and called McGuire for transportation, which arrived promptly. McGuire was found to be farther out than had been anticipated. Was greeted by the adjutant, CWO Larry Roffman, and by asst. adjutant, CWO George Vaeth, both most friendly. Saw Maj. Pepper, who was very kind, assigning me to the Isolation Section under Maj. Jack W. P. Love, another Penn graduate. Cpt. Bill Jeffers (from Penn) is in charge of cardiology. Would like to be in his section. Col. Percy Duggins, CO, is quiet, dignified, and quite obviously competent. Had a nice chat at the club with Maj. Morris Bowie, an altogether splendid fellow, who'd given us a few lectures in medicine at Penn but whom I'd never known personally. What a loss never to have really met him.

22 JUNE 44: HOSPITAL DUTY ASSIGNMENTS. No patients. Spent the day organizing the isolation setup with Lt. Foster (ANC [Army Nurse Corps]) of Baltimore. Remarkable how much an intern does not comprehend concerning the ward routine. The nurses did this at Penn. Maj. Bowie has asked me to help with the lectures to technicians. I am glad to oblige for several reasons: (1) I like Maj. Bowie very much; (2) good speaking experience; (3) there is nothing else to do. Subject is to be (infectious) isolation technique, with demonstrations.

26 JUNE 44: DECISION TO FLY. Went swimming in a lake this afternoon with Roffman, Vaeth, and a number of nurses. Saw a boy stunting in a cub plane. Think I'll look into the possibilities of taking flight instruction.

27 JUNE 44: HERMITAGE AIRPORT. Talked with one A. B. Lowery at Hermitage Airport today. Will begin flight instruction next week. He says he can teach me to fly an airplane but that I'll have to learn all the book courses on my own, since army cadet instruction has been closed. (He is pessimistic about my passing the written examination). Will buy books and use medical school study discipline.

30 JUNE 44: FIRST FLIGHT. First flight in an aircraft. Quite a thrill. Once up, it is truly remarkable how one can get back to the ground safely. Must study all alone to pass the rather comprehensive written examinations on CAA [Civil Aeronautics Authority] regulations, navigation, meteorology, and flight aircraft maintenance. It can be done.

Transportation to the field is slow and laborious. Must go after duty hours. Bus to town, then trolley, then bus. Takes over an hour at best. Ten-minute walk after all the riding (arriving about 1800). However, during the walk I can watch others land and take off, thereby noting certain points. (Being summer, adequate daylight lasted until 2000.) Then retrace journey and begin study.

Lowery seems likely to be a good instructor. Rolls, spins, power turns and endless sudden "forced landing" commands, for practice just in case.

15 JULY 44: ANOTHER HOSPITAL TRAIN AND CHICAGO. Made a trip to Schick GH at Camden, Iowa. First time to cross Mississippi River. Uneventful except for a return layover in Chicago of 24 hours. Enjoyed seeing U. of Chicago. Lovely grounds. Was in Professor A. J. Carlson's [physiology] laboratory but he was away in Canada for the summer. Photographed Chicago Lying-In Hospital and University clinics. Also Grant Park, aquarium, Field Museum (magnificent), art museum, and Lake Michigan.

In front of the officers club I bumped into a fellow Carlisle classmate—Walter Martin [we would later go overseas together].

Liked Chicago. Great for servicemen.

3 AUG 44: FIRST SOLO FLIGHT. Today was the day! Lowery and I went up. He said, "Circle and land." This was done. Then he got out and said, "She's all yours; take her up, circle, and land." That was about all. I was supremely confident. Had none of the anxiety pilots are supposed to have at first solo. However, it was an exhilarating sensation to realize overwhelmingly that you, and you alone, must land the aircraft safely if you're to walk away from it. Lowery watched from the field and when I'd landed and taxied over to him, said "Swell, Hardy. Take off and land a few times, and then we'll write you up as certified for solo flight."

30 AUG 44. Had a 5-day leave. Spent three days in Charleston with W. Then went to Philadelphia for two days. Talked with Dr. Miller and decided not to publish the Amigen absorption paper until further data can be collected. Dr. Starr, bless him, is keeping things going on the gelatin paper. What time HUP men are willing to devote to younger men! Teachers, all.

15 SEPT 44: MILITARY MELANCHOLY, ANATOMY OF. Back at Newport News but my train leaves tomorrow. Today several of us have taken temporary quarters in the Bachelor Officers Quarters (for transients). It is raining and I am melancholy. What *are* the anatomy and physiopathology of military melancholy? Why should a man be at times despondent, when he would not have been so in a civilian capacity? He is lonely out of all proportion to distance. It is probably because he is something of a

prisoner. His freedom is limited by a steel code which, while not a tangible ring, is none the less inflexible. Then, too, except in old units, he is essentially among strangers. His confidences must remain his own. Drinking a pastime and release for many.

28 SEPT 44: TRANSPORTING GERMAN AFRIKA KORPS TROOPS TO IDAHO. Back from a very tedious ten-day trip to Rupert, Idaho, as medical officer for a trainload of 500 German PWs. Mostly General Rommel's Afrika Korps. Was struck by wide range in ages. Some were eighteen and some were almost fifty. Enjoyed attempts at speaking German. Of the five hundred, twenty-five (8.5%) developed ankle edema from approximately 120 hours of the sitting posture (interrupted only by rare one-by-one to the latrine). One young boy went raving insane in Illinois. Probably schizophrenia. Put off at Camp Grant. Multiple furuncles and marked diarrhea were chief difficulties. Sanitation deplorable.

All of U.S. personnel in troop sleepers. Very hot and filthy. Was cold, though, out west. Went through Va., W. Va., Kentucky, Indiana, Illinois, Iowa, Kansas, Nebraska, Wyoming, and Idaho.

The PWs were unloaded in open country and were surrounded by heavily armed guards supplemented by huge, ragingly vicious dogs. Escape would have been impossible. (They were apparently to dig sugar beets.)

Some years later, Professor Ian Aird of London related to me a personal experience with General Rommel. In North Africa the Germans had overrun Aird's field hospital, and Rommel came in to inquire about one of his officers who had been desperately wounded in the chest and was soon to be operated upon. He asked about needs and sent morphine. A few days later the Germans had to retreat and a young officer on Rommel's staff came again. When told the colonel had died, the officer said he would like to collect his identification disc and valuables, including a gold watch and a gold cigarette case. With great apprehension, Professor Aird confessed that in the emergency these had been stolen; despite every search they could not be found. The German officer said simply, "This sometimes happens in war."

3 OCT 44: ANOTHER "DETACHED SERVICE" ASSIGNMENT (FROM McGUIRE). Here at Swift Creek Maneuver Area, out of Camp Lee, acting as medical officer for 1000 Negro quartermaster troops. At last—practicing medicine out of a No. 2 Chest. Julian will be amused. Not a very desirable assignment but, from some financial quirk, we get per diem. Living in a tent. Cold, often wet, and thoroughly uncomfortable. Have fired machine gun, though.

7 OCT 44: CAA PRIVATE PILOT WRITTEN EXAMINATION. Went to Richmond today and took written exam for private license. Feel sure I passed, though navigation and meteorology were plenty tough. The problems on gasoline consumption at different wind velocities were the most difficult. [Later passed actual Flight Examination with a CAA pilot inspector and got private flying license.]

12 OCT 44: REQUEST FOR OVERSEAS. Was at McGuire today and asked Maj. Pepper to send me along to Camp Ellis for assignment to overseas outfit. Want to get "over there" before war ends, preferably to ETO [European theater of operations].

17 OCT 44. ORDERED TO CAMP ELLIS, Illinois, along with Hal Barker. Many general, station, and field hospitals being organized there.

19 OCT 44: CAMP ELLIS, ILLINOIS—Nearest oasis, Peoria. Arrived at Camp Ellis and it is certainly no garden spot. Miles from any important town and transportation is practically nonexistent. What will assignment be? Probably a field hospital, possibly a GH, general dispensary, or a train company. Little known, apparently, of function of field hospitals, of which about 20 are being activated. Large numbers of medical officers here from all over. The assignment this time will be for the greater part of our overseas service.

22 OCT 44. Hal Barker and I were assigned to 81st Field Hospital (together, as requested) under command of Maj. Gerald Banks. "Hot" outfit, "overseas by Christmas." CO thinks European theater. Theme song seems to be, "You Always Hurt the One You Love." Chaplain Norris, Protestant, seems to view his army duties with an open and willing mind.

Major Gerald Banks was fairly short, sun-bleached, wiry, with close-cropped blond hair and a neat mustache. Regular Army, he exuded military spit and polish. The 81st had been activated on September 21, 1944. The table of organization (TO) called for 22 officers, 18 nurses, and 182 enlisted men (EM). This personnel could, and overseas probably would, be divided into three self-contained units from time to time. The combined units could handle 400 patients. A field hospital was the intermediate between the infantry's medical collection company on the one hand and the station hospital on the other. However, the field hospital could also function as a station hospital.

The CO and five Medical Administrative Corps (MAC) officers would carry the strictly administrative problems, though the medical and dental officers would be expected to share in the command activities at their various and appropriate levels.

We were favorably impressed with the CO. He had been in the army for almost four years, two of which had been spent on desert maneuvers. Moreover, he had just come from serving a year in the Surgeon General's office. Thus, when he guessed we would end up in the European theater, we felt fairly certain of not going to the Pacific.

The care with which the CO had selected certain of his key administrative officers was likewise reassuring. For his adjutant he had appointed Lieutenant Arthur Hurand, MAC, a swarthy, extremely energetic young lawyer from Flint, Michigan. Though as adjutant he represented all the authority of the commanding officer, never was I to see Hurand use this power unfairly. Selfless and sincere, he was trusted by all.

Lieutenant Russell ("Girls, just call me Russ") Lewis was supply officer. Having spent eleven years in the army, and having come up through the ranks, he was without doubt the most accomplished borrower I ever knew. For example, he had already acquired literally truckloads of furniture for the 81st offices without ever signing a single receipt. Such a man would be invaluable.

The other principal administrative person was Harold Williams, first sergeant. Tall, stocky, jovial, and sporting a black mustache, he was already a favorite with both the officers and the enlisted men. He too had been in the army several years. Formerly with an MP battalion in New York City, he had been, if memory serves, a salesman of feminine hygiene articles before the war. Leadership is where you find it, and he was a natural leader of men.

Despite the CO's assurance that the 81st had a good bunch of enlisted men, their morale was said to be low. To begin with, as many of them were former MPs, they resented having been transferred to the medics, a noncombatant service. Taunted by the jeers of "bedpan commando," they felt an acute sense of inferiority when around combat outfits. Moreover, Camp Ellis was said to have been poorly administered during the time these men were being trained (for hospital service) in the Army Service Forces Training Center, long before they were assigned to the 81st. Not only had their pay been irregular, but sometimes even the next meal had been in doubt.

Even so, the readiness date was not far distant, and all the officers were urged to dig in with a will at any problem that came up. One hundred tons of equipment was already on hand. Major Banks proposed a shakedown bivouac, but before this really got under way the 81st was ordered to Camp Lee, Virginia, for parallel training of the enlisted men in the regional hospital there.

Just before departure, Corporal John D. Head presented the mascot emblem he had developed for the 81st: "Heartless Herman."

The unit entrained on November 8 and arrived at Camp Lee a day later. The next six weeks was to be most important in achieving unity, efficiency, and a vast improvement in morale. First, we began to know each other. Soon the eighteen nurses had arrived, under the direction of a Regular Army nurse, Captain Eileen Donnelly, chief nurse. Most important, the enlisted men worked alongside medical officers and nurses in the Camp Lee Regional Hospital, promoting respect on all sides. Three units—A, B, and C—had been designated and had stabilized as functioning entities. I was assigned to C unit (or platoon) as the internist, by virtue of having had the medical residency. Captain Karl Corley (radiologist) was unit commander, and Ben Smith was the surgeon because of his one or two years of surgical residency. There were three other general medical officers, one dentist, six nurses, and one MAC officer. The other two units, A and B, were similarly constituted.

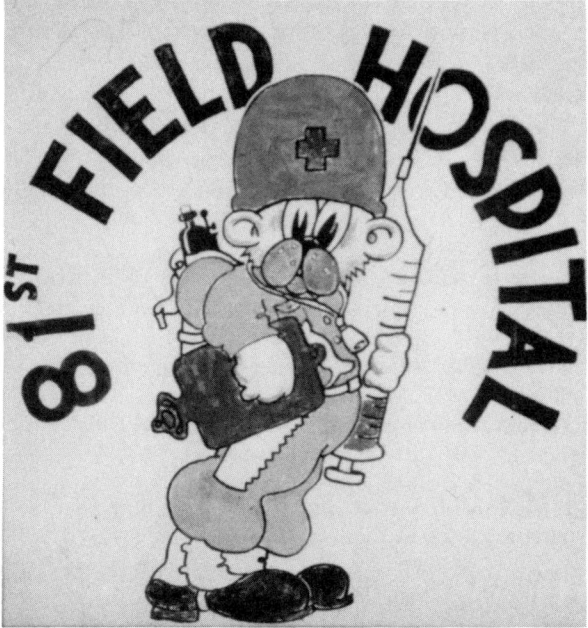

Heartless Herman, mascot of 81st Field Hospital

Presently, the 81st convoyed to Swift Creek Maneuver Area for a full shakedown, complete with tents, kitchen ranges, and latrines. When a surprise inspection by the inspector general (IG) disclosed specific deficiencies, I was assigned to lecture to the enlisted men on mines and booby traps; my presentations were embellished considerably with explosions set off suddenly in the back of the lecture hall by Sergeant Shaw, previously with the infantry. I was also assigned with Hal Barker to lay out a night compass- and map-reading exercise—this on the strength of my flight navigation using the compass. All officers, noncommissioned officers, and vehicle drivers would be required to complete this laid-out course at night under blackout conditions.

The 81st passed the next inspection satisfactorily. Actually, I personally had never doubted that we would be extended the privilege of foreign service, but Major Banks, being a career army officer, had been deeply concerned—and not without reason, for the CO of another field hospital at the station was reported to have been relieved for inefficiency. But this time the IG had sensed a difference in the 81st. The experience that the enlisted men had had in the regional hospital, their first with sick patients, had given them a new respect for medical officers and nurses, as well as for the importance of medical corpsmen (themselves) in the total scheme of things. A gratifying and indeed remarkable esprit de corps had developed in the 81st Field Hospital, though we had formed as a unit less than two months before. Clearly, the army had to be given some credit, somewhere!

17 DEC 44: CAMP LEE—ORDERED TO POE (PORT OF EMBARKATION). After a night of wine and song, we entrained and have arrived here at Camp Kilmer, New Jersey, about which we've heard since Carlisle days. Everyone rushing around attending to last-minute preparations. Rumors—all sorts—everywhere endless meetings—"sharp"! Passes to New York. Great variety of units. "Abandon ship" drill. Test gas masks.

Extremely cold, with deep snow.

Meanwhile, the course of war in Europe had abruptly taken a turn against the Allies. On December 16, with tactical surprise, the Germans had attacked in great force through the Ardennes, with massive early success. There was the very real danger that the armored spearhead could strike all the way to the coast, dividing the Allied armies. General Rundstedt had indeed struck a major blow and there was grim foreboding. Major Banks instructed me to review the situation with our enlisted men. It was the Battle of the Bulge.

20 DEC 44: THE LIST. Bombshell! The "list" is born! Reisman, Barker, Cummings, Martin, Tavener, and Simon are "elected" to go on ships other than the one on which the rest of the unit will make the crossing. Barker is most upset and overwhelmingly convinced that these separated men will never rejoin the unit. He really deserves better, for as P & T [Plans and Training] officer he's worked very hard. However, as lowly "baggage officer," my role has suddenly become important—logistics!

23 DEC 44: EMBARKATION! Loading officer with advance party. In the immortal words of the 81st, "What are we supposed to be doing? Snafu—can't get all the equipment placed in the railroad coach as it sez here in the manual in fine print." Everyone grumpy after being routed out at 0430 in the severe cold. Simon was so busy griping that he left his steel helmet in the truck. "Everyone sling equipment and prepare to dismount." We've arrived in New York. Damn! This duffel bag weighs a ton! Why did I bring all this stuff? The march from train to boat a nightmare of carrying equipment and belongings. Wringing wet with sweat, in almost zero temperature. Finally made it to the ferry and, after many stops, we reached the pier. Red Cross on hand. EM laughing at officers' huge duffel bags. Cpts. Scott and Bounds dragged holes in the bottom of theirs.

There she is! HMS *Vollendam*. Much smaller than the large liner we'd imagined—very much smaller. Probably doesn't carry more than 500 troops. Ship very new to us landlubbers, but we're informed that it was built before the First World War. Remarkably compact, a ship is. Officers' quarters clean and warm, with 15 men to each small cabin in our *overseas* travel, usually holding only two passengers going *abroad*. British stewards, rather low-class gents, exhibit a superior attitude toward us inlanders and it irritates.

Good heavens! Three thousand EM are to be packed into the lower compartments! Glad I'm an officer. The HMS *Vollendam* is, we're told by ship CO, very seaworthy. Two meals per day, even tomorrow on Christmas. Very little in form of recreation. Reading, letter writing, and bridge likely to be featured. Amusing incident when the many air corps officers were brought into line by Col. Nelson, troop commander, with, "There'll be no prima donnas on this trip. Many officers have expressed doubt as to whether you airmen would cooperate with the various assignments. You will, or else you'll answer to me." Incidentally, the air corps officers are a good-looking group.

Remainder of day spent in exploring the ship. Remarkable how much is packed into such a small space. Four years ago I saw the *Normandie*, the

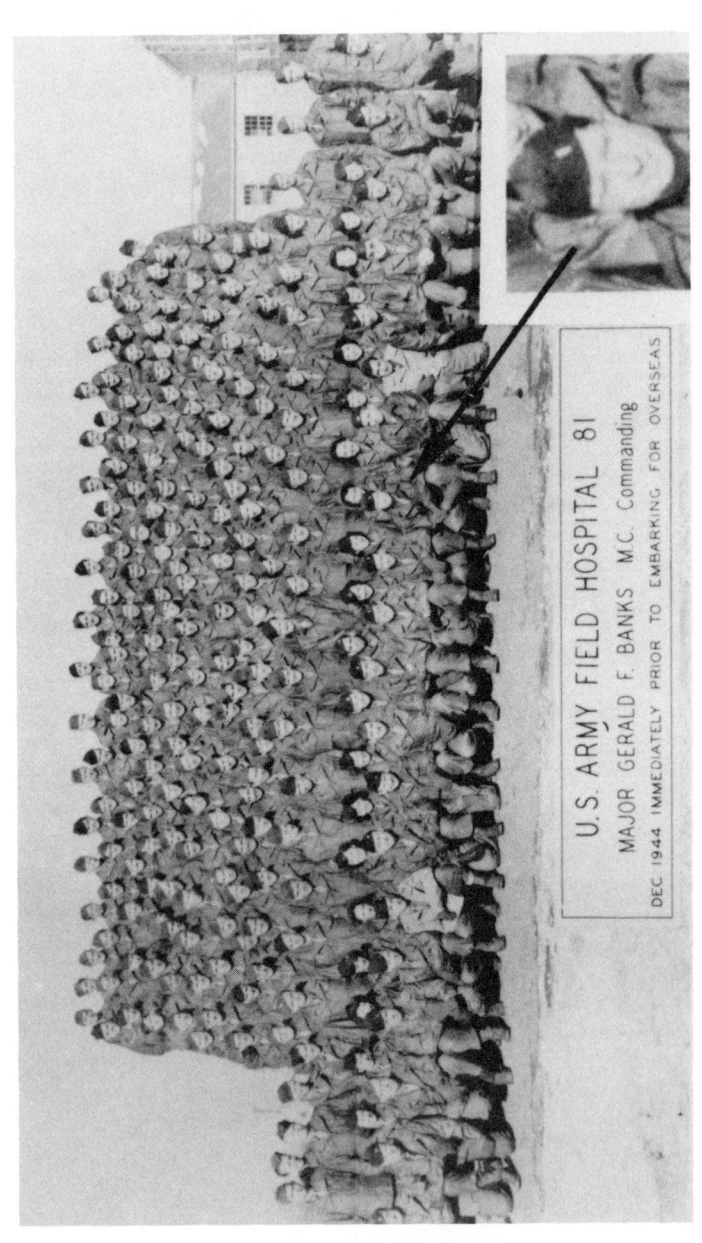

Complement of 81st Field Hospital. Arrow indicates JDH.

Queen Mary, and the *Rex* (Italian) docked alongside each other in this very place. Never did I dream that one day . . . !

24 DEC 44: THE ENLISTED MEN COME ABOARD. Another Christmas Eve away from home. "All loading officers report to lounge and prepare to load troops."

On they come, the American enlisted men, eager and in good spirits until—*bang*! They see their small compartment which must serve 250 men for eating, sleeping, and (?) playing. Most of them curse roundly; one yells out, "Lieutenant, I cancel my reservations." Another queries, "Lieutenant, is this trip really necessary?"

When the order "change into fatigues" is given, there is near mutiny. Against the first sergeant's advice, the CO had insisted that the men roll their fatigues into the pack and march aboard in uniform. Finally, though, the change was effected. Some will sleep on tables, some in hammocks, and the rest on the floor. It won't be a pleasure cruise!

25 DEC 44: MERRY CHRISTMAS! Christmas aboard ship tied up to the New York pier. What a situation! But this only serves to remind us once more of what an infinitesimal part of an enormous organization we are. Today has been long and the two meals very poor indeed. So, we write letters. Now to catch up on correspondence sadly neglected during recent weeks.

In late afternoon came the order over the speaker system. "Fill canteens before retiring; carry life belts at all times; no more smoking on the open decks." Thus we knew that the morrow would see us underway to the great adventure. Some wait up. Not I: we'll see water aplenty and I've seen the Statue of Liberty before.

Where are those bands we saw in all the movies of World War I? No one cares.

26 DEC 44: SUBMARINE PROTECTION. Got up and took a "turn about the deck." We were well out in the harbor, almost out of sight of land. Ships could be seen joining us from every direction. We noted our central position in the convoy with considerable satisfaction, and shed crocodile tears for those ships in the outside positions of the convoy. Subs seem far more real now than they did in the newspapers. [It was said, later, that this was the largest convoy of the war. Be that as it may, it was huge.]

29 DEC 44: ON BOARD. Same routine. Hallo! Hallo! Hallo! goes a voice over the speaker, followed by instructions in Dutch to the crew. Everyone has taken up the three signal words as a chant.

Tonight the calm sea, the scent of soft sea breeze, full moon, soft fleecy clouds, luminescent creatures down in the water, and the silhouettes of the ships on the horizon combine to paint a scene of breathtaking beauty. [All my life thereafter I was to picture this memory on first scenting a fresh sea breeze.]

30 DEC 44: ABANDON SHIP DRILL. Boat drills; action stations; ship inspection; physical training; sleeping; reading.

Sea has been very rough and many are seasick—miserable devils. [There were no anti-motion sickness pills in those days.]

31 DEC 44: TO ENGLAND OR COMBAT IN EUROPE? Rumors endless. Where are we bound? Italy? Marseille? Scotland? France? Liverpool? Most of us guess England—wishful thinking, perhaps, for if we land in France we may never see England. Major Banks ("Eager Beaver") is all for "straight to France." "We'll get back to see England later," he says. But several of us realize the hazards of such a plan; we're still in the army, and our time will have been planned for us when V-E day comes. Let's see England *now*!

2 JAN 45: DRAMA ABOARD SHIP. Murphy Bounds did appendectomy. "Murphy's first stage" but operation should have been done. Caused considerable comment aboard. Patient doing well.

7 JAN 45: LAND HO. Land in sight! What is it? At first we naively thought it the channel with France on the starboard, but we were presently informed that the land masses were Isle of Wight and England on port and starboard, respectively. Sailed into Portsmouth harbor, passing many ships of every variety, from gray battleships to destroyers camouflaged with a most deceptive paint scheme. Countless sea gulls. We feel safe from subs, after the many depth charges dropped by the escort last night, each jarring the *Vollendam*. Churchill and Roosevelt have just announced jointly that there has been an alarming increase in submarine warfare recently. "Scuttlebut" confirms this statement. Many troops have been lost in the channel crossing in the past few weeks. The Germans are trying to prevent U.S. reinforcements from halting Rundstedt's powerful drive in Belgium. No one of us has undressed for several days.

8 JAN 45: MONDAY. LE HAVRE, FRANCE. INFANTRY OFF. Le Havre in sight. Last night we rushed across the channel under very heavy escort. Depth charges all night long. All were uneasy; slept clothed even to combat boots. Very, very cold this morning. Strong wind with intermittent snow and sleet. We watched flights of bombers pass high overhead, leaving their streams of vapor trailing for miles behind them like tails of comets.

Late in the afternoon the *Vollendam* moved close into the harbor and from there we were able to view the staggering wreckage of what must once have been a splendid harbor. Almost everything in ruins. Ships half submerged. Buildings mere rubble. Many of us were watching for enemy aircraft, which never came. After dark the poor infantry were unloaded into LCIs [landing crafts], cold, wet, and packed like sardines. They were a somber lot and well they might be—for they were undoubtedly needed urgently to stop the German drive into Belgium, the Battle of the Bulge. These men—the infantry—are the ones for whom war is really hell.

9 JAN 45: TUESDAY. THE SUBMARINE MENACE. Lay in harbor all day. Evidently we go back to England. Boy! That was a close one! Maj. Banks outdid himself but could not get us ashore. When we come back to

France, my duffel bag will weigh little more than a feather. This business of carrying one's all on one's back is stupid.

We're on our own way again. Ship's crew indignant at prospect of remainder of troops having to cross the channel three times instead of once. Another night run under heavy corvette and destroyer protection. The submarine is effective not only in *sinking* ships but also in keeping them in ports, waiting for escort. Enormous waste of time. [Learned later, in Germany, that Julian's ship had been sunk in the channel. Rescued by a French fishing boat. A soldier hopelessly trapped in an air vent of the sinking ship had begged to be killed, and an officer had stepped forward and shot him through the head. Julian had left Oulton Park before the arrival of the 81st.]

10 JAN 45: WEDNESDAY. Portsmouth again. Thousands of gulls. Leave tonight.

11 JAN 45: SURVIVORS RESCUED. Pulled into Milford Haven harbor for safety. Two ships said to have been sunk just out beyond the submarine nets last night. Survivors have been coming in. Partly submerged vessels visible all about.

On a nearby hill stands an old castle surrounded by brilliant green slopes. Looks isolated and cold. Central heating preferred!

Left harbor once but were ordered back because of nearby wolf pack of subs. This Irish sea is infested with them.

13 JAN 45: SATURDAY: DEBARKATION IN SCOTLAND. Gourock harbor—at last! Very busy. Saw *Queen Elizabeth* [ship] leaving. We're finally to disembark.

Remarkably orderly and prompt movement. The train was waiting and we were gone in ten minutes. Coaches small, always swaying, but fast. Scotland countryside exhibits rolling hills, long stretches of water, and hordes of kids yelling, "Any gom, chum?" "Cigarettes, Yank?" Many soccer games in progress. No one seems to work on Saturday P.M.

Everyone's crabbiness, increased by unrealized tension occasioned by subs near end of voyage, is gone. Morale excellent in outfit.

The 81st was sent to Oulton Park Staging Area about thirty-five miles from Liverpool. There the equipment was to be assembled, reinspected, and preparations made to proceed to France. The officers who'd crossed on the other ships were already there, plus thirteen bags of mail. In quonset huts. The sleeping bag and air mattress bought in Chicago proved to be one of the best investments of my career.

17–18–19 JAN: WEDNESDAY, THURSDAY, FRIDAY. THREE-DAY PASS TO LONDON. Chaplain Norris, Barker, Lt. Cummings, Martin, and I visited

London. Went by train "third class," as this is only about one-half as expensive as "first class" with the accommodations the same, save for absence of arm rests with the former. We had a most pleasant and instructive outing. Massive numbers of prostitutes after dark. The Red Cross clubs saved us, since we could find no other lodgings. Went to see *Rigoletto* at the Princess Theater on first night; performance was good but not excellent. Next day we took a Red Cross taxi tour for ten shillings ($2.00). Places of interest visited were 10 Downing, the War Ministry, Admiralty, St. James Palace, Tower of London, Madame Tussaud's exhibits, Westminster Abbey, Fleet Street, Reuters, Lloyd's, Old Curiosity Shop of Dickens fame from which I sent Mother a card, and many other places of lore. Most impressive of all was Westminster Abbey, timeless. The names enshrined on the walls seemed to include many of the most famous ones of history. The immortals of England.

22 JAN 45: THE BRITISH PUB, COMMUNITY CENTER. Several of us spent the evening in a nearby Red Lion Inn, of which there must be hundreds in England. I see "Red Lion" pubs everywhere I journey on the bicycle, bought for 2½ pounds from a sergeant leaving with an engineer outfit. The notable incident of the three hours was the description of the buzz bombs and other bombings by the cockney proprietor. The very matter-of-fact serenity with which he described the destruction and hardships visited upon England by "Jerry" was inspiring. "What can you do? We'll stick it and someday we'll beat Jerry."

6 FEB 45: TUESDAY: ASSIGNED TO RUN POST DISPENSARY. Sick Call: (1) pediculosis, (2) pharyngitis, (3) poison ivy, (4) hoarseness for one month referred to 109th GH for ENT consultation, (5) insurance exams, (6) examination of food handlers, (7) anterior dislocation of shoulder in football, (8) painful feet. Engineers marched out at dark to build Bailey bridges. Ice and snow.

20 FEB 45. PNEUMONIA. Have been ill and quite miserable for several days. Chief symptoms are severe productive cough with hemoptysis, fever of 99° to 103°, anorexia—marked, severely tender gums, and intermittent abdominal pains not unlike those of peptic ulcer. A barracks is no place for one who is ill. Friends mean well and do their best, but the patient suffers. From now on all febrile patients will be sent to the hospital.

26 FEB 45: 109TH GH (PATIENT). Major Harvey, post surgeon and CO of dispensary No. 1, came by this A.M., found me still abed, auscultated, heard rales, diagnosed atypical pneumonia, and sent me here to 109th General Hospital. How extremely pleasant to have bed linen and an attractive soft diet. In camp, one eats the regular chow or he eats not. My sympathy for the ill will hereafter be increased. Imagine it: the hot water bottle at my feet is easily worth a £ note to me just now. Lt. Pinto, ward officer, did a careful physical exam. Found the moderate tonsillitis which I'd noted for the past few days. Also detected a possible sinusitis. Gums

are still so markedly tender that even to touch them with the tongue is exquisitely painful. Nurse administered a back rub—wonderful! Diagnosis in doubt. But, whatever it was, the disease is receding. (One thing learned here, and during detached service for a period at 68th GH, was that the best treatment for cold injury of the feet—frostbite, trench foot, immersion foot—was, essentially, to do nothing. Wait, and wait, for major gangrene, which was rare.)

2 MAR 45. Discharged weak but afebrile. About ten pounds lost. Even with suppurative tonsillitis, a leucopenia ranging from 3500 to 6000 prevailed. Sed rate was 80 mm/hr on admission but fell to normal.

Several comments on my hospital stay are in order. While it was restful to be in one of the private (isolation) rooms on admission, later, when I felt better, I thoroughly enjoyed being out on the open ward with the rest of the officer patients. I learned from a Lieutenant Elliott, who had been wounded in the foot during rapid retreat in the Battle of the Bulge, that he had run almost a mile and jumped into a foxhole to return fire before blood on his combat boot drew attention to the injury—bullet or knife wounds are not usually conspicuously painful, initially. Incidentally, he had found that a Garand rifle would stop an oncoming German, while a carbine bullet (issued to officers) might not.

The lieutenant in the bed next to mine had been wounded seven times and was now in the hospital for combat fatigue. Once, he told, when he was in a forward evacuation hospital, he had looked up to find General Patton standing beside his bed; jumping up, he came to rigid attention. "What's the matter with you, Lieutenant?" The answer, "Psychoneurosis, sir." Patton ordered, "Get up and go back to the front," and turned to leave. But abruptly he swung back and asked, "How long have you been a second lieutenant?" Then, upon hearing the answer, he departed. But when the patient had reached his outfit, he found a letter promoting him to first lieutenant.

12 MAR 45. MISFORTUNE! Severely sprained left ankle playing volleyball. Excruciatingly painful. Markedly swollen and ecchymotic. X-ray at 109th GH negative for fracture. Injection treatment a complete and painful failure. I shall never again use it on the patient with severe sprain. Hal Barker, surgeon, crestfallen.

13 MAR 45: OULTON PARK. Fever 102.6° F. General malaise; ankle still spontaneously painful. Anorexia. Severe abdominal cramps several hours after meals and relieved by food. The pains are most distressing and, once they've stopped, the anxiety one experiences, lest the pains recur, is

almost as bad as the pains themselves. No ulcer patient of mine will ever spend the night without food at his bedside, if I know about it. Here a loaf of bread serves the purpose.

14 MAR 45. Maj. Banks has twice insisted on my hospitalization but each time he's relinquished his stand. Having come this far with the 81st, I am determined to go to France with them.

20 MAR 45. Liefert, Cummings, and Barker are back from dispensary duty in Wales. All except Barker had a wonderful time. Crutches were secured from 109th GH and the appetite is better. Have lost 15 lbs. in past 6 weeks. Fever gone.

21 MAR 45: ANOTHER POE. This morning at dawn the 81st left Oulton Park and was transported by bus to Beaston Station. The sunrise was lovely, the meadows were green and rolling, birds were calling—and from nearby airfields fighter planes were climbing into the blue. The imperishable and the new, side by side.

During the train trip to marshalling area C5, near Winchester, we played bridge when not gazing at the receding countryside. On the way we passed through the city of Bath, from whose abbey Arch Fletcher had sent the simple but exquisite prayer. C5 is a typical staging area. Loudspeakers.

Hustle & bustle. Units arriving and units departing. Mess kits and long mess lines. Countless rumors. Primitive and dirty quarters. Unpredictable hot water. Poor food. George Maxwell [medical classmate and anatomy dissection partner] is here.

By this date the Allies had repulsed the massive thrust of the Germans in the Battle of the Bulge, brilliantly assisted by General Patton's armored divisions. In fact, troops of the American First Army had captured the still standing Remagen bridge and first crossed the Rhine in force on March 7. Clearly, the outcome of the war was no longer in doubt.

23 MAR 45. TO A SKYLARK. While awaiting a ball game's beginning this morning, I watched a skylark arise from a nearby field, and, ever circling and singing madly the while, he spiraled upward until out of sight. Even when no longer visible, though, his ringing cries came back to us as defiantly and clearly as Beethoven's chords on a fine piano. How lovely is Shelley's poem "To a Skylark," and how accurate.

25 MAR 45: RECROSSING THE CHANNEL. Left C5 by truck at 1200 and proceeded to Southampton. Under full field equipment, we return civilian waves with a ridiculously condescending air, as if these people had not suffered bombs of all types for the past five years. After a brief wait at the port, we boarded the well-appointed *Sobieski*, apparently named after an

ancient Polish king. How nice had we crossed the Atlantic in it in lieu of the *Vollendam*. Good food and pleasant lounge. Only complaint is that the E above middle C sticks on the piano.

(On crutches, I was told by the full colonel in charge checking the roster at the gangplank that I ought to be going in the opposite direction.)

Emergency drill was held promptly and in a most businesslike fashion. All are to sleep fully clothed.

26 MAR 45: LE HAVRE, FRANCE. Crossing quite uneventful. Here at Le Havre again. We're to entrain presently for Paris.

27 MAR 45: PARIS TO NANCY TO LUNÉVILLE. Night ride from Le Havre to Paris was most uncomfortable. Our next train, a Seventh Army leave train, left Paris at 1300. The long ride across France carried us past many names immortalized by World War I. Château-Thierry, for instance.

As for the Marne River, one could almost jump across it. Shell holes, trenches, foxholes, and shattered towns fade behind us. France has suffered more destruction than has England. The train arrived at Lunéville at 2300. All were tired, hungry, chilled by the drizzling rain. Our destination in doubt. Adjutant Hurand took over and soon had Seventh Army trucks on their way to transport us to the nearby 51st Station Hospital, which proved to be housed in a girls school. Most of us slept in empty beds on the wards; indeed, I awoke to find an amputee on either side.

Something new in toilet equipment has appeared. We found facilities boasting only of a place for each foot, with a flushing receptacle beneath. Poor arthritics!

28 MAR 45. TRUCK CONVOY. The 81st entrucked at 1045. It was broadly hinted that we would cross the Rhine before the day was over (though it developed that the Seventh Army had not yet taken Mannheim). Though we'd seen great destruction in localized areas of France and England, we were totally unprepared for the havoc we've seen this day. Our convoy passed town after town, formerly bitterly contested, and now mere rubble. So recently had American columns smashed through that the ruins were here and there still smoldering. Blasted Siegfried fortifications, wrecked vehicles, demolished guns, and dead horses lined the narrow forest roads. Actually, there must have been over one hundred dead horses in one short stretch.

The staggering wreckage was thundering evidence of the value of air superiority. Everyone was anxious to reach our destination, before darkness should allow German aircraft to steal out and strafe the roads.

So recently have these areas been battlegrounds that the natives are only now returning from the hills to their villages, pulling their pitiful belongings behind them in miserable little hand wagons. A woman pulls, an old man pushes, and a child is apt to be leading a goat along behind. There are very few able men to be seen.

Arriving within four miles of Mannheim at 1700, we were unable to find the proper route. To make matters worse, we had become enmeshed with a tank column on its way to aid in the battle for Mannheim. One could see and hear artillery fire down in the city. The ditches beside the road had not yet been cleared of land mines laid by the retreating Germans. The distance back to Kaiserslautern was too great for the convoy to return in search of further information. Gaining the autobahn, we moved aimlessly for a few miles under blackout conditions, when our convoy came abreast of the 59th Evac Hospital. There Maj. Corley discovered at 2100 that Mannheim was still occupied by enemy forces, and concluded that the orders had been meant to read *Marnheim*, not *Mannheim*, the former being a small hamlet not many miles away.

Prowling enemy planes, venturing aloft mainly at night because the Allies controlled the skies in daylight, effected anything but the simplification of our difficulties. It required blackout driving. Finally, and almost by accident, Lt. Elliott stumbled upon the 127th Evac Hosp. at 0500 and they put us up for the "night" in empty ward tents.

1 APR 45: SUNDAY: EASTER. There were only a few out in the cutting wind to attend the Easter sunrise service this morning. "Strong are the ties that bind." Even with our family scattered afar, I knew that each was preserving our family ritual of singing "Jesus Christ is Risen Today" and "Angels Roll the Rock Away" on Easter morning before breakfast.

4 APR 45: "LIBERATED" GOVERNMENTAL EXPERIMENTAL WINE STATION, NEUSTADT. Word had come that the infantry had liberated a huge agricultural station wine cellar, and today Liefert, Cummings, Barker, and I visited this wine cellar at Neustadt. Though the town proved far more distant than our informer had led us to believe, the trip was worthwhile from several points of view. Gradually leaving the destruction of war behind, we followed a road which presently carried us into the lovely Rhine Valley country. The villages were untouched and the German families tended the countless acres of grape vines quite as serenely as though they'd never been at war. Finally arriving at our destination, we were overwhelmed by the sheer beauty of the surrounding country. Neustadt itself nestled on the side of one of two long, low mountains which formed a valley stretching in either direction as far as the eye could see. Beneath a sunlit sky, studded occasionally by lazily drifting cumulus clouds, the farmers tended their vineyards, which appeared as settings delineated by the gorgeously blooming fruit trees' white and pink blossoms, which surrounded the red-roofed villages scattered at irregular intervals up and down the valley and hillsides. The war could nowhere else in Germany have seemed more distant than here.

Suddenly recalling our mission, however, we at once reconnoitered the agricultural experimental station whose basement housed the wine. So dark and dank was the cellar that we feared to make, at any moment, a false move that would set off a booby trap. We should have realized, nevertheless, that many had preceded us. With the light cast by the lighted match, one could see tier after tier of stacked bottles of wine. Often, the year of vintage and the type of the wine appeared somewhere about the individual compartment, each of which held about one hundred bottles laid horizontally; there must have been several hundred such compartments, at least half of which were still filled. Never before had the magnitude of the German wine industry been brought home to us. Two hundred sixty bottles of red and white wine were loaded into the ambulance and truck—and thousands, alas, had to be left behind.

This Neustadt foray has been presented in some detail because the experience afforded me one of the two special mental refuges which were to serve me often in the future, the other one being the infinite peace of a hillside in Wales years later. Each person needs a special retreat, to which he or she can withdraw momentarily for intellectual repose, amidst the vicissitudes of life, on rare occasions. And that vision at Neustadt, coming after all the utter destruction of most of Germany up to that point, was ever after one of mine.

Back at camp, Maj. Banks called a meeting of officers at 1700. Word spread that a court-martial was in the offing, that we had had no business taking an ambulance and a 2½-ton truck to get the wine while CO Maj. Banks [soon to be Lt. Col.] was off at Third Army headquarters. (Actually, it developed that we were not a part of Third Army, but of Seventh Army, which had been looking for us. Hence no mail for weeks.) However, we had gained permission from acting CO Adjutant Hurand. When all had gathered, the CO commanded, "Hardy, front and center!" I knew then that we should never have spent the better part of the day gallivanting around after wine. The heat was on! But, instead of "eating me out," Maj. Banks smiled, extended his hand, and said, "Congratulations, *Captain* Hardy."

After Martin, Cummings, and I had received the captaincies, Second Lieutenant Nurse Richards became first lieutenant, and then the important news of the day was broken: Tomorrow we move up and cross the Rhine. Units B and C will load and move up first. Unit A and headquarters will follow on the shuttle. Destination is Dieburg.

5 APR 45: A HEAVY LOSS. ALL WINE SMASHED. Though A and C units locked up all but a small portion of their wine, B unit issued all of theirs to the men. There followed considerable drunkenness, in which elements of all three units participated. So, this morning Maj. Banks ordered that all the remaining wine, some 150 bottles, be smashed. This was done with axes, to the accompaniment of great moans of anguish from all concerned.

The Rhine was crossed at Worms on a swaying and undulating pontoon bridge. The demolished original structure lay in the water some fifty yards downstream.

The excellent paved roads inside Germany are a great help to the U.S. now. Darmstadt is in ruins. [Thirty years later Darmstadt would become my daughter Louise's permanent home.]

6 APR 45: DIEBURG. PATIENTS AT LAST. Maj. Banks returned hurriedly from Seventh Army Hq. this morning with the instruction that the three independent units (A, B, and C) were to be combined into one immediately; that the 81st was to be prepared to receive patients as a station hospital on the morrow. Capacity 450 beds. Tentative lineup: CO—Maj. Banks; executive officer & ch. X-ray—Maj. Corley; ch. of surgery—Cpt. Bounds; ch. of medicine—Cpt. Hardy; ch. nurse—Cpt. Donnelly; ch. laboratory & pharmacy—Cpt. Cummings; A & D (admission and disposition)—Cpt. Martin.

The experience derived from the opening of isolation wards at McGuire General Hospital is quite useful, if for no other reason than that of reminding one of such details of ward equipment as thermometers, urinals, bedpans, sputum cups, etc.

7 APR 45. Miraculously, we were ready today to receive flocks of patients. Headquarters (Lt. Hurand), registrar (Lt. Elliott), and Maj. Corley have done a bang-up job. First patient was admitted, a Russian civilian freed by the advancing Allies, his right forearm and hand being markedly swollen from the infection of a hand wound.

8 APR 45: SUNDAY. Today approximately 170 patients, displaced persons all, were admitted. Variety of diagnoses. Chiefly Russians. Malnutrition, massive tuberculosis, hepatitis, peptic ulcer, arthritis, cirrhosis, bronchitis, pyorrhea alveolaris, pleurisy, diphtheria, leprosy, Hodgkin's disease, dysentery, gastroenteritis secondary to overloading half-starved stomachs, malaria, edema of undetermined origin, and idiocy.

9 APR 45. Long day of screening patients for tuberculosis by means of chest X-rays. Rest of time was spent in reviewing diagnoses by doing history and physical on questionable cases. What a criminal waste of the only real value in this world—human beings. Many French and British colonial troops have come in.

A shower! [A shower company had set up their equipment nearby. I learned in army that it is not necessary to take a bath every day—indeed, or every week?]

10 APR 45: Tuberculosis rampant. More patients in and many out. Several with tuberculosis have died.

11 APR 45. Walt Martin is as busy as a hound dog with fleas. Admitted seventy-nine more tuberculosis patients today. Were it not for Cpt. Cummings and his team of nurses and corpsmen, the badly strained isolation section would collapse in technic.

Lt. (nurse) Ruth Udy was to develop tuberculosis from this exposure and to spend several years with it after the war. Streptomycin, the first drug truly effective against the tubercle bacillus, was discovered by Nobel Prize winner Selman A. Waksman and was made generally available in 1948. After this discovery, the enormous and worldwide tuberculosis sanatorium industry gradually receded and eventually closed down.

13 APR 45. ROOSEVELT IS DEAD! Apoplexy. (Died April 12.) I first heard it from a liberated Russian soldier, on one of the tent wards: "Roosevelt ist todt." The radio at the tent headquarters confirmed it, and on and on.

14 APR 45. "Bed check Charlie," the German pilot who's given us several scares with nightly strafings of the adjacent highway, killed one man and very seriously wounded two others in a nearby convoy last night. Today he is reported shot down and is said to be a patient in the 27th Evac Hospital.

24 APR 45: TUESDAY: UNIT C TO HEILBRONN. RESERVE LAZARET—HEILBRONN. Today Cummings, Corley, 15 EM, and I came here to take over this large military general hospital, and to prevent the Germans who are being evacuated from removing equipment which is now the property of the U.S. government. Some 600 German patients are being moved to Bad Mergentheim. The U.S. Army clearing company effecting the move was one of the most undisciplined outfits of my experience. Their CO was perhaps the most obnoxious individual one could ever meet.

The Chefartz [senior medical officer] conducts us about the plant, often expressing the hope that he will be allowed to remain and work for us. The Oberschwester, or chief nurse, is a shrewd character who'll bear watching. "Alles ist kaput." "Es ist Hitler." "Es ist Krieg."

On 4 Dec 44 American bombers appeared, without warning, above Heilbronn, a town of some 60,000 inhabitants, and when they disappeared, after twenty-five minutes of bombing, between fifteen- and twenty-thousand people lay dead, buried under the ruins of their once proud city. (The total destruction was staggering. The wonder was that *anyone* had survived.)

Lt. Parker, commanding the company of Negro artillery troops guarding this hospital, has his hands full. One of his men raped a German woman out in the nurses quarters last night. This has happened often around here, the military government officers report. The German radio is making use of these shameful facts in the propaganda.

The German, Polish, Russian, and Italian civilians were treated most shabbily by the military, being crammed into the attic rooms, no matter how severe their illness. And there we found them, under the care of a tall, gaunt, civilian German physician. He treated Pole and German alike, and the patients' reverence for him shone in their eyes. The doctor himself was tormented by a peptic ulcer and appeared anything but well. He accepted the assistance of our nurses and later expressed amazement at the efficiency and training evidenced by American nurse personnel. Though free to remain with us, he preferred to follow his German patients to civilian hospitals, as soon as they could be moved.

The electricity is off, except for a few lights operated by a small generator in the basement. Most of the windows are shattered and the water supply from town is most unpredictable.

25 APR 45. Spent the morning lining up German civilians to remain in order to operate the laundry, kitchen, cleaning, heating plant, and other hospital machinery. Language *must* be taught with more realism and imagination. The civilians are anxious to eat and sleep, in this chaos. One's problem is not to secure enough help but to refuse work to individuals not needed. For instance, a blind masseur was led up by his wife. The poor chap was blinded in World War I and has earned his livelihood for the past twenty years by administering "scientific" massage to hospital patients. We can't use him. One gentlewoman who works in the laundry speaks English very well, having learned it in school, supplemented by travel in England and America. Now penniless, her husband was formerly a leading industrialist in Heilbronn. When asked if she wished to continue working in the laundry, she epitomized the situation obtaining in all of conquered Germany with these words: "One must eat, Herr Hauptmann."

At our command, the civilians were forced to bury three corpses that someone had discovered in the morgue. However, this occasioned no

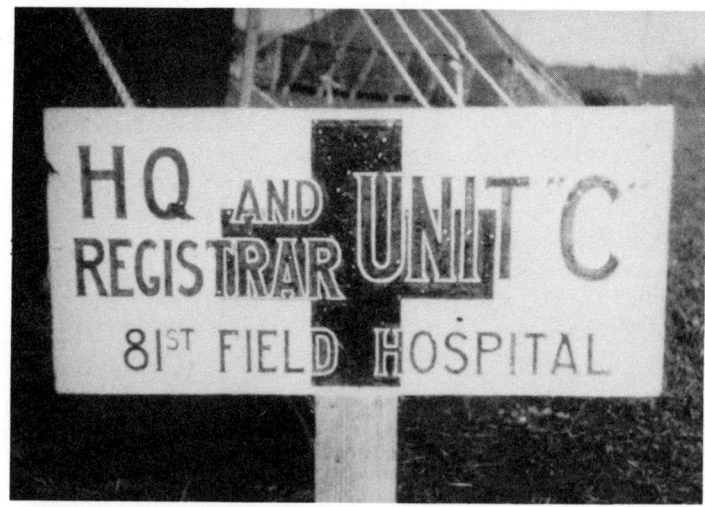

Sign at Unit C headquarters

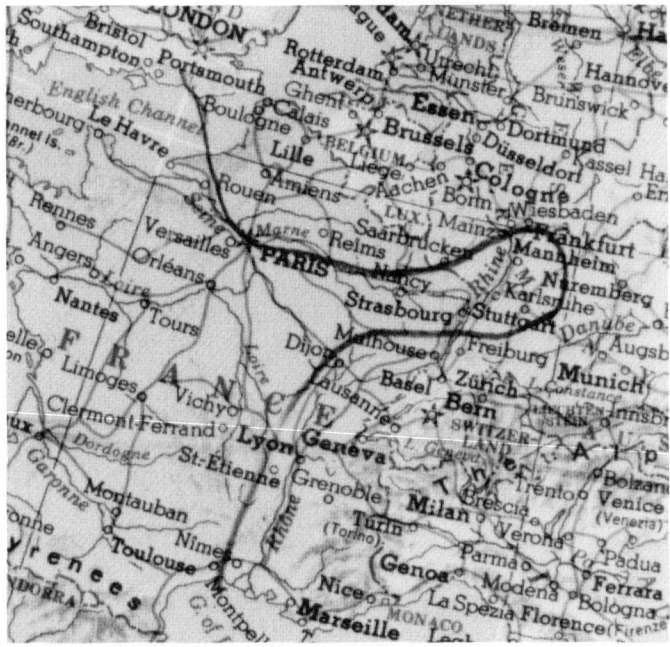

European movements of 81st Field Hospital

great problem, since the bodies were simply thrown into a common grave already containing fifteen others but only partially filled with dirt, and more sod was shoveled upon the newcomers.

It is surprising how many interrelated details must mesh in a smoothly run hospital.

Everyone has secured at least some small souvenir—or loot, if one must be blunt!

28 APR 45: GERMANS DIED TOO. A profoundly tragic drama was enacted in real life behind the hospital today. A few days before we arrived, a small boy had been killed while playing with a live grenade which exploded in his hands. Absent at the time, his family had now returned and had learned of the child's burial within the hospital grounds. Having received permission from Maj. Corley to disinter the body for reburial in the family cemetery, the father, mother, and young daughter trailed around behind the building [to] where the Germans had placed eighteen bodies in a common grave. As we watched from the windows, the family dug up two wrong corpses before the badly mutilated body of their child was located. The mother was overcome—and so were we all.

No mail for many days.

Days cold with frequent hailstorms. With windows out, the patients' rooms are like ice.

The German X-ray, laboratory, and operating room equipment is excellent. Particularly good is the photoelectric laboratory apparatus for colorimetric determinations.

Cpl. Wilson and I went several kilometers to see two Russian women said to have typhus fever. We found them in typical factory worker hutments, far back in the woods. They were both lousy but probably have typhoid rather than typhus.

The Heilbronn Reserve Lazaret bore huge red crosses on its roof and was untouched by a single Allied bomb, though all the windowpanes had been shattered. Our patients here consisted, again, largely of liberated Russians, Poles, and numerous other nationalities. In contrast to Dieburg, however, we now admitted not only chiefly men but also women and children from huge work camps in the area. In addition, numerous American troops, either wounded or injured in vehicle accidents, were brought in. Captain Smith, our surgeon, with one or two years of surgical residency, was heavily in demand. My job was that of triage officer and chief of medicine and laboratory.

Frau Elizabeth Wacker, a fair and buxom blond woman of about forty, ran the German X-ray equipment, thus sparing us from having to uncrate our portable equipment and generator. She was well educated. Her husband, a minister, had been killed on the Russian front. Her brother was a medical student at the University of Tübingen. With her, I had a chance to practice my German, for it was an army offense, with a fine of sixty dollars, for an American soldier to speak to a German civilian. One day I said to her, "Du bist wie eine Blüme" (You are like a flower). The next day, she brought in the full text of Heine's poem in a slender volume of poetry.

30 APR 45. German civilians say that Hitler was wounded yesterday by the Volkstrum. Fraülein Muller reports him dead. Looks like the war may end before too long.

2 MAY 45. Hitler is dead. Mussolini and daughter reported murdered by Italians and hanged by the heels.

More Russians were blasted while playing with grenades in Heilbronn DP [displaced person] camp. The vaunted Russian bravery would seem to be little more than an indifference as to whether he lives or not. How they hate Germans! They sit around with various assembled weapons and pot at German civilians.

4 MAY 45. SUPPLY PROBLEM has become most difficult. We have almost no intravenous fluids. Surgery, medicine, pediatrics, obstetrics and gynecology are all here. Lt. Smith has more than he can handle in the surgery, what with the Russians' quaint little pastime of playing ball with live grenades! Cummings is doing eminently competent job of pediatrics and isolation.

Rubeola, typhoid, typhus, scarlatina, pyelonephritis, pneumonia, tuberculosis, heart failure, methyl alcohol poisoning with blindness, scabies, postdiphtheritic paralysis, threatened toxemia of pregnancy—present on medical wards.

Herr Doktor Pobol, an Estonian physician, his wife, and a number of allied nurses of many nationalities—including Belgian, Greek, Hungarian, Lithuanian, and Austrian—have just arrived from Heidelberg, sent by the American military government to help us. We can certainly use them. The hospital census is running close to 200 patients, almost all of whom require considerable therapeutic and nursing care.

5 MAY 45. Had most unusual case today. Nicotine poisoning resulting from a Russian's handling a can of commercial nicotine and then picking his teeth with his fingernails. Comatose most of twelve hours. Clonic convulsions and intervals of mania interrupted the coma. Approximately one hundred twenty Russians in the Heilbronn DP camp, which houses 6,000 subjects, have been adding two drops of the pure nicotine alkaloid to 100 grams of crude crushed tobacco in order to give their cigarettes a "kick."

Herr Doktor Pobol is proving to be an internist of considerable training and no mean ability. In addition to his medical acumen, he has about him a sense of humor and an instinctive courtesy which make him a delightful colleague. Though he speaks no English, he is fluent in German, Estonian, Polish, and Russian. Our German improves daily. Too, Doktor Pobol is well grounded in Latin, thus greatly facilitating our discussion of drugs. Continentals use the metric system of weights and measures, of course. The Doctor is a past master at diagnostic thoracentesis. This morning he accomplished five such procedures without anesthesia and with very little obvious pain on the part of the patient, completing everything in 40 minutes.

6 MAY 45. Went over to the Heilbronn DP camp with the wife of the nicotine patient to secure the can of nicotine. The camp itself is enormous, having formerly served as barracks for German army personnel. After endless walking, we entered a large building, which simply teemed with human beings, and forced our way up three flights of stairs. The Russians, frankly surprised to see an American army officer there, stared quite openly. Finally, the guide indicated a doorway through which we passed, finding ourselves now in a room 14 feet by 20 feet by 12 feet. Cots took up most of the floor space. Russians of all ages and sexes

were lying or sitting on the cots. My female guide, after a brief conference in Russian with one of the young men, quickly passed to a place in one corner and produced a tin can down whose sides had streamed a black liquid. The can bore a prominent label marked GIFT, and below that the word nicotine. After thanking the guide I passed out cigarettes and questioned a young man of about twenty who spoke German. No, very few of the men and women in the room were married. At first he grinned, but then added more soberly that things could not be otherwise. When would they return to Russia? Very soon, he thought. Did he think Russia would fight Japan? Yes, he thought so. Four years, and no word from home. These Russians very obviously liked their American comrades.

7 MAY 45: MONDAY. The Germans have surrendered. Alles ist kaput! Tomorrow is "official" V-E Day.

8 MAY 45. V-E DAY. Churchill, King George, General Eisenhower, Bradley, Montgomery, Alexander, and Tedder have all broadcast this evening. We are so isolated here at Heilbronn that V-E Day has not changed things appreciably, except to pour a large number of drunk GIs into Receiving.

How soon to the CBI [China-Burma-India theater]? That is all that matters. We have little hope of getting a leave in the States, and even less of occupying Germany.

14 MAY 45. Twenty-seven today. Had hoped to have medical training behind me by age of 30. Not possible now.

28 MAY 45. What a pleasant surprise today. Billy Harris (medical classmate), having seen our hospital marker when his unit passed through a few days ago, found a chance to return and spend the day. He is with an artillery outfit which is presently down at Nordlington.

As we were passing the receiving office, a group of patients were sitting there, awaiting discharge. Suddenly a pretty, flaxen-haired young Polish girl in her teens who had had pneumonia stood up before me, extended her hand quickly, and blurted, "Wiedersehn, Herr Doktor!" Then, overwhelmed with what seemed to her a rash behavior, she abruptly sat down again, averted her gaze, and blushed in confusion. As we passed on quickly, in an effort to relieve her embarrassment by our absence, Billy said, "Jim, it's worth all the effort when you see things like that, isn't it?"

31 MAY 45: HEIDELBERG. Went to Heidelberg to locate German military medical personnel, after finding all but surgeons and nurses in the Heilbronn PW cage, which seems to stretch beyond the horizon and contains about 250,000 German troops. The route along the east bank of the Neckar River is exquisitely beautiful as it winds along, following the bends of the river through the mountains. Everything is sunny and green, and brilliantly red fields of poppies dot the landscape. Were it not for the occasional wrecked towns, the destruction of all bridges, and streams of liberated civilians who almost block the roads—afoot, on bicycles, and in

almost every other means of conveyance—were it not for these, one could almost forget the war. Only the bridges in Heidelberg were destroyed by the retreating Germans. It had been declared an open city and was not defended.

In Heidelberg I talked with a most stimulating young MAC of New York City, Lt. Hensel, who quickly made the desired personnel available.

Heidelberg itself is immediately captivating. As one drives in along the lazy Neckar, which divides the picturesque city into two halves, one is struck first by the number of well-dressed and otherwise attractive women. One senses at once the tone that seems to permeate all university towns. The predominance of feminine population so striking in most of Germany is not quite so obvious here. Heidelberg University is not one sharply delineated unit, but is composed of a number of units scattered all over the southwestern part of the city. The University Hospitals occupy several blocks in the center of the city and are surrounded by a high wall.

Heidelberg Castle is remarkably well preserved, and from its ramparts one gets an excellent view of the city below.

1 JUNE 45. UNIT ALERTED FOR DIRECT MOVEMENT TO CBI! It will be a long war for us. Returned to Heidelberg in search of billets for the 81st, but Sixth Army Group Hq says, *no*! Went with Murphy Bounds.

2 JUNE 45. Went with Maj. Corley to find billets somewhere along the Heilbronn-Heidelberg railway. After passing up Eppingen, Sinsheim, and Mosback we found Neckargemünd a likely spot and called upon the Bürgermeister of the town. He proved such a classic image of the obese, red-faced, stocky, "he-done-it" German, with hair clipped short and cigar in pudgy hand, that one could not suppress a chuckle, even though the situation called for a dignified firmness. After unsuccessfully attempting to persuade us to try another town, he asked how many houses we would need and, deploring the war, agreed to have the families moved out of ten houses on very short notice, a matter of hours, should we return the following day and request it. Had we been infantry, we would have simply given the families an hour's notice, but the medics can't work quite that way; the infantry's Garand rifle is a powerful persuader. *Heraus in ein Stunde* (out in an hour)!

6 JUNE 45: A TWIN TURNS UP. It finally happened! Informed that a captain wanted to see me in the receiving office, I knew at once that it would be Julian. "Is he an MC?" I asked. "I didn't notice, sir," answered the soldier. Hustling downstairs, I saw Julian standing there, looking like a million dollars. Well groomed, as of course he always is, standing erect, and wearing the dimpled smile, he was even handsomer than when we'd parted at Carlisle that Sunday at 1:23 P.M. in 1943. At first, peculiarly enough, we felt just a trifle like strangers, but before the evening was over we'd had a wonderful reunion bull session. Having had the advantage of the maps at 15th Army Headquarters, he'd known all along, as the 81st

FH made its various moves, and had been awaiting a chance to visit. All too soon, he had to leave this morning (7 June).

9 JUNE 45. Today we finished packing, said "wiedersehen" to Frau Wacker, surely a good German, and left Heilbronn Reserve Lazaret to the mercies of the German military medical personnel that we'd imported.

After arriving here at Schwetzingen in trucks, where Major Reisman, commander of unit B, had had civilians moved from a number of adjacent houses, my late arrival forced me to set up my cot and bedroll in the family library, a small room located on the second floor. I have been interesting myself with the clever way in which German propagandist Herr Goebbels has portrayed the United States as an imperialistic nation, making great capital of the Monroe Doctrine.

I instructed my enlisted men, very firmly, not to loot anything from the private home. However, one of the nurses, of course an officer herself, ingeniously, I thought, ran her index finger around in the Hausfrau's face powder box, and found her wedding rings, and, I suspect, kept them.

All the 81st is here together, once again.

10 JUN 45: SUNDAY. Was sent to Augsburg today on official business at 7th Army Hq. We traveled in open jeep for 400 miles. On the way down we crossed the beautiful Danube, *Der schone blaue Donau*, and halted to take photographs. The waltz surged into our minds. It was narrow and bluish green in color. The original bridge lay wrecked a few yards downstream from the present temporary one. The autobahn was a peerless road, suitable for, and actually used by, planes on the takeoff.

11 JUN 45: MONDAY. Moved out from Schwetzingen and began trip to St. Victorette staging area in southern France, near Arles of painter Van Gogh fame. On very old, wooden-seated railroad coaches. I threw my bedroll on the floor, blew up the air mattress, and slept.

Morale in the 81st FH is very low, as we begin staging for the long, long sea voyage through the Panama Canal to join the invasion of Japan.

14 JUN 45. Arrived at St. Victorette Staging Area at 4:00 A.M. Camp only 0.25 miles from railway station. Two officers to each sidewall tent. Dust hovers over the area in great red clouds. "Camp Barkley," the veterans call it. About 30,000 troops in this tent village. No mail for an indefinite period. Little work for MCs, much for MACs.

Appointed I & E [Information and Education] officer. Not particularly desirable, but suitable to my temperament and inclinations: (1) practice in public speaking, (2) precludes less desirable assignment, (3) Hurand works so hard that none of the rest of us can conscientiously complain; he's the backbone of the outfit, Hurand, and he has my profound respect. What he proposes I, for one, will gladly do. I am to read up on and lecture the enlisted men on Japanese army tactics.

19 JUN 45. Went to Marseille today. Considerable bomb damage. Everything dirty and ill-kept. The *marché noir* (black market) swarms about each entering GI truck in the form of persons of many

nationalities—Frenchmen, Senegalese, Moroccans, Syrians, and derelict Englishmen—and purchases anything offered for sale. [On a later visit, to see how the black market worked, I acknowledged an Arab, in full regalia, who had approached me. We entered a nearby bistro, where he paid me $14.00 (in francs) for a carton of cigarettes I had bought for 50¢ in the PX.]

The Russians are good fighters, yes, but will they cooperate? We'll wait and see. In this war we have merely shifted the balance of power. Russia emerges as a colossus, potentially a dangerous one. Let us hope for friendship. The English-speaking nations, combined in the matchless Churchill, are certain to be allied in any major war. Let's not forget!

21 JUNE 45. Mamma's birthday and wedding anniversary. Talked to the outfit on current affairs, tracing Japanese conquest from 1854 (Admiral Perry) to the present with MacArthur back in the Philippines. My delivery is creditably good and my manner self-assured. As Dr. Pepper always advised, the latter results from careful preparation. The next step is to strive for variation in manner and mannerisms of delivery. The men were satisfactorily attentive.

Went swimming in sea during afternoon.

Longest solar day of the year.

22 JUNE 45. Spent morning reading medical periodicals, washing clothes, and chatting with Hal Barker and Lt. Col. Banks concerning the unit history to be prepared for 7th Army Hq. Had cholera shot at 1500.

By great good fortune I met Arlette Saier and Michelle, a friend, at the Marseille officers club, and was invited to a party on the night of 30 June. A French affair! Girls always chaperoned by a younger brother.

25 JUNE 45: SUSTAINING PERSONAL MORALE. In maintaining personal morale, Osler's conception of the day-tight compartment is absolutely indispensable. One must detach emotional reaction from the mental realization of a slight, or be forever unhappy in the army. Thomas Jefferson has been credited with the remark that the art of happiness lies in the avoidance of unpleasant thoughts.

Had a letter from Dr. Bernard Comroe, in which he punctuated the importance that the Veterans Administration is likely to assume in postwar medicine. Tragically, Dr. C's young wife has just died of rheumatic heart disease. He's certainly a faithful friend to interns, residents, and medical students. Never too busy to discuss someone else's problems.

The enlisted men are in an extremely poor state of morale. It's bad enough for them to have to go direct to the Pacific, but the conditions under which they must live here are deplorable. As usual, the medical units are kicked around a lot. This situation, prevalent in all but combat outfits, is understandable but nonetheless destructive of the medical soldier's morale.

A day of bull sessions: (1) postwar medicine, (2) peacetime conscription—most are for it; we are all afraid the U.S. will forget too soon. Perhaps the English won't; certainly the Russians won't.

27 JUNE 45. Have just been censoring letters, the inevitable daily chore. What a virgin field for treatment by Robert Benchley, that of closing a letter. The excuses offered for ending a letter at a particular point often tax credulity. For instance, one closes, "Well, haven't much to do today so will close." Priceless! Help, Robert Browning or Lord Chesterton.

Clashes between French and U.S. soldiers are frequent and violent.

30 JUNE 45. Michelle's party was a brilliantly successful affair. Evening dresses and champagne, no less! Guests were three RAF officers, one French officer, two U.S. Navy officers, and four U.S. Army officers. Was impressed by: (1) Good will between Allied officers, (2) gracious hospitality of French hosts, (3) the Frenchmen's capacity for enjoying themselves in their homes, (4) the huge gulf between the educated French and the man on the street, (5) the meticulous supervision of the upper-class French girls by their mothers. One simply must learn French!

Madame Saier, doubtless by her daughter's request, has invited Tom Craven and me to dinner on July 4. Most appropriate, celebrating also French Bastille Day (July 14). Also to attend a birthday party to be given by Renée on evening of July 8. How different are these French girls from those who give France her unsavory reputation.

4 JULY 45: WEDNESDAY (MERCREDI). DINNER GUEST. Went to dinner at Madame Saier's, 133 Ave. du Prado. Lovely apartment, enchantingly arranged. While awaiting dinner, Arlette, about 20 and in college, and I played recordings by Liszt and, in addition, Beethoven's First Symphony; also something by Rimsky-Korsakov. Meanwhile we'd consumed an aperitif and I'd been introduced to Monsieur Saier.

Dinner began at 8:00 P.M., strictly a la carte. First came a deliciously cooked entree (what was it?) (appetizer), accompanied by a special wine. Next came stewed rabbit with *its* wine. Pommes de terre. De le salade. Apricot pie with new wine. Then pears. Coffee. And finally cognac in the salon.

Even more intriguing than the food was the discernment and tact evidenced by the seating arrangement. Monsieur Saier, who speaks very little English, sat at the head of the table. On his left was a male relative, who spoke *un peu* English. On his right was son Freddie who, too, speaks English *un peu*. Next on Papa's left (my immediate right) was Arlette, my immediate hostess who of course speaks good English, if a bit picturesquely! On my left was Madame Saier at the foot of the table; on her left was Captain Tom Craven, an engineer officer from Maine. Next Michelle, and then Freddie. In short, seating arrangements were designed to minimize language difficulties. Everyone had a most pleasant evening. Later, Madame Saier, Tom, Arlette, and I drove to the magnificent Delta Base officers club and danced.

In astute self-appraisal, Madame Saier characterized the French people as always searching for something to revolt against—but just a little, not

4 July 45: Wednesday; (mercredi) Aust to dinner at Madame Baier's, 133 Rue Ave. du Prado. Lovely apartment enchantingly arranged. While awaiting dinner we listened to Baier's recordings by Dinu, and in addition, Beethoven's first symphony, also something by Rimsky-Korsakoff; meanwhile we all consumed an aperitif, and I'd been introduced to Monsieur Baier.

Diary entry from July 4, 1945

too much! Madame Saier, herself, perhaps 38, appears no more than twenty-eight.

7 JULY 45. A DECORATION. The 81st received a second battle star for central Germany. Why?

True, we had been there, but never as part of a real battle. But then, relatively few troops in a war actually ever see the immediate combat area—the firing line, as it were. For the most part, troops are in support, or in reserve, or not even in the war zone. We had done what we were ordered to do, and to the best of our ability. To the extent called upon, then, we had participated in the "storm and stress" of our generation.

Astute observation of the day: One of our EM's letters contained the following message to his mother: "If the war with Japan only lasts long enough, I will get out on points." At least a new point of view!

Dust in clothes, bedding, mess gear, food and lungs.

9 JULY 45. The hospital equipment is to be packed in three days.

Had dinner with the Saiers last evening. British consular official, Michelle's uncle by marriage, startled me out of a trance by asking whether or not Alabama beat Georgia Tech last fall. It turned out that he'd been stationed in Atlanta some years ago. Later, the conversation turned to the book *Jeeves*, which I'd just finished. The Englishman, Monsieur Saier (brother of the host), and I had a good laugh. M. Saier, too, has traveled in the States and reads the *Readers Digest* at every opportunity.

Later Freddie, Arlette's younger brother, Arlette, Michelle, and I went to Mon Rêve for dancing. Freddie, only about 17, is so amusingly French!

11 JULY 45. Lt. Col. Banks, CO, was wounded seriously in the right parietal area by a bullet accidentally discharged by a Luger being cleaned some distance away. Struck and dazed while sitting on his bunk, he staggered out of his tent calling for Major [Karl] Corley. The bullet itself had passed through the tent wall and lodged in Corley's bedroll. Col. Banks suffered a depressed skull fracture, with subdural hematoma, resulting in weakness of the left arm. We'll doubtless get a new CO.

23 JULY 45. Carl Leifert leaves tomorrow. Good man. Transferred out. No reason given, as usual in army. The composition of any unit over even a brief period is truly kaleidoscopic. Officers Lewis, Walter, Hippenstiel, Leifert, Scott, Scimeca, Tavener, Tuttle, and Lt. Col. Banks are gone from the originals who left the U.S. with 81st in December. Haunting melody: "Some day I'll meet you again. Don't know where; don't know when."

26 JULY 45. Talked on Japanese tactics. Churchill's government fell. What a colossal crash. Stalin alone of Big 3 remains "in." [Shocked by the results of the British election, I had asked a group of British officers at the

Marseille officers club one evening, "How on earth could the British have dumped Churchill after all he's done?" They replied, "Easily, old chum. Churchill was a war leader. We now need a leader who can rebuild the country." Just as simple as that. This harsh treatment of Churchill, in his moment of triumph, always thereafter served me as a firm reminder that no one is essential, especially when I was tempted to take a position which political strength might not be sufficient to sustain.]

By late July there had sprung up extremely persistent rumors to the effect that the 81st would be sailing before long. If so, it would not be too soon. The high prevalence of venereal disease in the Marseille area had begun to be reflected in the 81st's sick book. Before the unit reached St. Victorette, not one man had ever contracted VD. (At least, no one had reported it.) But during our stay in southern France a number of the men had come down with gonorrhea, syphilis, or chancroid. It was extremely discouraging to have medical troops expose themselves, when they knew perfectly well how to employ the simple but effective precautions.

30 JULY 45. Held last orientation conference with the enlisted men. The fall of Churchill's government, the portent of the enormous Red Army, universal military training in the United States, tropical medicine, and the Japanese soldier were among the topics considered in the rough and tumble discussion. But I reserved the closing moments of the hour for a few remarks on VD. In them, I gave what I hoped was an alarming description of the ravages and heartbreaks that could result from such diseases. Neither penicillin nor arsphenamine would cure *all* syphilis, and it was still a frequent cause of heart failure and insanity. Likewise, a simple "dose" of gonorrhea might possibly prevent a man from becoming a father.
Men, for heaven sakes use a pro!

The new CO had arrived. He was Major John B. Moring, Regular Army. A close-cropped brunette, he was stocky, ruddy-complexioned, and had a refreshing sense of proportion. The two Negro enlisted men from his former command who had driven him down from Germany characterized him as "GI" but eminently fair in all his dealings. And we, too, were to find him so.

7 AUG 45. "Atomic bomb" dropped on Japan! How in hell could such a small object do such damage? Even more incredible: How had the United States, of all nations, managed to keep the bomb so secret? Had the

power of the atom really been harnessed? And the U.S. had done it!

WEDNESDAY, 8 AUG 45. Russia declares war on Japan! What a day! Give 'em hell, Bama! Surely the war could not last long now. What did it all mean? More precisely, what did it mean to the 81st Field Hospital? If the war should end in the next few days, would we go on to the Pacific, or would we go to the States? No one could sit still, even for a minute. The hour was too momentous. And the camp was in an uproar. Loud laughter, backslapping, betting—in short, the urge to *do* something drove men from tent to tent.

THURSDAY, 9 AUG. Rise and shine! This was it! Everyone was awakened at 0430 hours and told to get ready to move out. Still dark. Breakfast (cooked by German PWs) was eaten in fading darkness. Trucks arrived at 0630 hours. The 81st was checked out at the post entrance at exactly 0700 hours.

As we moved away from the gate, a chilling breeze was sending spasmodic flurries of red dust about the camp. The red sun was just peeking from behind the low mountains, lazily contemplating his unavoidable upward journey. The sky was cool and serene, with not a cloud to be seen, not even a little one, not even one the size of your hand. In other words, this was where we'd come in. In short, the 81st was a veteran outfit.

The trucks moved to within fifty yards of our ship. She was the *General George O. Squier*, a navy troop transport. By 1000 hours the unit was aboard. Unlike the *Vollendam*, the *General Squier* had individual lockers in the officers' staterooms, and thus the gear was not a problem. There were eighteen officers to each cabin. Having claimed our bunks, we went back on deck and watched as the troops were loaded, all day long, until there were almost three thousand aboard.

At 1700 hours, the anchor was weighed and the vessel put calmly to sea. As we stood on the decks, watching Marseille fall behind the horizon, we knew that an era had passed. Now—at last—we must wrench our minds away from the ETO and anticipate the Orient.

The two novelties that the *General Squier* presented were the navy lingo and the superb food. On the *Vollendam* the orders had always been given over the "speaker" in an unintelligible (to us) jargon that was said to be Dutch. Hence, such terms as *the smoking lamp, lay below, turn to, sweep and wash down*, and *change the watch* were new and engaging. And all such broadcasts were prefaced with an alerting "Now hear this," not the "Hallo! Hallo! Hallo!" of the *Vollendam*.

And the Food! Though everyone had groaned when it was announced that only two meals would be served each day, we needn't have worried. Those two meals that the Negro stewards *did* serve—they were a dream! Fresh eggs, fresh meat, fresh vegetables, fresh fruit, good coffee— everything the army had *not* had in the ETO. And what with the ice-cream and cakes (not *Nabiscos*) that one could purchase in the canteen at the noon hour, we were perfectly, so perfectly, satisfied. Next time, we'd join the navy!

SATURDAY, 11 AUG. Passed the Rock (Gibraltar). Africa visible on port side. The fortress did not appear nearly so formidable as the enemy must have found it. As we passed through the narrowest part of the strait, a number of sleek porpoises raced playfully along beside the ship.

The next few days were ones of countless rumors. Had the Japs really offered to accept the Potsdam terms? And had President Truman actually refused the Japanese proposals? [On one single day (13 August) I listed no less than seven different rumors. Each spread like wildfire, and, of course, each was "straight from the bridge." They ran thus: (1) the captain was steering a course midway between New York and Panama—just in case, (2) the captain was certain we would go to the States (this in spite of his repeated denials of any such thoughts), (3) the ship was proceeding to the Azores for further orders, (4) the war ended yesterday and everyone in the United States was now celebrating, (5) the Japs were now determined to fight to the last man, (6) the *General Squier* would continue to Panama in any event, (7) if ordered to the States, the ship would put in at Frisco. And these were just the ones that I heard personally—there were many others. Aboard such a small ship, among men whose every waking thought was of home, each of these rumors struck with a terrific emotional impact.]

TUESDAY, 14 AUG 45: THE JAPANESE HAVE SURRENDERED! So what? So we were still bound for the CBI. Hadn't the ship's radio picked up a flash to the troopship behind us, directing that it alter its course and proceed to the States? And had we received such orders? *No!* Quite obviously, then, we were to go on to the Pacific.

However, opinion was divided and absurdly large bets were made. ("If we go to the CBI I won't need it, and if we go to the States I'll be glad to lose.") Every scrap of information, no matter its source, was seized and devoured, wrapping and all.

It was late the afternoon of August fifteenth. The moody vessel wallowed along through a glassy sea so smooth that not even a ripple scarred the gently rolling ground swell. The enlisted men's long mess lines were feeding down into the mess halls and out the other side. The officers listened listlessly for the first dinner call, as they watched a taunting sun inch toward the West they longed to see.

And then it came!

Suddenly a voice came over the speaker system: *"Now hear this! This is the Captain speaking. All passengers aboard will be interested to learn that this ship is altering its course and will dock at Hampton Rhodes."*

Interested? God! We were wild! A great spontaneous roar began in the very bowels of the ship and tore right to the heavens above. We had never before known such joy! *It was the happiest day of my life.* Everyone was yelling—no one knew what he himself was saying—no one cared. He had to DO SOMETHING. Men ran from deck to deck, insane with emotion, yelling with inane monotony, *"It's over! It's over! We're going to the States! We're going home!"*

HOME. Yes, we were going home. It was almost unbelievable. It was too good to be true. It *was* too good to be true. Something would surely happen. The army would snafu it some way—it always did. Yet, how could they? The captain of the ship had said we were going home, and he got his orders from the navy.

Let's have a drink! As if by magic, bottles ("prohibited aboard ship") appeared on all sides, and some got drunk. But I did not want any liquor. I was already drunk—drunk on emotion. We were going home—home two years before anyone would have dreamed we would be there. What would it be like? Would it have changed? Probably not in the nine months the 81st had been gone, but some of the men aboard had been away three years. But sure it had changed—hadn't everything?

(A person away thinks that some great thing must have happened, while to those at home there seems to be only a continued monotony and lack of incident.)

By late evening the frenzied jubilation had subsided, and everyone went blissfully to bed. But sleep was long in coming to the eighteen officers in our cabin. Long after the lights were out and all was quiet, cigarettes glowed in the darkness. And from time to time the silence would be broken by a long, suppressed sigh. Too, whenever the light from the hall chanced to follow a latecomer through the doorway, it invariably betrayed some pair of thoughtful eyes fixed silent upon the darkness above. The gazer was thinking of home—home which he'd idealized during long months of impatient waiting. His thoughts were not of such sordid and commonplace details as rents, or jobs, or the other humdrum vexations of everyday life. No! He thought of rosy paradise, which neither bombs nor starvation could reach—a place for two, or three, or more. For he knew she'd be waiting there, as always. And his happiness would be complete. Truly, his cup runneth over.

The ensuing days were luxuriously idle ones (for all except the unit clerks, that is). Hordes of fancies, long suppressed, were now allowed to enter the conscious mind—the parlor, as it were—like naughty children who heretofore were not to be trusted. Anticipations of delights were leisurely contemplated, toyed with, mentally fondled—much as one might savor a sip of champagne. As always, girls were the main topic of banter. But this time it was not just any girl—English, French, or Italian. No! This time it was *the* girl. It was *"her."* And ribald innuendoes were carefully avoided when one man ribbed another about "her."

The privacy of monotony was by no means boring, so filled were our minds with private contemplations. Nevertheless, the daily gun practice drew a good audience. The procedure seldom varied: A balloon would be released and then, after the wind had wafted it far and high, a designated gun crew would begin firing at it. While one should not like to give comfort to the enemy, I am bound to relate that most of us were gratified to know that the ship would not be called up to repel hostile attack!

Meanwhile, everything was being readied for debarkation. Camp Patrick Henry had radioed detailed instructions as to what records must be completed. In turn, a consolidated report of the number of men desiring leave from each of the numerous induction centers in the United States was flashed to headquarters at Patrick Henry.

MONDAY, 20 AUG 45: THE 81ST CAME HOME. The Pacific still loomed beyond the thirty days of temporary duty at our homes, but for the present we were back in the United States—the "Promised Land."

There was little horseplay aboard the *General Squier* as she came to berth at Newport News. Indeed, it was with considerable effort that the men forced an indifferent smile and wave for the gratification of a press photographer who stood down on the pier, snapping pictures of "the wildly cheering troops."

Everything was beautiful, as the waiting train departed for Camp Patrick Henry—even the Negro shacks along the tracks. Home was wonderful! Absolutely no place like it! Every neck was craned, lest its owner miss some little glimpse of America. All the civilians waved. The Negroes waved too—but timidly, furtively, almost as if they were afraid. Yes, we were back in the States.

Patrick Henry was well organized. Immediately after detraining, we were marched a few hundred yards to a movie theater where an "on-the-ball" major gave a brief, bang-up orientation talk: "Please salute the second lieutenants around here; they're doing the best they can. And please, men, don't forget to tip your hat before striking a lady!" And more of the same—meaty advice being couched in terms the soldier would remember. After this came the steak dinner.

And at long last—the telephones!

I returned home to find Mother dying of metastatic cancer. Before I left for Europe, she had called my attention to a wheeze she could produce on deep inspiration, clearly audible to anyone in the room. Remembering the dictum "not all that wheezes is asthma," I had insisted that she get a chest X-ray and it had shown a probable tumor in her chest. The family doctor urged that we be frank with her, saying that she was an intelligent woman and knew she had cancer, but this honesty was not yet generally accepted. I wished later it had been, for then we could have communicated so much more. As it was, her last words to me were, "James, I'm sure you are a fine doctor, but you're not much of a nurse." The next time I was summoned, she was gone. Though long anticipated, her passing was a heavy loss. We had always been close, and her noble spirit had been the major force in developing my intellectual orientation.

15 DEC 45: OBITUARY: HEARTLESS HERMAN IS LAID TO REST. After forty-five days leave, the members of the 81st not discharged reassembled at Camp Sibert, Alabama. But things were not the same. A number of the officers and many of the key enlisted men had left the ranks. And, instead of filling these men's empty places, the faces of the new replacements only rendered the loss of our old friends more poignant. The old 81st, as we'd known it, was disintegrating before our very eyes. And to watch a seasoned unit die was not a pleasant spectacle.

Now Herman had grown listless; daily he became weaker. He no longer cared for the wild and strenuous parties as of yore. Rather, he seemed to prefer sitting quietly at home, surrounded by a few of his old friends from back at Camp Ellis, reminiscing about the old days, perhaps sipping a quiet beer. He seemed to sense that the end was near, though I do not recall that any such allusion was ever made.

On the first of November, the outfit moved by train to Crile General Hospital at Cleveland, where the personnel would live in temporary barracks but work in the hospital. There, on 14 December 1945, deactivation orders were received. Then the 81st Field Hospital of World War II made its final move—this time into the pages of history.

Herman was tenderly laid to rest. Only his immediate family attended.

On February 11, 1946, orders transferred me from Crile General Hospital to the U.S. Army General Dispensary, the Pentagon, Washington, D.C.

The assignment at the Pentagon was an opportunity to learn something about our capital city and to become addicted to the *Washington Post*. My specific duty was to assist in caring for officers in the Pentagon, where General Dwight D. Eisenhower once sent down for nose drops. One day a young air force full colonel came in with the complaint of substantial weight loss. "Colonel," I told him, "you have either hyperthyroidism or diabetes. Your relative youth and your ravenous appetite weigh against cancer, and since you have no goiter, you must have diabetes."

"I can't have diabetes: I'm a West Point man!" What he meant was that diabetes would ruin his military career. However, within minutes we had demonstrated sugar in his urine.

But my most diverting assignment was as chief of ENT. The colonel called me one morning to say I was now in charge of that service; the ENT specialist had just been discharged. I remonstrated that I had hardly looked in a throat since internship, but he offered me a

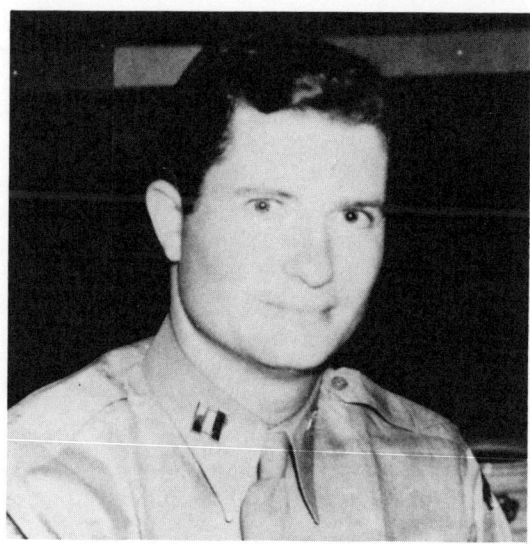

JDH, the Pentagon, 1946

book and said there was a general waiting in the chair. Going around to the ENT section, I told the nurse to go in and turn on everything that shone or moved, and said that I would look over the patient's old chart and then enter with a flourish. But it was a *General Simmons*—could he be the head of the army's Preventive Medicine Program and an oft-mentioned friend of Dr. Miller at Penn? The general said he was there to have his antrum punctured again for sinusitis. "General, are you a friend of Dr. T. Grier Miller in Philadelphia?"

"Why, yes, Captain, Grier and Sarah have been good friends of mine for over twenty years."

"General, I'm going to level with you. I was appointed chief of ENT only minutes ago. I've had little experience. I suggest you go over to Walter Reed Army Hospital."

The general scuttled down the hall as if exposed to hostile enemy fire. But the ENT service was now covered by an appointed chief (me), who was enveloped with all the prestige and authority accompanying the office. This ENT experience was to provide an ironic twist in a prolonged struggle far in my future.

I had definitely decided to specialize in surgery instead of internal medicine. This decision had been brought about perhaps by the subtle influence of the research in wound healing I had done as a medical student, but *definitely* by experience in the field hospital (the wounded I had to turn over to a surgeon), and by discussions with friends. In the 81st I had the feeling, in the presence of wounded men, that I was something less than a complete physician. I needed a field to which I could devote, with complete dedication and without mental reservations, whatever abilities I might have. The great German surgeon Theodor Billroth had written, "The surgeon must become an internist and something more, not something less."* Certainly surgery was a discipline of *action*, whereas there had been so little that we could do in internal medicine for arthritis, renal failure, heart failure in many, liver failure, and leukemia.

From Europe I had written the medical chiefs, Drs. Miller, Pepper, and Starr, that I did not wish them to hold open a postwar residency position in internal medicine for me any longer. They had replied graciously, a vast relief to me. Although I did not know it at the time, each wrote a strong note to Dr. Ravdin, who returned from India and now was to be chairman of the Department of Surgery.

I had written Dr. Ravdin to ask for a residency in surgery several times. On each occasion he had been noncommittal about my application but had suggested I get in touch again after I knew when I would be getting out of the army. Finally I wrote that I would be discharged on July 8 and would come to Philadelphia from Washington to hear his decision, whether it be positive or negative. I was walking up the hall of the first floor of the University Hospital when I came upon Dr. Ravdin and his entourage waiting for an elevator. I was introduced, "Dr. Ravdin, this is Jim Hardy."

"Yes," said the chief, "I remember Hardy. He's gained weight." (Which I had.)

Then there was a long silence. I really had nothing further to say. At this point I simply needed an answer; my whole future depended on it, one way or the other. For a momentous interval Dr. Ravdin gazed out the window toward the Wharton School of Finance across the street. Then he turned back abruptly, looked at me squarely, and said, "When do you want to start to work?"

"September the first."

---

*Theodor Billroth, *General Surgery, Pathology and Therapy: 60 Lectures* (Reimer: Berlin, 1863).

The day I was to be discharged at the Pentagon the colonel called me in. "Hardy," he said, "the army has a place for you."

"Colonel, I respect the army very much. I value my experience and especially the experience in command. But now, after going on three years, I have not really found my place in the army."

He laughed. "Good luck, then, but regulations say I had to ask you."

CHAPTER 7

The 1940s: The Rise of Physiologic Surgery

"Now that surgery has been made safe for the patient, the patient must be made safe for surgery."

This quotation, attributed to Lord Moynihan around 1935, clearly states the attitude that began to pervade surgical thought at that time. It had become increasingly evident that larger and larger, and longer and longer, operations could not be imposed successfully on patients who were not prepared to withstand them. Hence the watchword became "preoperative preparation" or "preoperative and postoperative care," at times to the extent of almost denigrating the clearly preeminent importance of a good technical operation itself.

Wars traditionally advance the field of surgery in one context or another. Most often dire necessity has spawned invention, always based on knowledge gained beforehand. For example, the high amputation rate in World Wars I and II following injury to the popliteal artery was essentially halved in the Korean War by immediate direct artery repair, though the rate still approached 70 percent when the artery was simply ligated.

Similarly, the emergency management of dire chest wounds in World War II afforded many surgeons operative experience they could never have obtained so rapidly in civilian life. They were operating under circumstances where there was nothing to lose and possibly a life to be saved. These surgeons then returned home and served as important leaders in the advancement of lung and heart surgery, made possible, to be sure, through rapid advances in endotracheal controlled-ventilation anesthesia, improved blood replacement, and antibiotics.

But the forces generated by World War II went much deeper than this. First, the American Board of Surgery had been established in

1937 to certify that surgeons allowed to take and then pass its examinations had had specified formal residency training and related credits. These certified "board men" were then accorded special assignments in the military and later in the Veterans Administration hospitals. Clearly, the apprentice system of surgical training was dated, and young physicians soon perceived that to have a secure career in surgery it was going to be necessary to take a formal residency and get one's boards.

Thus, when World War II abruptly ended, thousands of young physicians were discharged, and a great many of these sought additional formal training in surgery. And chiefs of surgery in hospitals approved for residency by the board wanted to help. Whereas there might have been only four residents in general surgery before the war, as in the Hospital of the University of Pennsylvania, this number was promptly increased to ten or even twenty. These men were usually highly selected. Many in this developing vast reservoir of surgical manpower had had, or soon gained, experience in disciplined research as well as in technical surgery. Many of them would become academic surgeons, with a lifelong dedication to improving surgery and investigating surgical problems. Incidentally, this great increase in residency training positions had not been cut back significantly almost forty years later. The Hill-Burton Act provided community hospitals all over the United States. Medical schools increased in number apace. Hence, the manpower pool was in place to develop the next surgical era.

Equally important was the change in basic scientific orientation that began to permeate the field of surgery more generally in the late 1930s and the early 1940s. There had always been physiologic surgeons, or surgical physiologists, but they had been few in number. The "father of modern surgery," John Hunter of Great Britain, had worked in the 1770s, his advice being "don't think, experiment." However, it was only with the seminal influence of a relatively few physiologic surgeons in the 1940s, extended through their residency training programs, that the full flowering of the new metabolic and other investigative techniques was brought into mainstream surgical thought and practice. Such techniques included the demonstration that all atoms and molecules of the body are in various and varying states of dynamic equilibrium, not in fixed and stable body compartments as heretofore believed. This perception had been derived from research using the newly available radioactive and nonradioac-

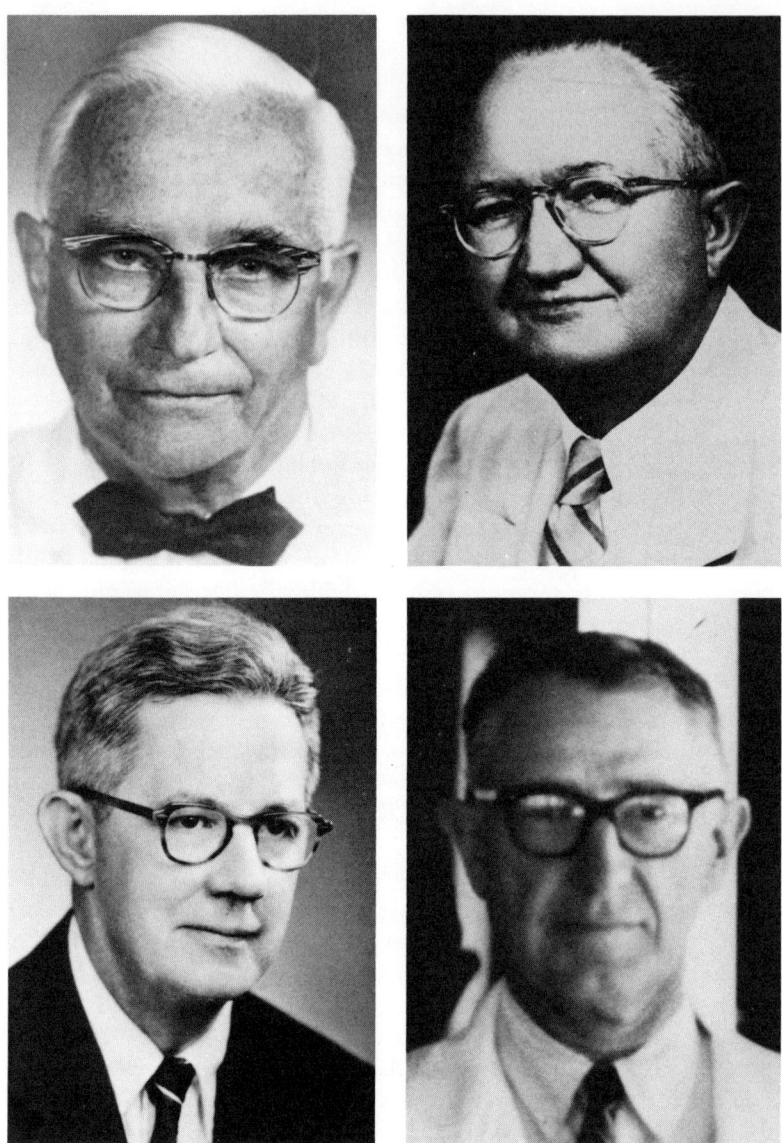

Physiological surgeons: Owen H. Wangensteen (top left);
Lester R. Dragstedt (top right); *Alfred Blalock* (bottom left);
Francis D. Moore (bottom right).

tive isotopes available from Oak Ridge and other nuclear facilities.

But even before that, my old medical chief Dr. Pepper had called me up to his office one day and said, "Jim, I've just come across an article that is going to revolutionize our approach to body composition and metabolism." A man named David P. Cuthbertson in Great Britain had shown, with metabolic balance studies in rats, that simply breaking the femur resulted in a loss of nitrogen and calcium in the urine for weeks. This loss was often far greater than could have derived from the fractured bone itself. But even before this, John Hunter had written in 1794, "There is a circumstance attending accidental injury that does not belong to disease, namely, that the injury done has in all cases a tendency to produce the disposition and the means of cure." Enter endocrinology.

The stage was thus set, in 1945, for surgeons to move from their all-too-common previous role of simply being technicians, to the high ground of becoming leading clinical physiologists as well. They had the inestimable advantage of being able to make important observations, not only in the many laboratories required by the American Board of Surgery for resident training, but also in their own private domain, the hospital operating theater.

Lastly, there came an increasing flood of financial support for research. The American public, thoroughly impressed with the research success that had made penicillin generally available and developed the atomic bomb—this public now wanted diseases conquered and they were willing through Congress to pay for it. Everything was now in place—the experimental approach, manpower, newer investigative resources and techniques, and large financial support. These permitted formal invasion of the thorax, with the special physiology and diseases of its numerous anatomic structures. Routinely successful blood-vessel surgery would later lead to successful organ transplantation.

CHAPTER 8

Isidor Schwaner Ravdin

I. S. Ravdin ("Rav" to his peers) was one of the truly outstanding surgeons of his time. He was born on October 10, 1894, in Evansville, Indiana, where his father, also the son of a physician, practiced medicine. After local schooling he took his bachelor of science degree at Indiana University, where he also completed two years of medical training. He then transferred to the School of Medicine at the University of Pennsylvania as a third-year student. Graduating in 1918, he took a rotating internship in the University Hospital and in 1919 was appointed instructor in surgery and became chief resident in the University Hospital. In 1921 he married Dr. Elizabeth Glenn, who was the first woman to intern in the University Hospital.*

In 1927 he went abroad to the University of Edinburgh and worked with Sir Edward Sharpey Schaefer and Sir David Wallace and later with Sir Henry Dale in London. Thereafter, Isidor Ravdin was always to approach surgical problems from a physiologic point of view and, in doing so, he was a leader in the rise of physiologic surgery in the United States. His laboratory, in the 1930s and thereafter, was always involved in hepatobiliary problems, nutrition in surgical patients, wound healing, and other research. Major staff collaborators in this work were Drs. Cecilia Riegel, Harry Vars, Samuel Goldschmidt, Jonathan Rhoads, Otto Rosenthal, and still others—in addition to a continuing stream of residents and research fellows who were thus indoctrinated with the investigative approach to unsolved surgical problems.

One feature of Dr. Ravdin's research deserves special comment. This was his respect for, and appreciation of, the basic and major role that scientists with the Ph.D. degree can play in the research of

*Brooke Roberts, "Memoir of I. S. Ravdin," *Transactions and Studies of The College of Physicians of Philadelphia* 41 (1974):237.

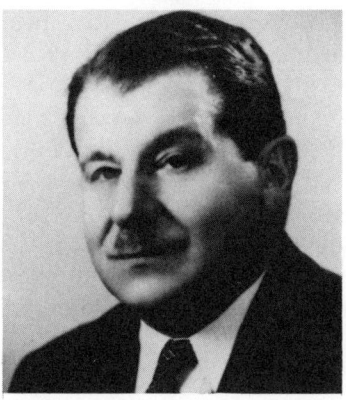

Isidor S. Ravdin

a clinical department. This relationship between clinicians, especially surgeons, and Ph.D. chemists and physiologists in a clinical department can be an uneasy and indeed a fragile one. The chemist or physiologist in a department of surgery may not receive from those in the medical school departments of chemistry or physiology the respect and professional advancement they deserve. Therefore, if they do not receive sympathetic support from the M.D. members of their clinical department, much is lost all around. But here Dr. Ravdin was at his best. As an investigator himself, he fully realized the great value of able basic scientists in a clinical department—scientists deeply versed in biochemical and physiological investigative techniques and analyses who knew how to *do* things. He respected and nurtured these scientists, and in turn they accepted him as one of their own. He went to *them*, was at home in *their* laboratories.

In 1940, Dr. Ravdin developed acute cholecystitis, and he chose for his surgeon Jonathan Rhoads, who himself had completed his training with Dr. Ravdin only months before. True, Allen O. Whipple, chairman of the Department of Surgery at Columbia, and Eldridge Eliason, chairman of the Department of Surgery at the University of Pennsylvania, were both present. But Rhoads was the surgeon. Such demonstrations of confidence did much for young men; for example, when I was his chief resident, he would at times simply sign out his service to me when he left the state on a speaking engagement. What he was saying was that he had confidence in my judgment to call in one of the senior staff members immediately if some problem were to arise with one of his patients. Obviously I did no surgery in his absence. Incidentally, the story, possibly apocryphal, was told that at his own gallbladder operation, while under spinal anesthesia (which he vastly preferred for his patients), he was awake and could see the operative maneuvers reflected by the mirror-effect of the light above the operating table. Thus, he began to make suggestions to Rhoads as to how to proceed. Finally, Dr. Whipple said firmly, "Rav, either *scrub up*—or *shut up!*"

A major period in Dr. Ravdin's career was his participation in forming, and later as commander of, the University Hospital's 20th General Hospital army unit in India. Returning a brigadier general (and later major general), he accepted the chairmanship of the Department of Surgery at Penn with the understanding that there would be one unified organization. Before the war there had been two separate services, the Eliason and the Ravdin units, with considerable rivalry and at times more than that. Everyone in the department would now be on a full-time basis, with one central office handling all the finances. For the first time, this afforded the chairman and his senior associates access to pooled financial resources, which gave them much greater flexibility than had been possible before the war. The salary support of the full-time clinicians and the department was derived almost entirely from private practice; Dr. Ravdin once told me that he received as salary only about 10 percent of what he brought into the coffers from his personal private practice. There still remained two general surgical services, one run by Jonathan Rhoads and the other by Julian Johnson. The former had conducted the Ravdin service during the war, but the latter had been with Ravdin in India. Nonetheless, Dr. Ravdin was the single person in overall command. He once told me that he had asked Dr. Eliason, who was retiring, to tell him frankly which man he would select to run the second service, Julian Johnson or Kreer Ferguson, both Eliason trainees. I was intrigued that Dr. Ravdin had asked, for in teaching conferences Eliason had often taken what appeared to be unnecessarily sharp issue with some opinion voiced by I.S.R. In fact, we students were impressed that Ravdin always remained calm in these encounters. Eliason replied that he would sleep on it, and would give his opinion the next day. He then recommended Johnson.

My most personal contact with I.S.R., one on one, was probably experienced when I was first back from the army and still on surgical pathology. I was then much more free to leave the hospital on short notice, having no clinical duties, and one day he asked if I would like to drive up to Bethlehem, Pennsylvania, on a consultation. On the way, he began to ask my opinion of various middle-level members of the Department of Medicine, their personalities and relationships with personnel, clinical and teaching ability, and research activities. He knew, of course, that I had been a medical resident before the war. He particularly asked about Drs. Isaac Starr and Francis C. Wood. I did not know it then, but I.S.R. was apparently on the committee to select a new chairman of the Department of Medicine. In due course Francis Wood was appointed.

When we arrived at the Bethlehem hospital and had examined the patient, Dr. Ravdin passed smoothly by the clustered relatives, taking the consulting surgeon by the elbow and moving to the solarium. He closed the door and then laid out his full opinion of the clinical situation and possible future therapeutic measures. Thus he had done the other surgeon the courtesy of discussing the case privately, one of the many dimensions of professional courtesy which all of us too often neglect in the busy day. However, Rav knew he also had an obligation to the family, to let them, too, know what he thought ought to be done, lest his opinion never be conveyed fully to them. Accordingly, he proposed that we invite the relatives in so that they might ask questions. (Though several years later he was called down to Washington to operate with Surgeon General Leonard Heaton on President Eisenhower for small bowel obstruction, he always downplayed his role.)

On at least two occasions, "the Professor," as we called him, sent me on scientific missions he could not attend. One morning I was rushed abruptly down to Baltimore to join Dr. Everett Evans of the Medical College of Virginia and Dr. Margaret Sloan, Executive Secretary of the National Research Council, for a project site visit. The committee was to inspect some clinical studies at the Fort Howard Veterans Hospital involving two new enzymes, streptokinase and streptodornase. We were then to recommend whether or not the National Research Council should extend substantial financial support for large-scale commercial production. We were impressed with the way these enzymes, applied locally, had cleaned up infected wounds. However, we decided to recommend only that the investigator be invited to report his results to a meeting of the full National Research Council in Washington.

My second assignment was to drive across Philadelphia one rainy night to meet an inventor who had had the novel idea that blood could be stored in plastic bags instead of fragile glass bottles. In fact, he had produced such bags, which he filled with water and then dropped on the concrete floor of his garage from a considerable height. They did not burst! I duly reported this back to the Professor. I don't know what he did with my report, but it was to be some years before plastic bags were generally accepted for blood storage.

The Ravdins had three children. Bob, who became a surgeon, was of much help to his father near the end of his tenure. Sadly, Bob died abruptly of a coronary at an early age. Elizabeth (Betty, "Sis") entered nursing school and eventually married a U.S. diplomat. Bill entered the business world.

Dr. Ravdin relinquished his chairmanship of the Department of Surgery at sixty-five and became vice-president for medical affairs. But soon he began to develop significant complications of atherosclerosis. Always moderately obese, he was a long-term smoker. In addition to angina pectoris, he developed severe ischemia of the right leg, which threatened the loss of this extremity. However, to the informed, it was his progressive loss of memory that was most apparent. My first exposure to this problem came on the evening of October 10, 1962. I had been invited up to Philadelphia to give the annual Da Costa Oration of the Philadelphia County Medical Society. The topic selected by the program committee was "Problems Associated with Gastric Surgery." Incidentally, while Da Costa (once head of surgery at Jefferson Medical College, a post then held by John Gibbon) had been a "household name" when I'd been in Philadelphia years before, I realized that I really knew little about the man. I would be in an awkward position if my introducer at the meeting did not himself make the usual few felicitous remarks about the honoree of this named lecture. Therefore, leaving Jackson early, I stopped off in Washington at the National Library of Medicine and found reams of material on Da Costa. However, it was one particular statement by Da Costa that instantly bonded us as kindred spirits: He had said, approximately, that "when leaving for a new position, many men say they were called by the Lord; but, more often, they were called by the Board!" My hotel that night was the ill-fated but then venerable Bellevue-Stratford, site of the outbreak of Legionnaires' disease years later.

At the University Hospital the next morning, Dr. Ravdin explained with regret that he had an unbreakable commitment for the evening and could not be at the dinner. This was not surprising, for his executive assistant, Miss Lucas, had once explained to me that the regular residents' dinner could not be scheduled immediately—she had promised Mrs. Ravdin the professor would dine at home at least one evening in the next six weeks. However, he insisted that my sponsor, Henry Moss, and I come around to his home on Delancy Street after the Da Costa affair; we would have a drink and chat before I took the midnight plane back to Jackson. He had Miss Lucas call various hospitals on our itinerary, throughout the day, to repeat the invitation. Well, when Henry and I showed up at his door about ten that evening, he was completely dumbstruck and exclaimed, "Jim Hardy, what on earth are you doing here, in Philadelphia, in a tuxedo, at this hour of the night?" Sadly, his condition progressed inexorably.

In an environment where anti-Semitism was not unknown, I never heard Dr. Ravdin even acknowledge it but twice. The first occasion was at a staff meeting, where he sternly ordered that race was not to be stated on the hospital record. Actually, the writer of the offending record had intended no slight; we had all been taught in physical diagnosis and history taking to make presentations as descriptive as possible, in any informative way. On the other occasion I was in Dr. Rhoads' office late one afternoon, catching up on patient visit dictation. Unavoidably, I overheard Dr. Ravdin and Miss Lucas exchanging humorous Jewish jokes in the vernacular. He had a large and devoted following of Jewish patients.

It was acknowledged that Rav was tough. In fact, there were those, at a distance, who said he was ruthless, this being the reason given for his nonelection to a major surgical society. This notwithstanding, he was eventually president of virtually all the others. He was a master at preserving, at least to outward appearances, equanimity in the face of considerable provocation—a policy I tried to emulate, though much less successfully.

He was a precise speaker, reading his remarks at any important occasion, and he was a great showman in the best sense of the word. For example, he had performed an abdominoperineal operation for rectal carcinoma in a physician, who had the common temporary complication of difficulty in voiding; he was finally discharged still wearing a catheter. The next day, down at Atlantic City, Dr. Frank Lahey of the Lahey Clinic was presiding at a panel on colorectal cancer at the American Medical Association meeting when the proceedings were interrupted by a man who stood up in the huge audience. He yelled that Dr. Ravdin had made a bad mistake in his case—it was the physician patient! Dr. Lahey turned and asked, "Rav, do you want to reply?" Rav said he would and strode to the podium: "Yes, I did make a mistake in the doctor's case—I discharged him a day too soon!"

On other occasions, the Professor would get advance but brief notice that some research agency was coming for a survey of the facilities; whereupon he would call me (and, of course, others), and I would speed over to the Medical Laboratories Building and, in twenty minutes or so, set up charts and procedures and prepare for the visitors. (Not that we did not work at other times.)

A major facet of Rav's extraordinary leadership was his sensitive perception of human motivation, of just what would be most appropriate to enlist the affection, loyalty, and performance of each individual around him. Rav set great store by loyalty. Much later, at a memorial service for him, it was said that he never fired anyone. Be this as it may, he was certainly supportive. Julian Johnson once remarked that if one had a bad complication in a patient, Dr. Eliason would say, "stew in your own juice," whereas Rav would say, "*we've just got to get out of this.*" On one occasion, I urged the Professor to fire someone because she exhibited truly extraordinary ineptitude. "Now, Jim," he replied, "have you ever seen her unpleasant?" No, sir, I hadn't. "Have you ever seen her call in sick?" No, again. "Have you ever seen her fail to come in, somehow, no matter how deep the snow?" Once again, no. "*Jim, she's loyal!*"

After he had relinquished the chairmanship of the department to Jonathan Rhoads, I had written Dr. Ravdin, suggesting firmly that now was the time for him to dictate his memoirs, while memory was fresh and materials were at hand. He had replied:

February 16, 1961

Dear Jim:

    I suppose you will never know how deeply your recent note touched me. I have always questioned the value of an autobiography because all too frequently we do not see ourselves as others see us and we have too great an idea of our importance in the whole realm that we have lived in.

    I was chosen as one of the two surgeons to prepare a type of autobiography for the Nicholas Murray Butler Library at Columbia University. One copy, as I understand it, will go to the Library of

Congress; one stays in the Nicholas Murray Library, and one I would receive. One of these days when it is all finished I will go over it with you and then the two of us will decide just what to do with this.

Sadly, poor health overtook him, and, to my knowledge, this autobiographic project was never completed.

Suffice it to say, Rav, forever *the Professor*, was the ablest boss I ever had.

Isidor S. Ravdin died on August 27, 1972, at the age of seventy-eight.

CHAPTER 9

Resident in General Surgery at Penn

The three senior surgeons principally involved in training residents in general surgery were, as noted previously, Drs. Ravdin, Jonathan Rhoads, and Julian Johnson. I came to think of them as overall commander General Eisenhower (Ravdin), General Bradley (Rhoads, deputy commander, with many varied activities), and General Patton (Johnson, a pure surgical warrior).

The American Board of Surgery had informed me that, to fulfill the five-year training requirement, one year of credit would be given for the prewar internship–medical residency and one year for the years in the army, but beyond this, three solid years of clinical surgical residency would be necessary.

When I reported for duty, I found that I was to be assigned to surgical pathology for the next four months, to begin actual surgical rotations in January. Dr. Ravdin then asked, "Doctor, what do you plan to investigate?"

Without hesitation I answered, "Cachexia, sir."

He looked nonplussed and said, "But that is a blank wall. What will you actually do?"

"Well, sir, when I was a resident in medicine before the war, I was always fascinated with and mystified by the way cancer patients lost their appetite, wasted away, and died, when no specific body organ was blocked or grossly interfered with. I plan to pass a tube into the stomach and feed these cancer patients when they have no appetite, to see if they can thus be made to restore lost body tissue and regain strength."

These studies would clearly continue along the lines of the body fluid relationships that I had pursued before the war. But it would be necessary to know whether the cancer patients who gained weight on the tube feedings had actually manufactured new body tissue or had simply gained water. After all, even lean body tissue, such as muscle, is normally approximately 70 percent water, and fat contains very little water (as we, and others, were to confirm several years later). This ultimately proved far more complicated and difficult than I had ever imagined, but more about this later.

Right now my assignment was to surgical pathology. It was an informative service, and I had always liked pathology.

One episode at the beginning of this pathology rotation humbled me considerably and brought home to me just how little I knew about surgery. One morning I received an urgent call from the operating suite. Dr. Ravdin wanted me to come down from pathology and scrub in the operating room right away! The chief was performing a ligation and stripping of varicose veins on both legs, simultaneously, of an obese lady. I hardly knew what to do, but of course I rushed down as summoned. I scrubbed, gowned, and managed to get into the operating room, which was the scene of furious activity. Though swarming over the operative field, the team was still considered to be short handed, and I was told to sew up the various skin wounds left behind by the team. Here I was, absolutely green of even such elementary human surgery; having been an internist, I had no idea just what I was supposed to do. Mortified, I was immobilized, afraid I would do something wrong, when John Howard (a fellow resident) told the scrub nurse firmly to "give Dr. Hardy the absorbable *subcutaneous catgut* suture, with which to close the deeper layers of the skin." Taking the hint, I began placing deep sutures and would probably have been placing sutures still, just to stay out of trouble and avoid detection by the furiously operating Professor, when John chanced to look at the number of sutures I had placed and, startled, then quickly told the nurse to *now* give Dr. Hardy the silk sutures with which to sew up the skin itself. She muttered loudly that "some of these new military residents couldn't operate their way out of a paper bag; how did we ever win the war," but finally the operation was over. As my old German professor used to say, now that I knew I did not know, I was certainly ready to learn.

Rotating off surgical pathology, I began clinical training. I went to Dr. Ravdin's large private service and was to remain there for perhaps six months. He gave his best on all occasions and we gave ours. We did a world of surgery, with remarkably few complications and almost no deaths, except in far advanced cancer. He spoke constantly of the need to develop a "surgical conscience" and to have compassion. "Always remember who you are and what you represent." He had an astonishingly good memory for patients' and their relatives' names. He demanded that his residents not come to the operating room without having had breakfast. He required that paste tubes be rolled from the end rather than squeezed in the middle. Like most good surgeons, he reduced the details to meticulous routine, addressing thereafter the major decisions inherent in the infinite variations of the individual patient's pathologic condition.

My routine, almost unvaried, was to get up around five, see all our patients, with special attention to those scheduled for surgery, then get a quick breakfast and be in the OR by half past seven for the day's schedule. Lateness to scrub was absolutely not tolerated. The schedule would contain anywhere from five to fifteen cases (usually about ten), and included the usual range of general surgery cases, such as thyroidectomy, mastectomy, cholecystectomy, gastrectomy, colon resection, and herniorrhaphy. After the operations, we saw every patient again with the chief. Then we residents did work rounds to perform tests and work up new patients, perhaps an emergency appendectomy, then rounds again in late afternoon and again around nine o'clock. Then we would call Dr. Ravdin with the "evening report," with every pertinent detail about every patient's condition carefully at hand.

One evening he was extremely annoyed. He had called me about eight o'clock to tell me to expect a private patient with an acute gallbladder. I was to see the patient in the emergency room, assess the situation, and then call him at home.

Well, I kept calling the ER but the patient did not come. So that Dr. Ravdin could go on to bed, I called about ten to give the evening report and to say that the patient still had not arrived, though Dr. F.'s office was only a few blocks from the University Hospital. "I don't know what happened," Dr. Ravdin said, "but you go to bed and get some sleep."

Unfortunately, he had called me after considerable delay, and in the interim the patient had come to the emergency room without a note from her physician. Assuming she was a charity case, and there being no remaining charity beds on general surgery, the residents had sent her down to Graduate Hospital. After finally discovering what had happened, I called Dr. Ravdin and he was very disturbed.

Thinking the matter over, I decided that if the 81st Field Hospital could admit well over one hundred patients in one day to tents in Germany, it should be possible to get this one patient back from a hospital twenty blocks away. A strategic plan was activated. The surgery resident at "Graduate" was extremely doubtful, but he finally agreed.

But by this time it was pouring rain and I could not get a taxi, so I called Quinnie, the night operator who made the wake-up call each morning. She was a wonderful institution, though I never actually saw her during the five years I lived in the hospital. She knew every doctor's voice. For example, when I returned to the hospital after two and a half years in the army, she said instantly, "Why, hello, Dr. Hardy. It's great to have you back!"

On this rainy night Quinnie took over, leaving the switch key open so I could listen in. "Hello, Yellow Cab. We have a matter of life and death out here at the University Hospital. A patient must be moved immediately from the Graduate Hospital. Pick up Dr. Hardy at the University emergency room and he will support the patient during the trip." Yellow Cab responded at once. Taking along University Hospital bedding for a linen exchange ("the patient's husband has taken her clothes home"), I brought the somewhat startled lady back.

Storming in the next morning, I.S.R. was astonished to find his patient resting comfortably in a borrowed bed on the tonsil ward.

We usually worked long hours, but late-night emergencies were not terribly frequent. Gunshot wounds and knifings were usually delivered to adjacent Philadelphia General Hospital by the ambulances. Back then I could work all day, stay up all night, and then work through the next day without any problem. It was not until I was fifty that a night of operating left me a bit jaded the next day. If I felt tired back in the residency days, I knew I was getting sick. One thing a surgeon needs is good health and stamina for long days and sometimes twelve or more hours of operations.

The senior resident on Dr. Ravdin's service was Archibald Fletcher of internship and army days. He'd had a year of surgical residency before entering military service. I was the junior resident. With little authority to announce specific treatment decisions to the patient, I was left to check on the patient's condition and progress, and to create a pleasant and light atmosphere. One day as he was leaving, an elderly Jewish man who'd been seriously ill said, "Dr. Fletcher, thank you for taking care of me. Dr. Hardy, thank you for the jokes." I did not forget the implications of this distinction.

Mammography, as a new diagnostic modality, was brought to our attention during these months. One day Dr. Ravdin said he was going to admit a woman for breast biopsy, but he did not want us residents to accuse him of doing unnecessary surgery. He went on to say that Jacob Gershon-Cohen, the radiologist at Graduate Hospital, had been following about seventy-five women for several years, taking X-rays of their breasts periodically—this was in line with some work he had seen in South America, as I recall. In any case, Gershon-Cohen was convinced that the woman to be admitted had a cancer at a specified site, though no lump could be felt in her voluminous breast. We operated, and to the impressed surprise of all, she *did* have a cancer at the precise point predicted. Even so, it was to be some years before many, if not most, radiologists were convinced of the value of mammography.

When Arch Fletcher rotated off Dr. Ravdin's private service, I became the senior resident, with a former classmate as the junior resident. One day we were operating when a call came that there was a private patient for Dr. Ravdin in the ER, appendicitis suspected. "Drop down and size up the situation," the chief told me. Meanwhile, he and the other resident continued, operating next on a little boy for an inguinal hernia.

Later that afternoon, as we were making rounds, the boy's mother said, "Doctor Hardy, my son's hernia was on the left side but the bandage is on the right side." Startled, I took the junior resident aside.

"Which side did you operate on? The mother is right. How did this happen?"

"Well, Dr. Ravdin asked which side and I said the right." (He was a very bright man, usually right, but never able to say he did not know.)

"I must tell Dr. Ravdin at once," I said, but he begged me to let him tell the chief, saying otherwise he would never be named a chief resident. Against my better judgment I agreed, but Dr. Ravdin called me up to his office and gave me a severe dressing down. "You are senior resident. You should not have let me operate on the wrong side. It is your fault, you were in charge!" Finally he subsided. (He was right, of course.)

"Well, Professor, I accept the principle that the senior resident bears full responsibility. But I did know which side the hernia was on, and I would have been there had you not sent me to the ER." Actually, as is true in about one-half the cases, the boy had had bilateral hernias; hence the mistake had not been suspected during the operation. The hernia on the other side was repaired a day or so later without event.

I would not want to leave the impression that working for I.S.R. was a grim activity. It wasn't—it was fun. He was just volatile. His explosions, usually in the operating room (again, understood by every surgeon), were like a summer thunderstorm, impressive momentarily but soon gone.

The monthly mortality conference was approached with some trepidation. Each patient who had died following operation was discussed and the cause assigned to one or more of the standard classifications: Error in operative technique? In judgment? In diagnosis? In postoperative management? In anesthetic management? Or was death due primarily to the patient's disease, or to an unavoidable complication such as a heart attack? Rarely, the classification of TBG (trying to be God)—that is, trying to accomplish with an operation more than could reasonably have been considered humanly possible—was irreverently assigned.

The Professor presided over these conferences fairly but firmly, with all staff and residents in attendance. The sessions could be painful to the responsible surgeon or surgical service, but they established truth and did instill the essence of a "surgical conscience." (Would you yourself have had this operation, Doctor, or would you have permitted it on your wife?)

I next progressed to the Rhoads ward ("charity") service. (The sharp distinction between the private and ward services was to become blurred years later, with the advent of Medicare, Medicaid, and many other types of third party coverage.)

Jonathan Evans Rhoads had been born in 1907 in Quaker Philadelphia of long Quaker lineage. After graduating from Haverford College, he took his medical degree at Johns Hopkins University and then trained in surgery with Dr. Ravdin. A man of extremely varied interests and capabilities, he ultimately became president of most of the major surgical organizations in the United States and a number of international groups as well. He shared large credit for rendering total parenteral nutrition clinically feasible. His major participation in civic activities culminated in his being named the recipient of the extremely prestigious Philadelphia Award. A tall and Lincolnesque figure, he treated everyone with unfailing quiet courtesy. I was never to hear him raise his voice, on any occasion, regardless of the circumstances. He was apparently only the second physician ever to serve as provost of the University of Pennsylvania.

I had been "senior" on Dr. Ravdin's private service because there was no chief resident there, but now I was a junior resident again,

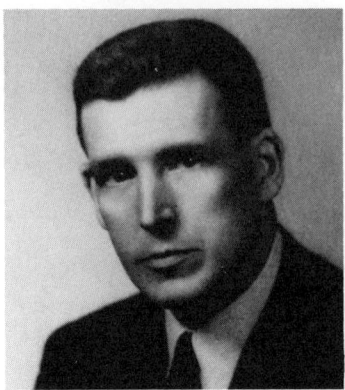

Jonathan E. Rhoads

allowed to perform supervised herniorrhaphy, appendectomy, and other operations of similar magnitude. The first day I was allowed to perform a gastrectomy, I sent a wire to Weezie in Charleston. Actually, it came as a surprise to me, for the junior resident was often not told ahead of time just which operation he would be allowed to do. Rather, the hopeful resident knew to be prepared for the big chance. When Quinnie, the night operator, rang me at 5:00 A.M., I would switch on the bedlamp, reach for Orr's *Operations of General Surgery*, and once again read over every operation we had scheduled to be done that day. At the beginning of each operation, there was a brief paragraph in fine print entitled "Errors and Safeguards." This was my target, for I had long since learned the major operative steps, but I had come to know that in most major operations there are only a few places where the surgeon can inflict serious and potentially irretrievable harm: to the laryngeal voice nerves in removing the thyroid gland, to the ureter draining the urine to the bladder in the course of colon resection, to the common bile duct near the liver. I had reviewed gastric resection many times, and I sailed through my first stomach.

One day the chief resident played a practical joke that momentarily gave me a severe start. The junior resident was allowed to begin some rather simple operations, such as routine leg amputation, by himself—this while the chief resident was doing his ten-minute scrub. The suture nurse had the patient all prepped and draped and the scalpel waiting in her hand for me to start. The lower legs—both the one to be amputated for foot gangrene and the normal one as well—were already wrapped and covered. I knew the patient well, and knew that it was the *right* foot that was gangrenous. So, with a flourish, I made the standard long and deep amputation incision. Just then, backing through the swinging door to keep his hands sterile and ostensibly talking to an invisible medical student outside, James Donald (the same one who had recommended Penn to me in Tuscaloosa nine years before) said loudly, "Now when amputating it is obviously important to amputate the correct leg. It's this patient's *left* foot that is gangrenous!" My heart skipped a beat, but thereafter I never operated on any paired organ—arm, leg, or lung—without first checking personally.

In the spring of 1948, the chief resident on the Rhoads Service told me privately that he had been directed "to pour the surgery to Hardy," and that in his opinion this meant I would be named one of the two chief residents to begin in July. This was good news indeed, for the residency was a "pyramidal" residency, and there could be only two chief residents—one for the Rhoads ward service and one for the Johnson ward service, the two chiefs changing services at mid-year. Those residents who failed to make chief resident were usually made eligible to take the American Board of Surgery examinations, but obviously it was a sore disappointment. The major authority, prestige, and independent operating went to the chief.

And I was appointed one chief resident, Arch Fletcher the other. We ran the teaching services, under the umbrellas of Drs. Rhoads and Johnson, and did most of the big operations on the ward ("charity") services, though always under appropriate supervision. There is no substitute for the sobering, disciplined maturation that a chief resident in surgery experiences. He also learns to run a team and to expect performance.

My next rotation, now as chief resident, was to the Johnson service. Julian Johnson was born in 1906 at Cox's Creek, Kentucky, the son of a Baptist minister. After graduating from Maryville College in Knoxville, he took his medical degree at the University of Pennsylvania and his surgical training under Eldridge Eliason at the University Hospital. Following his war experience with the University Hospital unit in India, he was assigned to develop the new field of thoracic surgery. Dedicated to perfection in surgical operative technique and patient care, he made many contributions to practical problems in cardiothoracic surgery. The Johnson and Kirby thoracic operative textbook was to become the standard of its time. His achievements were to be recognized by his election to the presidency of the American Association for Thoracic Surgery.

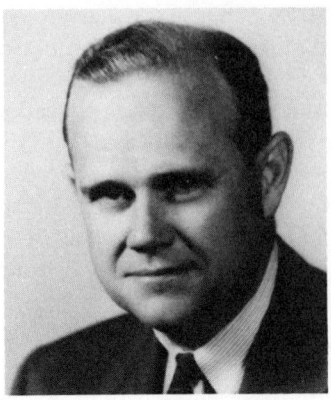

Julian Johnson

I began on Dr. Johnson's ward service as chief resident in July 1948. I was frankly uneasy. The discipline on that service, which covered not only general surgery patients but also the rapidly developing lung and heart surgery, was legendary. By some quirk of the rotations, I had never been on the Johnson service before—and here I was, his chief resident. I had asked others how to conduct myself on J.J.'s service. "Do your work and say nothing unless called upon, and then you'd better be right!"

Having thus far had no thoracic surgery, I did no independent chest operating. His staff deputy, Charles Kirby, rightfully did what J.J. did not want to do himself—and J.J. was not generous. A technical error during an operation could all too suddenly result in sudden, massive, and possibly fatal hemorrhage. J.J. felt the responsibility heavily, but he was a superb surgeon, with utter self-criticism and honesty, and painstaking with infinite detail. These qualities would become ever more important when open heart surgery came along several years later.

I got along with Dr. Johnson well enough. I did my work and volunteered nothing during the first few weeks. During the following two years, when I was to serve as thoracic resident, the crucial importance of the discipline he exacted was to become ever more apparent, day by day. The surgery I learned from J.J. was what made my later career in thoracic surgery possible. He used to say he didn't want a surgeon who'd "never had a complication"; he wanted a surgeon who'd had the inevitable complications and knew how to get out of them. He always demanded we "fight for the patient's life."

One day we had scheduled a man who'd had a gallbladder operation at another Philadelphia university hospital, in which his common bile duct had been injured. Incidentally, the operative note from the other hospital read, "The common duct was identified and *divided.*" What joy to the heart of a malpractice lawyer had he seen that statement, though malpractice suits were rare in 1948.

In any case, J.J. said, "Jim, has the Professor [Dr. Ravdin] ever helped you do a case?"

"No, Dr. Johnson, since he of course does not cover a ward service." As chairman of the department, Dr. Ravdin had many duties and thus covered only his own private patients.

"Well, I think he would be tickled pink if you were to ask him to help you do Mr. X tomorrow. He specializes in common bile duct injuries. Why don't you ask him?"

I did ask him. He was obviously pleased and was a perfect assistant, somewhat to my surprise, for it is one thing to be the surgeon and tell the assistants what to do, but it is quite another thing to be the assistant and refrain from endless suggestions. We found the bile duct promptly, in all the old scar tissue, and we made an excellent repair. Well-placed sutures afford aesthetic satisfaction.

With the end of my general surgery residency in sight, I had to make plans for July 1. Although it was clear that thoracic surgery was going to be an important new field of surgical advancement, and I hoped that I might get further training in it, I was reluctant to ask Dr. Johnson if he could take me on, since Charlie Kirby, his junior staff man, was all the help he really needed. Also, I suspect that part of my reluctance was due to a concern that I might be turned down.

But necessity forced my hand; I had to either be asked to stay on at Penn or find a place somewhere else to support my forthcoming marriage. I had saved some money during army days, but we were paid only a hundred dollars per month as residents plus the GI benefits. The staff took under advisement my informal request to stay on for thoracic training and after several months offered an arrangement. I would help Dr. Rhoads with his private service and office hours on Tuesday, Thursday, and Saturday, and work with Dr. Johnson on Monday, Wednesday, and Friday, all with considerable overlapping. Meanwhile, I was to apply for a Damon Runyon Clinical Research Fellowship which paid five thousand dollars per year. This I did on the basis of considerable research done before the war, and my application was successful, giving me more freedom

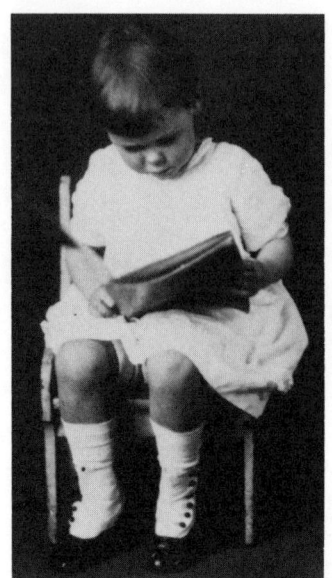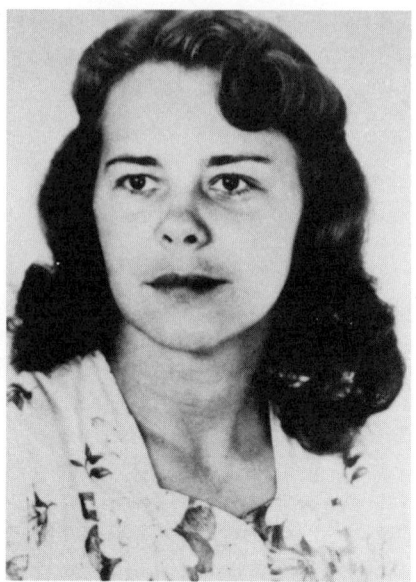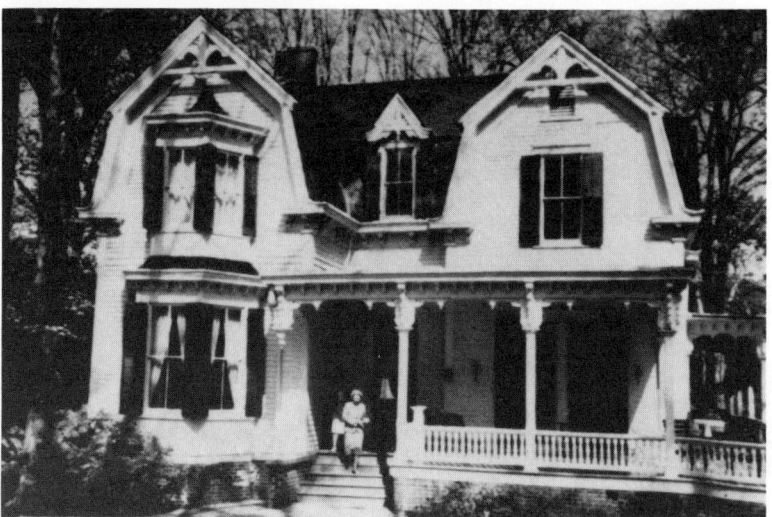

Louise ("Weezie") S. Hardy: at age 3 (upper left); *at marriage* (upper right); *at centennial ancestral home* (bottom)

to do research the next year. Actually, during the general surgery residency, I had put in a lot of time trying to develop the exquisitely elegant falling-drop method for determining heavy water to within three parts per million as a means of measuring heavy water concentration in plasma. To measure the total amount of water a human body contained, a measured amount of pure heavy water would be injected intravenously, then allowed to equilibrate with all the water in the body; the volume of water in the body was then determined by how much the injected heavy water had been diluted—the dilution principle. It was crucial that I be able to measure total body water in my investigations of body fluid shifts in health and disease, but as yet I had no results to show. In fact, Dr. Ravdin remarked one day, "Jim, you've done little research."

To this I replied, "Yes, Professor, but I *am* chief resident!" But to myself I promised to get my research really moving after I returned to Philadelphia a married man.

The marriage, on July 1, 1949, was a traditional one in the Presbyterian church in Decatur, Georgia, with Bach's "Jesu, Joy of Man's Desiring," Handel's "I Know That My Redeemer Liveth," and the wedding march from Wagner's *Lohengrin*. Julian was my best man.

Weezie and I had planned to go all the way to Acapulco but, after leaving Mexico City, we liked the beautiful city Taxco so much that we stayed right there until it was time to drive back to Philadelphia.

CHAPTER 10

Resident in Thoracic Surgery and Surgical Staff at Penn

Weezie and I set up housekeeping and soon reached the next clear turning point in my life. The clinical load was not so heavy that I could not get to the laboratory for a part of many afternoons and most evenings. I once lamented to Weezie that I wished I had just *one* person to direct—a remark she was to remind me of, from time to time, in later years.

In the spring of 1950, we were robbed one night by a cat burglar, immediately after we had got into bed. We actually saw him and called the police. Eating peanuts and dropping the hulls on the floor, one officer said, "Doc, we see you were in the army. Take this permit and go down tomorrow and buy yourself a pistol. Next time shoot the son of a bitch. We can't cover every house in West Philadelphia." I bought a .38-caliber revolver, still have it after thirty-five years, and probably haven't fired it more than ten times. Incidentally, the burglar got none of our valuable possessions: my microscope and Weezie's wedding silver.

My office work with Dr. Rhoads gave me the opportunity to see him quite differently than when we had been making rounds and operating in the hospital. My job was to see both his old patients and the new patients: I would take a history, do a physical examination as the situation required, and then brief Dr. Rhoads and lead him to the examining room. One particular patient was a spectacular brunette of perhaps thirty years.

"Dr. Rhoads," I said, "that patient is an absolute knockout!"

"I take you to mean, Jim, that you find her attractive. Well, let me tell you something about her. Women like that require a great deal of attention. I happen to know that her husband is a very frustrated and unhappy man. The most important thing in a wife is that she be loyal to the common enterprise."

I was a bit startled that he placed beauty in considerably less than first place, but then I remembered what my senior brother-in-law, Douglas Thomason, had once said about my sister: "Agnes is a wonderful woman. Why, I've seen her get out of bed with fever of a hundred and four and dress the chillun, feed 'em, and get them off to school."

Heavy water successful

Finally, the three principal elements of my elegant heavy water (D_2O) measuring apparatus, which would permit the measuring of the total amount of water in the human body, were all coming together. To achieve the necessary accuracy to three parts per million, it was necessary to release serial drops of exquisitely purified water (from plasma or urine) of absolutely reproducible size through a vertical cylinder filled with ortho-fluoro-toluene in a water bath maintained within 0.001 degree centigrade. The water bath was a ninety-liter aquarium bought from a tropical fish dealer in South Philadelphia. The exquisitely sensitive glass thermoregulator, filled with acetone and placed in the water bath, was blown by James Graham, the medical school's widely recognized scientific glass blower. The dropping cylinder apparatus was duplicated by Charles Gobel, master machinist in the School of Engineering, from one loaned by a chemist at Columbia University, David Rittenberg.

When at last all components were functioning smoothly, I one day had the immense satisfaction of seeing the progressive known concentrations of D_2O samples fall on a straight line. This demonstrated the accuracy of the complex apparatus in measuring D_2O concentrations to within three parts per million. The long, sustained discipline and intensity required had been perhaps the greatest intellectual challenge of my life thus far, but it had led me from a swamp of uncertainty and self-doubt about my research to the paved road of basic physiological research which was publishable anywhere. I had set up the apparatus in one of the laboratories of Dr. David L. Drabkin in the Department of Physiological Chemistry over in the medical school; he had kindly given me space and had staunchly supported me during many discouraging times. This day, as we calculated and plotted the concentrations of the "unknown" control D_2O on graph paper and got the straight line, he was as excited as I was. He hastened up and down the hall, insisting that the other chemists rejoice with us.

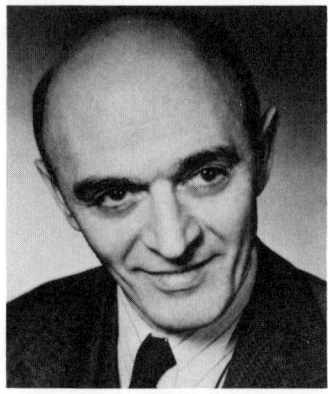

David L. Drabkin, chairman of Biochemistry, Graduate School of Medicine, University of Pennsylvania

At that particular moment, we had the only falling-drop D_2O method in use anywhere, since Rittenberg in New York had discontinued his metabolic studies which had required it. Francis Moore at Harvard had measured total body water in man using a gradient tube method, but this had required so much of the scarce and expensive heavy water that he was in the process of converting to the falling-drop method. I had succeeded in obtaining two twenty-five-gram sealed tubes of heavy water from Norway.

We could now measure blood volume, extracellular fluid, and, with D_2O, total body water in normal people. I had had the heavy water injected intravenously into myself, in the first experiment, for there was still some question about its toxicity. As with all dilution principle measurements of an unknown volume, the injected molecules of heavy water slowly equilibrated with all the water molecules in my body. Again, since the number of heavy water molecules (the concentration) was known, a subsequent measurement of the concentration of heavy water in the plasma taken from a vein would reveal the total amount of water (in my body) throughout which the injected heavy water must have been diluted. As German scientists had found some years earlier in the study of a single obese man, most of the heavy water was excreted in my urine in nine to eleven days, almost all the rest by twenty-nine days, and presumably a few circulating molecules of isotope escaped excretion indefinitely. Of normal obesity, my body was 60 percent water. A very obese physician who volunteered was only 43 percent water by body weight, and the leanest surgical resident we could find was 72 percent water. Thus, fat contained little water, but muscle and other lean tissue contained about 70 percent water.

One day Dr. Ravdin brought Dr. Owen H. Wangensteen, chairman of the Department of Surgery at the University of Minnesota, around to see my apparatus and results. This visit was to prove important to me in the future.

In rapid succession, I presented these and related studies before the Philadelphia Physiological Society and the Philadelphia Academy of Surgery. As we were leaving the academy that night, J.J. said, "Jim, that was pretty heavy stuff. I think I'll keep estimating how well hydrated my patient is by seeing how moist his tongue is."

But the big research meeting of the year was the annual meeting of the American Physiological Society, always held in Atlantic City in those days. My heavy water results were on the program and I practiced and practiced giving the paper to Weezie and to the mirror. We drove down to the meeting and stayed at the Lyric Hotel. As I was registering, the desk clerk saw Dr. P. K. Sen and Weezie unloading the car. Dr. Sen, from Bombay, had been assigned to work with me in research. "He can't come in here," she said, "even if he does have reservations."

Doing a doubletake, I suddenly realized the problem. "But he's an Indian," I said.

"Then why didn't you say so!" And, somewhat unsettled, we got in. Incidentally, Dr. Sen, a brilliant young surgeon, had been brought over by the Rockefeller Foundation. The foundation then set up a heart surgery program and laboratory for him at the Seth-Edward Hospital and Medical School in Bombay. It became a model in India.

The big day came and I was very pleased with the way my ten-minute address had come off before the large audience. However, our paper was followed by a paper from Dallas in which the author reported that, in an animal study, some dogs' body weight was 90 percent water. Preposterous! Such an animal would have been flowing around like an amoeba. Clearly, since my humans and his dogs were both mammals, either his results were wrong or my results were wrong, and I was determined to have the audience know that I doubted the dog work. At the question and answer interval, I arose and asked, "Mr. Moderator, I would like to inquire of the essayist as to the character of his dogs." To this the speaker replied, "Sir, I'll have you know that the character of my dogs was unimpeachable!" The audience roared. And from this I learned to phrase questions more carefully.

All the Damon Runyon Fellows were invited to New York's Memorial Hospital for Cancer and Allied Diseases to put on a scientific program. Walter Winchell, Leonard Lyons, and Sherman Billingsley would host a luncheon at the Stork Club. Winchell stood up at the microphone and, in his characteristic staccato delivery, extolled the fight against cancer and the Damon Runyon Fund's participation in this fight. The syndicated columnist Leonard Lyons, who was seated beside me, leaned over and said, "If Winchell's done nothing else, he's sure scared the hell out of the American people about cancer."

At lunch on the second day, in the enclosed roof garden of the hospital, I was seated beside John Teeter, executive director of the Damon Runyon Fund. Making conversation, I asked how the fund raised its money and how the research grant awards were decided. Donations came from famous entertainers, he explained, and a scientific committee appraised the scientific value and promise of grant requests. However, he continued, he held back a small percentage which he himself could assign as seed money to young investigators just getting started—*venture capital*, he liked to call it. This bit of information later became most significant to my future as a research scientist.

That evening we all went to a costume ball for TV celebrities at the Waldorf-Astoria. Weezie, who had become pregnant the previous fall and was now very large, had rented an academic cap and gown. One doctor at our table remarked, "You know, your costume would be a fine idea if one were pregnant." Weezie just smiled. During the evening Mary Martin rushed over from *South Pacific* in her sailor costume and sang several songs from the musical. We had a memorable experience.

By this time I was doing more thoracic operating and was allowed to have private surgical patients, though they were rare. For one thing, my name and admitting priority were at the bottom of all the ten or so surgeons in the group, and it might take six weeks to get my patient admitted, by which time he or she might have grown impatient and switched surgeons. However, two patients were signally instructive.

One had been discussing with me her forthcoming gallbladder operation. As she stood up to leave, she asked, "Doctor, how much will your fee be?" I was so caught off guard by the fact that, after a college degree, four years of medical school, an internship, a medical residency, and five years of surgery, someone actually expected to pay me, that my mouth must have fallen open. My appearance apparently flustered the lady, for she became embarrassed and blushed, and then blurted out, "I mean unless complications set in,

Doctor. Then I know it would be more!" (Actually, I thought to myself, if complications set in I probably would pay *her* to leave town.)

But it was I who was at a loss for words. I muttered that the receptionist at the front desk would give her these charges. I had absolutely no idea what to charge. Alas, I soon heard Miss Betty Smith up front telling the patient emphatically, "Dr. Hardy knows perfectly well I don't set the charges. We'll just have to get back in touch with you later."

Miss Marjorie Lucas, the office business manager and a marvelously capable woman, had heard all this, and she called me into her little office, put her feet up in a chair, lit a cigarette, and said, "Now, Dr. Hardy, sit down and let me give you the facts of life. First, you should always be ready to answer the patients' questions about fees. After all, these are private patients, they expect to pay, and they want to make plans for their hospital costs. Next, you should have in mind an average fee for each common operation—removal of the gallbladder, thyroid, colon, or whatever. I will give you the average and reasonable fees the rest of the staff charge. Then, if complications do set in, or if it is an extraordinarily difficult case, you can modify your fee accordingly. Finally, some patients have little but their pride, and these we charge less."

My other private patient presented a painful problem that almost every young surgeon just starting out must suffer through. Just after I had gone "on the staff," one of the urologists, being kind to a newcomer, referred me a "hemorrhoid." Like any surgeon, I took much pride in the fact that I had been referred a private patient. The man had had a prostate operation a day or so earlier, but he had been anemic.

I examined the patient. He did have hemorrhoids, but they did not look to me like an adequate cause for the significant anemia. Lo and behold, I found he had a mass in the right lower portion of his abdomen which I thought was probably a colon cancer. This was readily demonstrated by X-ray. Pleased with myself and the prospect of a nice colon resection, I called the urologist and told him the news. Startled, he said hastily that he would get back to me. The next call I got, however, was from Dr. Ravdin.

"It seems you did a careful physical on a very private patient and discovered an overlooked colon cancer," he said. "I know how awkward it is and how you will feel about it. However, if I don't do the operation, his doctor will transfer the patient to Temple University—he says he just cannot risk having an immediately ex-resident doing a colon resection on this particular patient. Let's do this. I'll scrub in, you do the operating, I'll assist you, and everything will work out." And it did.

The Professor was a genius at perceiving and protecting other physicians' sensibilities. For example, a large sponge had been left in a woman's abdomen at another hospital in Philadelphia. When the wound did not heal after numerous drainage operations, the patient's family physician told the surgeon that he was going to send Mrs. X to the University of Pennsylvania Hospital. At this the surgeon threatened to get the family physician kicked off their hospital staff. As chief resident, I explored the wound and found a large sponge just inside the abdomen. I notified Dr. Ravdin and he told me to call the outside surgeon. The surgeon did not believe me and sought confirmation. The Professor said, "Yes, Hardy has the sponge. Now, do you want to call her family physician, or do you want me to call him?"

"Rav, I've made an ass of myself. I want to call the doctor myself and apologize."

I learned a lot from "the Professor" that could not have been expressed in milliequivalents.

Meanwhile, I was working with Dr. Johnson on the thoracic service, where Charles Kirby was the assistant chief. Back in those days, thoracic residencies were not formalized as they were later, hence my opportunity to have the occasional private patient. Unfortunately, Charlie developed cavitary pulmonary tuberculosis, of the right upper lobe as I recall, and eventually had surgery. This left Dr. Johnson and me, to cover Philadelphia General Hospital as well.

I felt that I had won my spurs in thoracic surgery following my "worst case" in Philadelphia. The patient, a seventeen-year-old girl, had an abscess in the upper lobe of the right lung and a lobectomy was planned. J.J. insisted that we always operate lung abscesses with the patient positioned face down on a special operating table that supported the shoulders and the pelvis. No sooner had I opened the chest than the nurse anesthetist said we would have to take the patient off the operating table and put her back on the litter on her back so that the defective endotracheal tube could be replaced. Any thoracic surgeon will appreciate my predicament, but somehow we kept the wound sterile and the patient ventilated.

That accomplished, the anesthetist next announced that she had almost run out of oxygen and that the new tank had not arrived. It soon did arrive, but by now my nerves, in a very difficult and bloody operation at best, were becoming a bit frayed. I then told the anesthetist to start one of the six bottles of blood stored for transfusion. To my consternation no blood was available, despite preoperative assurance to the contrary, and there was none in the hospital. By now I was desperate. Halfway through a difficult operation, past the point of turning back, J.J. out of town, and no blood. What an appalling situation. Just then I spied a telephone on the wall. I said furiously to the circulating nurse, "You get Dr. Brooke Roberts over the fence at the University Hospital on that wall phone this instant!" Mercifully, he answered at once.

"Brooke," I said, as the nurse held the phone for me to protect my sterility, "I'm in a desperate situation over here at PGH. No time for details but bring me six bottles of O-negative blood from the University Hospital blood bank at once." I had immaculate confidence in him.

Within five minutes, or ten at the most, Brooke panted up the stairs with the blood. I finished the operation and the patient survived. The University Hospital blood bank authorities were extremely exercised by this transgression, but just imagine J.J.'s reaction if I had lost this patient in his absence!

Another year for decision

I was embarrassed, among my physician friends, to have taken Weezie to the hospital with false labor, before true labor set in. Our first of four daughters was born on July 29, 1950. Seeing Louise Scott Hardy actually born was deeply moving, and every father who so desires should have this enriching experience. Our firstborn, her mother, and her grandmother, all were named Louise Scott. The new arrival altered our life style far more than we had imagined it would. I had tended many babies, but not my own baby. I did not know what to say to her, but Weezie said, "Just say anything, so that she will learn to know your voice."

I now had to make a choice, at least between academic surgery and pure private practice. My research program was active, I was publishing papers regularly, and I had a research grant of my own from the army in Washington. I was confident I could go to a new place and do all my own research chemistry and other procedures if necessary. True, I would lose momentum in my research and probably not have such interdepartmental support as I had had at Penn. I felt comfortable doing general surgery and most routine chest surgery, but not heart surgery, though heart operations (closed mitral valve commissurotomy, resection of aortic coarctation, division of patent ductus) were just becoming common and I had helped with a good many. Open heart surgery was still in the future.

I did have the option of staying at Penn, perhaps, though the staff had now grown large and I would of course rank at the bottom. Dr. Ravdin had a deputy in William Fitts (later to be chairman), Dr. Rhoads had Cletus Schwegman on his ward service, and Dr. Johnson had Charles Kirby on his ward service. To move to a less crowded department of surgery, in a lesser school, would mean more freedom for self-expression and growth and a more satisfying service in surgery; but if I left, my friends would cluck, assume I'd fallen from grace, or question my sanity.

At first it looked as if something could work out; it was said that a surgical service might become available at Episcopal Hospital. The hospital was all the way across Philadelphia, but my labs at Penn would remain intact and active, and I knew I would have more prestige at Penn than at most southern schools. In 1839, a friend had written Dr. Oliver Wendell Holmes, who was considering an anatomy-surgery post at the University of Maryland, as follows: "New England is the place for you to acquire a reputation and Hanover [New Hampshire] in the chair of anatomy is the best place to begin. New England candour is worth a fortune to a young man. A small affair that would ruin a man at the south and west would not ruin the same man here."* Unfortunately, the Episcopal Hospital position fell through.

Curiously, for some reason I was reluctant to move west of the Mississippi River (my father-in-law was to chuckle when we ended up in Memphis, on the bank of the river). Perhaps I did not want Weezie and the children too far from the supportive matrix of our relatives in Alabama and Georgia. (*Sie alles gehen heim.* [They all go home].)

Dr. Ravdin was cool when I told him I wanted to look for a smaller school that had more available patients and really needed whatever I had to offer. Thus he was not very forthcoming with advice. He did, however, steer me to Dr. Michael E. DeBakey, who was organizing a new department of surgery in Houston, and Dr. Carl M. Moyer, who was doing the same thing in Dallas. Both suggested a

*G. E. Gifford, Jr., "Five Unpublished Letters to Oliver Wendell Holmes in 1839 Concerning the Offer of the Chair of Surgery at the University of Maryland School of Medicine," *Bull. Hist. Med.* 38 (1964): 260–270.

possible position, but each job presented its own special problems.

I then went to Jonathan Rhoads, who had come to be a man with whom I knew I could talk frankly and who would give me sound advice. I can still see him, with one foot up on a small steam radiator under the window in the surgeons' dressing room. The scrub suit pants were always short for his tall frame, and the pant leg hit him well above the ankle. I was going to Dallas to see about joining a private clinic there.

"Well, Jim, you should go on down and look the situation over. But let's say you make fifty thousand dollars the first ten years and put it in the bank. What are you going to do the next ten years, the same thing? I've watched you since you were a medical student. You're at home in the laboratory, a rarity in a surgical resident, and I don't think you will be satisfied just to operate on patients for the rest of your life. If you can have your heavy water work going, you'd be valuable to a good many departments of surgery around the country. But go on to Dallas and see."

Suffice it to say that, financially attractive as the tentative Dallas offer was, it was not for me. My decision to stay in academic surgery was made. There was to be just one other moment of doubt regarding the academic career, in Memphis three years later.

Meanwhile, I had begun to write my first book. Each year a course entitled "Advanced Physiology in Medical and Surgical Nursing" was offered through the nursing school of the University of Pennsylvania, and I had been asked to give the instruction in *surgical* physiology. There was ample reference material to cover most topics of interest to surgeons, but on endocrine or hormonal aspects the literature that was available was often inaccurate. For example, a standard anatomy textbook stated that "all four parathyroid glands together weigh scarcely more than a gram." I weighed parathyroid glands in the autopsy room and found that in fact each weighed only about thirty to forty milligrams. I recognized these inadequacies simply because my research now involved the adrenal, thyroid, and pituitary glands. This research had evolved because it was increasingly clear that hormones profoundly affected total body water, body salts, and most other metabolism. I wrote Dr. Ravdin a note proposing a small monograph to fill the obvious need. He endorsed it with his usual enthusiasm, "Go ahead!"

Not all projects went smoothly, however. For example, I needed the chemical analysis of cortisone-like steroids in patients' urine to validate and complete certain elements of the research I was doing. Dr. Ravdin and I drove over to Rahway, New Jersey, to make arrangements with a chemist at Merck Laboratories to store and analyze the samples. I laboriously collected and refrigerated complete twenty-four-hour urine collections from many patients over a period of months, and shipped well over one hundred liters of the stored urine to Merck. However, I became more and more concerned when I got no response to either letters or telephone calls.

One hot summer day, as I was helping the driver load the refrigerated urine onto the truck, I said, "You will of course store this urine again under refrigeration as soon as you reach Merck?"

"Doc, ain't no urine been stored since you started shipping it months ago. It's all sitting out there in a hot old warehouse. Never been touched."

The unrefrigerated urine was now worthless for steroid analysis. All that time, work, and expense was down the drain.

The Decision for Memphis

I knew almost nothing about the Medical College of the University of Tennessee before I made the swing through Texas to talk with Dr. Michael DeBakey and Dr. Carl Moyer, whose schools were in their formative stages. As I was planning the Texas trip, Dr. Rhoads suggested, "Why not stop off in Memphis on the way back from Texas. My friend Harwell Wilson was appointed chairman of surgery there about a year ago, and I think he could use a man like you."

He wrote to Dr. Wilson, and I arrived at the William Len Hotel one rainy Sunday afternoon on the way back to Philadelphia. Monday morning we met and talked, after he had finished his morning operating schedule at the Baptist Hospital. Earlier, I had strolled in adjacent Forest Park and heard a mockingbird singing for the first time in years—the faraway call of my origins?

Dr. Wilson showed me the series of empty laboratories assigned to the Department of Surgery in the new Pathology Building which was just being completed; they were connected through a short corridor to the John Gaston (charity) Hospital, where I saw surgical problems of such numbers, range, and severity as I had never seen in Philadelphia. No one was doing serious clinical metabolic studies on any of the surgical patients. There was a "dog lab" where some very limited animal research had been done.

I met the short and wiry dean and vice-chancellor, Dr. Orin Hyman, an anatomist who had run the Memphis units (medical school, dental school, pharmacy school) in his autocratic but effective way for many years. A possible salary of nine thousand dollars per year was mentioned. The position was attractive.

Back in Philadelphia, Dr. Rhoads told me: "The one requirement you must insist on is specific and regular rotations on the ward service. Without this you'll never be able to show yourself as a surgeon, and they will label you as only a dog surgeon. Remember, if they really want you, they'll make room on the ward service. And you should agree on some amount of private practice, even if quite limited. Finally, if you do move to Memphis, try to see Harwell every day, if possible."

Apparently, my wide range of prospective plans for research at U.T. was somewhat unnerving to Dr. Wilson, for he cautioned me by telephone, "Now, look, Hardy. Don't come down here and tell Dr. Hyman you're coming to save it for him."

I returned to Memphis. This time the ice had been broken by the previous visit and letters, and we got right down to business. After a decent amount of small talk, Dr. Hyman turned to me abruptly and asked, "Doctor, what do you plan to do with your life?"

"Work like the devil until I'm forty-five, and if I haven't got a chair of surgery by then, go into private practice."

"My, but you are an opinionated young man for your age. How old are you?"

"Thirty-two, sir."

There followed some talk about salary, limited practice, space, teaching assignments, and so forth. Then, preparing to leave, Dr. Hyman said, "Well, is there anything else to be covered?"

Here was the sticky point. I had told Harwell ahead of time that I would need six months ward service on general surgery each year and three months on thoracic surgery, and Harwell was over a barrel. The young surgeons who had been covering the general surgery did not want to give up time to some interloping stranger from Philadelphia, and the chief of thoracic surgery did not want a general surgeon (me) doing thoracic surgery in Memphis (which he had managed to keep as a private preserve for "pure" thoracic surgeons).

Dr. Hyman turned to Dr. Wilson and said, "Harwell, I think Hardy would be useful to us. Why don't you talk with your staff again tonight and see what can be worked out about the ward service. Hardy doesn't leave until tomorrow and perhaps we can give him something definite by then."

Harwell gained reluctant approval from his staff, but I was never actually to get the ward service in thoracic surgery (although I managed to achieve this later in another way).

I will never forget my arrival back in Philadelphia. It was already dark at the old Philadelphia airport. As the propeller plane taxied toward the restraining wire fence with its lights on, I saw a smiling Weezie against the wire holding a baby girl, Louise, in a little red coat and cap over ringlets of blonde curls. I told Weezie we were going to Memphis the next August.

I had already passed the written and oral examinations of the American Board of Surgery. The written exam, back then, consisted of ten discussion questions instead of the extensive "none-of-the-above" test now, and four of the questions had been on a list of topics likely to be asked that Arch Fletcher and I had studied specifically.

I had little concern at the oral examination some months later, in which I had three pairs of examiners. One examiner, however, was especially severe. Finally he eased up a bit and asked, "Now, Doctor, what would you like me to ask you?"

"Why not just throw one across the plate?" I replied.

I had found a replacement for Merck and had had a sufficient number of analyses of urinary steroids run to correlate with and validate a number of other related metabolic studies I had been doing, resulting in a number of publications in major journals. In fact, I later presented an overall survey of these metabolic studies as the opening paper at the 1952 annual meeting of the American Surgical Association at the Greenbrier Hotel at White Sulfur Springs, West Virginia.

Two studies in particular gave me much satisfaction. Way back when I was on Dr. Ravdin's service, we had had a wealthy patient, I think from New York, who had promised the chief "a boat" if he did well after removal of his colon cancer. After the operation, the long tube that had been passed far down into his intestine to keep it decompressed and thus protect the colon anastomosis failed to drain more than a minimal amount of fluid. Dr. Ravdin was upset.

"Doctor," he said to me sternly, "that tube had better drain. Did you inject fluid through it before passing it down?" I did. "And did you suck back?" I did. "Well, I'm going home now, but you call me at ten o'clock—and that tube had better drain." It did drain, the next day.

I had observed other patients whose tubes had not drained but who had done well. I surveyed the charts of fifty such patients and showed a consistent reduction of tube suction drainage, as well as urine output, during the first postoperative day. The Professor was surprised but delighted when I left the manuscript on his desk. I was also able to correlate these findings with an increase in adrenocortical activity. One report was published in the *Annals of Surgery* and the other in *Surgery*, both very promptly. Such is the stimulus for many research projects—"clinical inspiration."

A disappointing affair was the competition for the Markle Award, a substantial five-year grant support to a promising young physician in academic medicine. I had first learned of this grant when I was casting about for some type of research support for work I planned to do in Memphis. Candidates from all over the East met with the selection committee and the committee members' wives in Williamsburg for several days—morning, noon, and night. We dined with various selectors at different meals, and also had one-on-one interviews. I left feeling that, compared with most of the perhaps twenty-five other candidates, I had made a good showing. But I was unsuccessful. A common question put to me was, "Why are you leaving the University of Pennsylvania?" Also, I later found that Tennessee had never sent in all the material stating how well I would be supported at that school, always an important consideration. Tennessee hardly knew me, and they were not helpful.

At all possible moments and late at night I had been working on my proposed monograph. I had said nothing to Dr. Ravdin after getting his initial go-ahead back in the fall, but one day in May I placed on his desk the complete manuscript of *Surgery and the Endocrine System*.

He called me to his office the next morning and said, "Jim, this is remarkable. I had no idea. I want you to take this down to the president of the W. B. Saunders Company. I've already called him. I think they just might be interested in publishing it." They were. It apparently proved, in later years, to have been the first book ever written on surgery of the endocrine system.

In the early months of 1951, Dr. Drabkin told me one day that the Committee on Graduate Studies was much impressed with my research with heavy water and other modalities in studying body composition. If I would write a thesis on the work, submit it for approval, and pay a fee, he believed I could be awarded the degree of master of medical science in physiological chemistry. I received the degree at the Penn commencement, 1951.

I had brief concern that I might be called back to the army, as the Korean War was just getting under way. However, I had not remained in the reserves, and thus an act of Congress would have been required to recall me.

The last day in Philadelphia

How well I remember the last day in Philadelphia, home for thirteen years. It was a somber time. Reluctance at leaving, yes. Doubts about the future, yes. Aware of falling from grace in the eyes of friends and acquaintances, yes.

I went up to pay my respects to Dr. Ravdin last. It was after five o'clock and the secretaries had gone. The door to his office was partly ajar, and I saw that a barber was cutting his hair. Not venturing to go in and intrude, I simply said through the doorway, "Goodbye, Professor."

He cut his eyes to the right toward me, as the barber snipped here and there, and said, "You'd better stay."

"No, sir, but thanks."

The car was packed and I was out of the apartment. Weezie and Louise had gone ahead. There remained only to take the final, corrected book manuscript to Saunders before the doors there were locked for the night. I drove down across the Schuylkill River (here my Rubicon) and got inside the publisher's building. Once there, I continued correcting the manuscript. When the final occupant left, she put on the night lock and told me to pull the door closed firmly behind me when I left.

I had finished the manuscript. I tilted back in the swivel chair for a moment, looked out at the lights and skyline of Philadelphia, thought of all I had learned and experienced there over the past thirteen years—my whole adult life thus far—and asked myself: Why am I really leaving?

The answer, I knew, was that I did not really fit the mold. I did not think my personality would be spiritually successful in the system, which was too regimented, too pyramidal. I needed more room to grow as an operating surgeon over the next ten years. It was important to me that these years be employed to the fullest. I walked out, closed the front door, got into the black Oldsmobile, and drove south through the rain toward an uncertain destiny.

CHAPTER 11

The 1950s: Cardiovascular Surgery Comes of Age

The 1940s had represented a decade of preparation for the huge strides that cardiovascular surgery made in the 1950s. André F. Cournand, Dickinson W. Richards, and Werner Forssmann received the Nobel Prize for their introduction and use of heart catheterization for many physiologic studies. It was used later, by others, for the diagnosis of heart defects. Incidentally, Forssmann, a German surgeon, had first performed catheterization on himself (after his animal work), to the consternation of those around him. This had followed similar studies in animals by the great French physiologist Claude Bernard in the 1860s. A parallel achievement of similar magnitude was the visualization of blood vessels and the chambers of the heart by injecting intravenously a radiopaque medium containing iodine (angiocardiography).

In 1938, Robert E. Gross of Harvard had successfully closed a congenital shunt from the aorta to the pulmonary artery (the patent ductus arteriosus), and both Gross and Clarence Craaford of Stockholm had operated successfully to remove the congenital blockage—coarctation—of the aorta, which otherwise caused high blood pressure with its serious early or late complications. Alfred Blalock at Johns Hopkins, at the suggestion of Helen Taussig, had pioneered the "blue baby" operation for the tetralogy of Fallot, in which a branch of the aorta, in the systemic circulation, was anastomosed to the pulmonary artery to shunt more blood through the lungs for better oxygenation. Following earlier attempts, Charles P. Bailey of Philadelphia and Dwight E. Harken of Boston had pioneered opening the obstructed mitral valve by introducing a finger into the left atrium through a pursestring suture and actually fracturing the valve leaflets blindly.

Most of the thoracic surgeons operating at that time had come up the hard way, often as tuberculosis or "thoracoplasty" surgeons. Actually, little thoracic surgery had been done, and what there was had consisted of either introducing air into the chest on the side of the diseased lung (pneumothorax) to collapse and thus rest the organ, or of removing ribs (thoracoplasty) to collapse the lung permanently. At other times, the phrenic nerve on the involved side was crushed to allow the diaphragm to rise. It was not until after 1945 that single or multiple lobes of the lung were individually resected routinely. It was not safe to do this for tuberculosis until streptomycin became available in 1948, lest the infection spread to more lung or be made worse. However, this large group of early thoracic surgeons was poised to undertake further operations in the chest, specifically on the heart, when it became possible. Many of them soon took up heart operations which did not require the as-yet-undeveloped heart-lung machine ("the pump"), but relatively few made the long jump from tuberculosis surgery and closed-heart operations, on the one hand, to full-scale open-heart surgery when the field was rapidly developed after 1954.

Open-heart surgery demanded a new breed, surgeons thoroughly familiar with cardiac and pulmonary physiology and management, with a high degree of technical expertise in addition. After John H. Gibbon had developed the heart-lung machine and used it in the first human case in 1952, C. Walton Lillehei, Richard A. Dewall and

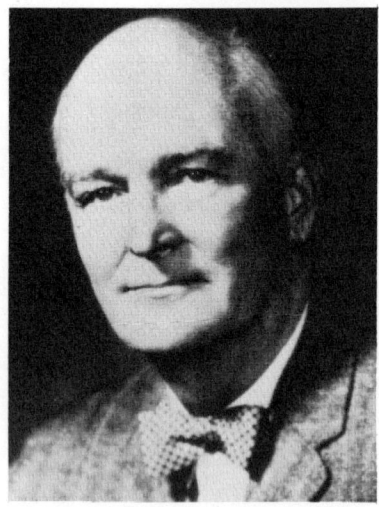

John H. Gibbon, Jr., chairman of the Department of Surgery, Jefferson Medical College, and inventor of the heart pump-oxygenator

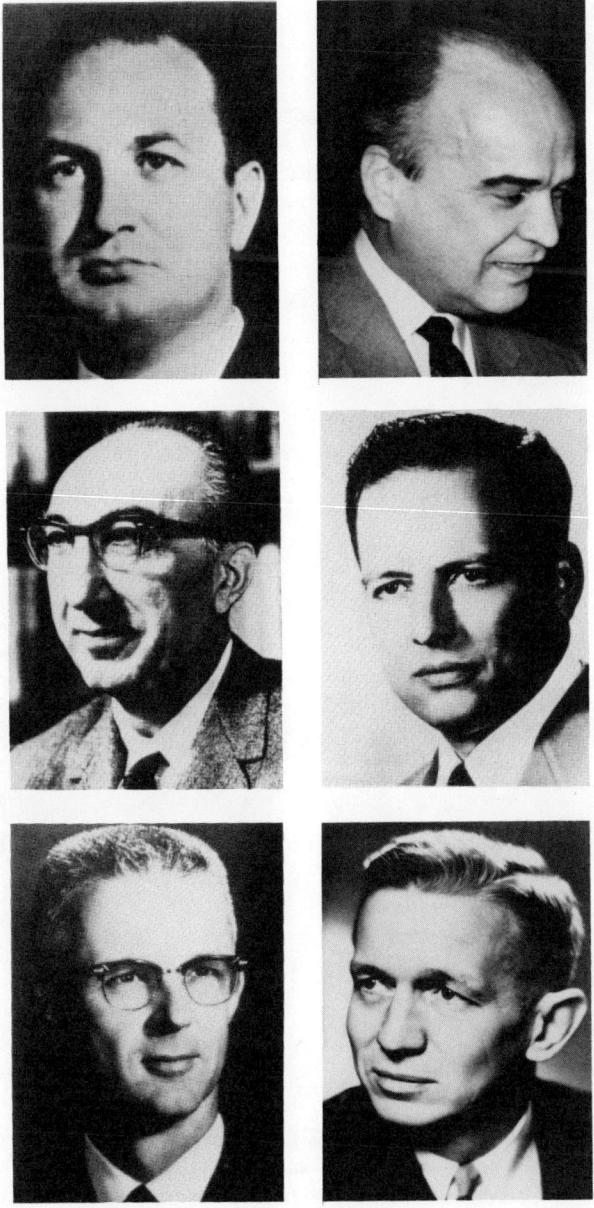

Some American leaders in development of cardiac surgery:
Robert E. Gross (top left); *C. Walton Lillehei* (top right);
Michael E. DeBakey (middle left); *Denton A. Cooley* (middle right);
John W. Kirklin (bottom left); *Henry T. Bahnson* (bottom right).
Alfred Blalock is pictured earlier.

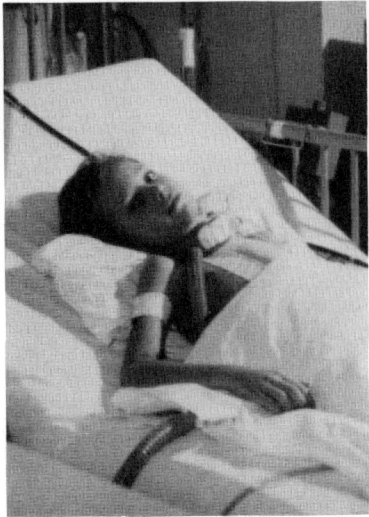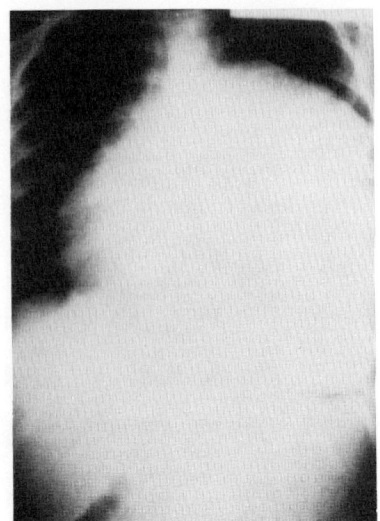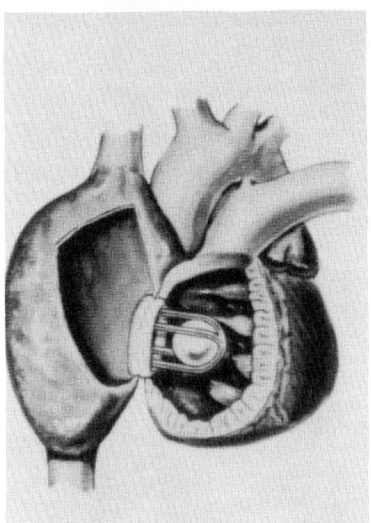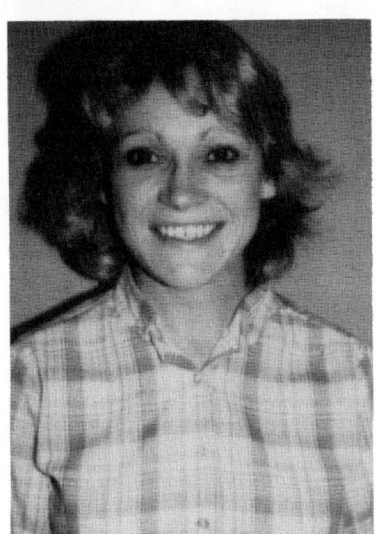

A triumph of open-heart surgery. C.J.K., age 10, in preterminal cardiac failure (top left); *massive cardiac enlargement due to Ebstein's anomaly* (top right); *replacement of defective tricuspid valve with Starr-Edwards ball valve* (bottom left); *C.J., age 29, working daily, original artificial heart valve in place* (bottom right). *From Timmis, H. H.; Hardy, J. D.; and Watson, D. G., "The Surgical Management of Ebstein's Anomaly,"* Journal of Thoracic and Cardiovascular Surgery 53 (1967): 305.

others at the University of Minnesota truly moved the field ahead by introduction of the vastly simplified "bubble oxygenator." Many thought Gibbon should have won the Nobel Prize, and years later, before Gibbon's death, many of us were asked to write letters of support to the committee, but to no avail. A person close to the Nobel committee told me privately that Dr. Gibbon was considered seriously, but in the end, it was concluded that, important as his contribution was, he had used *known* information; to receive the prize the information had to be new. Meanwhile, John W. Kirklin, then at the Mayo Clinic and later at the University of Alabama, enhanced sophistication and elegance in open-heart surgery. Michael E. DeBakey and Denton A. Cooley, in Houston, made advances in the course of establishing the largest volume cardiovascular center in the United States and probably in the world. Albert Starr was the first to develop a dependable and widely used artificial (ball) heart valve.

Of much importance to the field was the development of a wide variety of new surgical instruments and suture materials, for in few other surgical disciplines is it so important to have available the special instrument for the special situation. There was also great progress in anesthesiology, blood banking, intensive care units, and the management of lung function.

Last but by no means least, arterial surgery. There came in the 1950s a veritable explosion in the knowledge and the practical clinical application of surgery on the arteries. Even as late as 1950, injury to a major artery was usually treated by simple ligation of the vessel above and below the point of injury. If the part became gangrenous—the leg, for instance—it was removed. To be sure, Alexis Carrel had clearly demonstrated at the turn of the century that either an artery or a vein, from the same or even another animal, could be substituted for a damaged artery with routine success. This followed his perfection of the technique of arterial anastomosis, and for such work he was awarded the Nobel Prize in 1912. However, this work was ignored clinically until in 1948 Robert Gross successfully used segments of aorta taken from cadavers to bridge otherwise unresectable lengths of coarcted aorta. Then, in the Korean conflict, a number of young American surgeons, after practicing on animals, performed immediate repair of injured arteries with remarkable success, thus markedly reducing the incidence of leg amputation.

In 1951 Charles Dubost, in Paris, successfully replaced a large aneurysm of the aorta in the abdomen with a homograft from a cadaver, providing for the first time an effective treatment for these otherwise fatal lesions. Henry Bahnson at Johns Hopkins was a leader in early resection of aneurysms of the aortic arch. But so common were aneurysms, so great the need for grafts, that the supply from cadavers soon proved inadequate. A massive search for synthetic arterial substitutes gradually produced acceptable materials, Dacron being a very good one.

Thus, the time came when it was routine to replace or bypass defective arteries. It became inappropriate to amputate a leg for atherosclerosis without first obtaining an arteriogram to assess possible remedial surgery. Vessels only one to two millimeters in size, such as the coronary arteries or arteries of the brain, came within reach of microsurgery using extremely fine needles and improved, fine suture materials, often with the use of operating lens magnification or the operating microscope. Such progress in vascular surgery would pave the way for organ transplantation.

PART III

Memphis
1951–1955

CHAPTER 12

The Medical College of the University of Tennessee: Surgery Staff Member and Director of Surgical Research

By driving most of the night, I arrived at Bristol, Tennessee, the next morning and assumed that Memphis was almost at hand. But Tennessee is almost five hundred miles from east to west. I arrived at the Peabody Hotel in Memphis late in the afternoon. There, waiting in her room, was a round-faced, brown-eyed, brown-haired, lovely, and very pregnant person in a pink slip. Elysian fields.

Recollections of our first house, way out on the edge of Memphis, are of roads not yet paved and very dusty, neighbors of all pursuits and stations in life, floor furnaces which left burn prints on Louise's little hands when she fell on them, and elephant-eye–high Johnson grass (Jimsonweed). Harwell Wilson, bless his heart, came out to see us in his new Cadillac, bringing a roast duck; but his car slipped into the ditch, and by the time we got it out, the high spirits of his visit had somehow been dissipated.

The surgery laboratories had been finished, but they were completely bare of instrumentation. I went to Harwell to ask if the Department of Surgery could buy the basic laboratory equipment from its budget. He replied that there really wasn't much of a formal budget but that he would ask Vice-Chancellor Hyman. He did. Nothing happened.

Meanwhile, I was flooding the mails with research grant requests to every possible granting agency—army, navy, National Institutes of Health, American Cancer Society, National Science Foundation, and still others. All too often they replied that "the research proposal is interesting, but it does not appear that the University of

Tennessee would supply even the basic laboratory equipment one might reasonably expect a university to provide."

Finally, I asked Dr. Wilson if I might go see Vice-Chancellor Hyman myself. I asked for a few hundred dollars, just to get glassware and a few chemicals and so forth.

Dr. Hyman listened to me briefly. He then held up his hand and said sternly: "Hardy, we pay your salary. It is *your* job to get the money for research." I learned later that he'd had many disappointments with research support. (And, incidentally, later on he insisted that he would pay a research fellow who wanted to work a year without pay: "Hardy, you don't get something for nothing.")

I went back to my office-laboratory, empty except for a desk and a chair. Things looked pretty bleak, and I began to wonder just what I had got myself into. But just then an idea flashed into my mind: The Damon Runyon Fund! John Teeter's *venture capital*. "Seed money."

Within several weeks my grant application for more than four thousand dollars of equipment was approved. I have always considered this small grant of Damon Runyon venture capital the most strategically important research grant I ever got. I then bought the basic equipment, listed it in the previously unsuccessful grant requests, and mailed them off again. Within months I had received grants from the NIH, the American Cancer Society, and the Research and Development Section of the army Surgeon General's

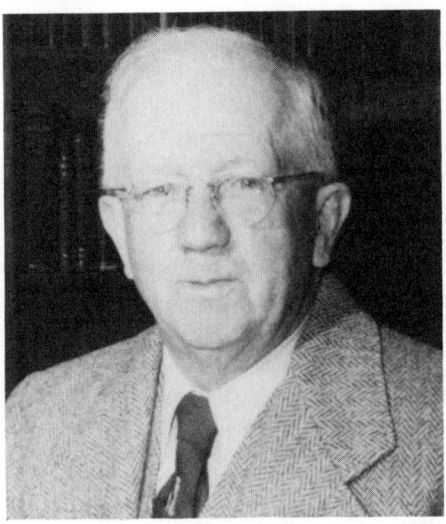

Orin W. Hyman

Office. Once a pauper, I was now overwhelmed with more money than I could use efficiently. I told Dr. Wilson that I was going to decline the money from one of the granting agencies, that even though I now had several technicians and two research fellows, I could not cover the third grant effectively. Dr. Wilson was concerned, because the university received considerable money for overhead from research grants. He said I had better go talk to Dr. Hyman before I did anything so rash as to send back money.

Dr. Hyman didn't like it. He even proposed that we pay my own salary from the grants. I told him, as diplomatically as I could, that if the university itself were paying me absolutely nothing, I could hardly feel appreciated. Besides, I wanted to use research money wisely and effectively, and thus build a reputation for dependability and productivity with the national research-granting agencies.

I sent back the money.

I also learned something about grantsmanship in connection with the successful American Cancer Society request. Dr. Douglas Sprunt, chairman of pathology at Tennessee and a member of the ACS research award committee, came down to my laboratory one morning and asked, "Hardy, how do you know Owen Wangensteen?"

"I wouldn't say I really know him. He once came to my laboratory at Penn, where I was running heavy water measurements." (He was with Dr. Ravdin, who was moderately obese, and he asked me what percent water the Professor was, since I had told him fat contained little water.)

"Well, you sure made a convert out of him. Frankly, your grant request was poorly written and was about to be turned down there in New York yesterday. But Owen stood up, said he knew you personally, and that in time you would learn better the technique of writing grant requests, but that you must certainly be supported. And you got the grant!"

Julia Ann Hardy was born October 30, 1951, a brunette duplicate of her mother, whereas Louise had been a blue-eyed blonde like her father. The obstetrician and I were standing in the hall chatting, and the night nurse would not believe Weezie when she insisted that the baby was *coming now*. Weezie never forgave the obstetrician and would not have him again, despite the fact that he and I were good friends.

With a growing family, we bought a spacious, old, two-story house not far from the university and close to the zoo. In fact, Weezie's visiting sister swore she'd heard a *lion* roar during the night. It was in this house that we had another burglar. One night I heard heavy footsteps ascending the squeaking stairs in the dark. I quietly awoke Weezie, but just then Louise's little piping voice from across the hall called, "Daddy, is that you?" The steps then descended and went out the front door. After that I kept the pistol I had bought in Philadelphia at hand. When we again heard the same noise one night, I got my gun and was poised. Just then a little voice on the stairs called, "Daddy?" It was Louise!

Meanwhile, I was busy supervising resident surgery in the John Gaston Hospital, where the patients often had more extensive disease, larger tumors, and worse traumatic injuries than anything I had attended in Philadelphia. The volume of surgery at the hospital was impressive, especially trauma cases. About six younger surgeons covered the night service in rotation, supervising the surgery residents. On the rotation soon after my arrival I received a call about 6 P.M. I asked Weezie to hold supper, promising to be back in about an hour, but I walked in the next morning at 6:00, having operated on one emergency after another all night long.

I also covered a "colored" men's ward (about eighty percent of the patients in "the Gaston" were black.) A strapping day laborer of about thirty was brought in with a severe lower leg wound, shot by the police. He said that the police claimed he had "stole a turkey," but that those who had stolen the turkey had got away. The patient, who had "done nothing," did not run and so had been shot. Orthopaedics was consulted and recommended immediate amputation, in order to get the patient fitted with a prosthesis promptly. I objected vigorously, remembering the case of Jimmie Lee Johnson from my childhood, plus others, and I proposed that the case be presented the next night at the quarterly staff dinner meeting: orthopaedics could debate in favor of immediate amputation, and I would debate to accept long hospitalization and try to salvage a useful foot. But heavens! Little did I know Memphis medical politics. I got an urgent telephone call from Dr. Wilson: "Hardy, what are you trying to do to the Campbell Clinic (which covered the Gaston in orthopaedics)?" I explained. "You're new here," he said. "If you won't amputate, then transfer the patient to orthopaedics." He was transferred.

The problem of the lack of opportunities for thoracic surgery continued to rankle, for despite my written memorandum of understanding before I left Philadelphia, Dr. Wilson had never been able to persuade Dr. Duane Carr, chief, to put me on the thoracic ward rotation. I realized the political delicacies involved. First, Dr. Wilson was not all that much in control of the Department of Surgery.

Second, he and Dr. Carr were friends of long standing, and Dr. Carr referred Dr. Wilson numerous private patients, which Dr. Wilson needed since he was paid only a nominal salary by the university. Third, Dr. Carr was a strong medical political force both in Memphis and in national circles. Furthermore, he was an able thoracic surgeon.

When I had brought the employment agreement up one last time, Harwell said, "Jim, it's embarrassing and I'm sorry. I know we promised, but I simply have not been able to get Dr. Carr to give you the rotation. This is the one promise to you that I just can't keep." I knew this was true, and that Harwell really had tried.

"Dr. Wilson," I said, "I have a solution if you and Dr. Hyman will agree. They need help at the [immediately adjacent] West Tennessee Tuberculosis Hospital. They would give me a contract to perform one or two lung operations each Wednesday."

Dr. Wilson was relieved, Dr. Hyman agreed, and I began a useful and productive association. Moreover, Dr. Francis Cole, assistant chief surgeon there, and I got heart mitral-valve surgery started in Memphis. Our first mitral valve (closed, of course—the heart pump was yet to be developed) caused us much consternation. The operation itself had gone smoothly enough. We had passed the gloved index finger through a pursestring suture in the wall of the left atrium. Then, after the inside finger had explored the deformity of the valve, its lumen was forced open more widely by "fracturing" the now fused commissures at each end. The result was considered excellent. The next morning, however, the patient, though clearly

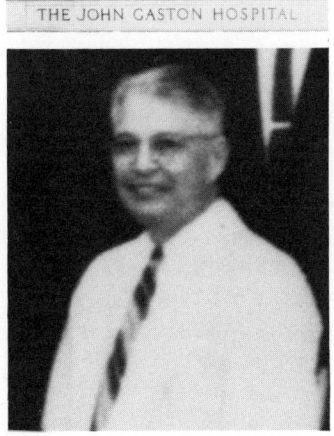

Harwell Wilson

not comatose and staring wide-eyed at the ceiling, apparently could not move a single muscle. What a start in Memphis! Fortunately, the cardiologist realized that she was in conversion hysteria. He soon brought her out of it and she made an excellent recovery. We found that before coming to the hospital she had made a will, giving everything away and donating her body to science postoperatively. We also did aortic operations, but these had previously been done occasionally by others. I passed my thoracic board examination in 1952, the day before the election that made Eisenhower president.

It was at the West Tennessee Hospital that I had one of my most poignant cases. The patient was secretary to Dr. Frank Alley, surgeon-in-chief with vast experience in tuberculosis surgery.

"She has not been really well for months," the chief told me. "She's been seen by all sorts of doctors. You're the only one of us here who's not only a thoracic surgeon but also a general surgeon. Would you be willing to give E. a good going over?"

I took E. into an examining room and began to take the history. I noted she had sort of a husky voice, and asked her if she had a cold or sore throat. No. She did mention that her menstrual periods had become irregular. Not much else.

Next I called in the nurse and examined the patient from head to toe. I noted nothing special except that her pubic hair was a bit more male than usual, extending upward toward the umbilicus rather than in the usual female transverse pubic hair line. There seemed to be a fullness in the right upper quadrant of the abdomen, but I decided that her liver was just a bit prominent, since she was thin. She said she had a gynecologist and that he had recently examined her, so I omitted the pelvic examination—I knew her as a daily friend and I knew she would be embarrassed.

I went to write up the history and physical, but as I was walking up the hall I said to myself, "You didn't do a complete physical examination, the first requirement of a good doctor." I whirled around, hastened back, got the nurse, and asked E. to undress again, saying that I wanted to do pelvic and rectal examinations.

No sooner had I sat down to do the pelvic examination than I noted a substantially enlarged clitoris. I touched it gently with the gloved finger and said, "How long has your clitoris been enlarged?"

"Oh, I've been so embarrassed. It's been enlarging for months."

"Now, when we first began the examination, I asked about your husky voice. Has your voice changed?"

"I've been thinking about that since you asked. Now I remember that I had to drop out of the church choir because my voice range had decreased so markedly. I used to sing soprano."

"E.," I said, "I think you may have a masculinizing tumor of the adrenal gland, probably on the right. We can be certain by analyzing the steroids in a twenty-four-hour urine collection."

We soon established the expected diagnosis. The masculinizing steroids, androgens, in her urine were in enormous concentrations—forty times normal for a female—indicating a masculinizing adrenal cortical malignancy. I removed a large malignant tumor of the right adrenal gland beneath the liver.

The urinary steroid levels fell at once to normal, but I warned her that we would need urine specimens at six-month intervals for years. When she returned in September, the steroids were up again, indicating fatal tumor metastases.

Dr. Alley, her caring boss, had bet her fifty cents that she was cured. Now he could not bring himself to tell her. He entered her room, looked at her silently for a moment, placed a fifty-cent piece on her bedside table, and rushed out. It was left to me to tell her that she had recurrent cancer, but I realized she had known already.

"E.," I asked her, "just when did you know that the tumor was malignant?"

"Well, I'd suspected it from everybody's long faces, the nurses' whispered conversations, and what *you* did *not* say after my operation. But when Tom said, 'Honey, I don't think we ought to go to Colorado when I finish with dental school this year; let's just practice here in Tennessee,' then I knew."

Looking back, the year 1951–52 was particularly important. I began to get research grants and to continue to publish research work that had been done in Philadelphia. In the early spring, the slender volume *Surgery and the Endocrine System* appeared on the bookstands. Dr. Douglas Sprunt had urged me to become a surgical consultant to the Oak Ridge Institute of Nuclear Studies. My occasional visits to Oak Ridge gave me a considerable insight into the rapidly expanding use of isotopes for many research, diagnostic, and therapeutic purposes. (I remembered the course in "Atomic Structure" from college days.)

My laboratory was now the scene of increasingly vigorous activity. When I looked at what types of patients were in greatest abundance and might lend themselves to clinical research, it was apparent that the hospital received many burn patients. I reviewed the charts of five hundred consecutive burn patients to learn why some had died. I had expected to find that a good many had died in shock due to inadequate fluid treatment or kidney failure, but this was rarely the case. Actually, some years earlier, Blalock, then at Vanderbilt but later at Johns Hopkins, had shown that burn shock in animals was due largely to inadequate fluid treatment. He did this by the simple expedient of lowering one-half of the anesthetized animal's body into hot water for a period of time, and then later at sacrifice comparing the weight of the burned side with that of the unburned side. He found that the burned side weighed considerably more than the unburned side, showing that a massive fluid shift (and thus fluid loss from the circulation) had occurred into the tissues of the burned side. This had been widely accepted and now human patients rarely died of inadequate fluid replacement following a major burn. Nowadays, with adequate fluid therapy, even the very severely burned patient usually survived for the first week or so, only to develop the curious "toxemia of burns" and gradually die from this, or to linger still longer and finally die of general weakness and malnutrition.

We developed a research project, "The Cause of Death in Thermal Burns," and submitted a proposal to the Research and Development Section of the Surgeon General's Office, Department of the Army. After considerable revision and refinement of the proposal, this research was supported substantially by the army. By studying burned patients, we and others showed changes occurring in these patients that could be treated more effectively. Specifically, the major cause of death eventually proved to be infection due to bloodstream invasion by bacteria.

Meanwhile, I was helping the residents with a lot of major operations in the John Gaston Hospital, choosing an adult general surgery ward service for three months and then the children's service for three months, with continuous weekly thoracic surgery at the West Tennessee Tuberculosis Hospital.

I missed the openness of peer discussion and constructive criticism to which I had been accustomed at Pennsylvania. There was no death and complications conference in Memphis that compared with the rigorous analysis at Penn. Since virtually every surgeon was in private practice, open criticism of peers who might refer a private patient was necessarily muted. My outspokenness was perhaps excessive at times. For example, when Dr. Wilson came each

Wednesday for rounds with the staff, he did encourage discussion, but the discussion often did not reach a candid conclusion. In one patient, the surgeon had done an operation on the gallbladder and common bile duct that obviously would necessitate a second operation later, although the entire operation could have been done at one sitting. Surprised, I made bold to ask why the surgical team had stopped short of removing the large gallstone from the lower portion of the common bile duct, when it was known at the time of the operation that it was present. The answers were not very satisfactory, but it was clear to me that I had said all I had better say on that occasion. On thinking the matter over later, I decided that I would offer an editorial on this subject to *Surgery, Gynecology and Obstetrics*. I did this with the title of "Duodenotomy for Common Duct Stone." I pointed out that, in fact, opening the duodenum to remove the stone from the lower duct had been recommended by Dr. Charles McBurney, of appendectomy fame, as early as 1898. He had been a pioneer in surgery for appendicitis. The editor accepted the piece and it caused a number of chuckles among my acquaintances.

On another occasion, I was asked to present the program for the monthly staff meeting at the beautiful, new Le Bonheur Children's Hospital; the program was always held late in the afternoon after the physicians had been working since seven that morning. Attendance by staff physicians was required, which occasioned something less than ecstasy. The elderly patriarch of Memphis pediatrics was always the chairman, and after a frequently extremely dull presentation, he would invariably congratulate the essayist on one of the most outstanding presentations that it had been his privilege to hear in years.

I insisted on a free hand. I arose at the beginning of the hour and said loudly, "I am presenting these two cases of intestinal obstruction in children because, in my opinion, they were grossly mishandled."

There was a noticeable ripple through the audience and everyone sat up and began to pay attention immediately. I went on to say that the gross mismanagement was not entirely the fault of Dr. David Dunavant, since he had not been on the service the entire time these two patients were in the hospital. This really galvanized the attention of the audience, as I had actually named names. I included the name of a radiologist and implied that he had made an inadequate X-ray diagnosis.

In the middle of the session Dr. R. L. Sanders, the best-known surgeon in Memphis with a huge private practice, stood up and stalked out of the lecture hall. I went on, and there were many questions and spirited defenses at the end. For example, Dr. Dunavant pointed out to the audience that he had certainly not been on the service the entire time, that he in fact had not been on the service for some years. (I noted dryly that this was what I had said.) Moreover, the radiologist got in a telling blow, to the delight and vigorous applause of the audience.

The next day, over in the Baptist Hospital, Dr. Sanders encountered Dr. Dunavant in the hall. "Dunavant," Dr. Sanders said, "that performance by that fellow Hardy yesterday was the most disgraceful attack I've met in forty years of practice. If you want to sue him for slander, I'll back you."

At this Dunavant laughed and said, "You must have left early. At the end, Dr. Hardy turned over the final sheet on the big easel, which stated that 'all participants were warned in advance.'"

The upshot of this was that Dr. Sanders called my boss and told him that he thought I ought to be put up for membership in the Southern Surgical Association and that he would like to be one of my supporters.

Late in 1951 Dr. James H. Hendrix, a young plastic surgeon also interested in the management of burns, told me that he was planning to move to Jackson, Mississippi, where a new medical school was being formed. He would be the only plastic surgeon in Jackson and probably in the whole state of Mississippi. He thought it was an outstanding opportunity to get in on the ground floor. He did make this move, and in 1952 he was already getting enough surgery to pay his expenses.

In the spring of 1952 I was elected to membership in the Society of University Surgeons, and with this and progress in other areas, I no longer had serious doubts about being successful in academic surgery.

There were, of course, discouraging moments. As Jonathan Rhoads had predicted, I was virtually quarantined as a full-time university employee, somehow slightly tainted with socialism, compared with all the others who were in private practice. I was, in fact, the only full-time person that the Department of Surgery had ever had, though I was allowed a minimal private practice. This situation was not going to be satisfactory forever.

On the other hand, I really was not interested in doing a lot of time-consuming private practice there, for private patients require a lot of private attention, such as frequent discussions with relatives beyond the real clinical need. Once when things were at a rather low ebb, after I had completed my boards in thoracic surgery, two prominent internists came into my office one afternoon and made a proposition.

"Hardy," they said, "we have been following your chest work. If you will come over to the Baptist Hospital and rent an office, severing connections with the university, we will send you our chest surgery for as long as you need it to be successful. We are tired of one group's having a complete monopoly on thoracic surgery. We would like for them to have some competition. We should add that we represent several other internists."

I said I would like to think about it, of course, and discuss it with my wife. It was an attractive offer. However, it had several drawbacks. First, it would require that I become a pure thoracic surgeon. This was not in line with my long-term goal of being chairman of a department of surgery. Furthermore, my research involved not only the chest but most other organs of the body.

Second, it would almost certainly end all academic aspirations. It is easy to leave a university for private practice, but it is difficult to return from private practice to a university career and be truly successful.

Third, I had been treated fairly by the university, despite the minor vexations that will always pursue any endeavor, and I felt I would be disloyal to Dr. Wilson and the university to move out in quite this way. In addition, I had finally established a genial relationship with Dr. Duane Carr, head of thoracic surgery in the Baptist Hospital and the university, the "competition." It would not be a particularly happy professional relationship, to say the least.

As so often has been the case, in her own quiet way, Weezie was an important influence. "We have put in too much effort to abandon our objective now, Jim," she said. "You would never be satisfied outside of academic surgery. It's very nice of the doctors to make the offer, but let's stick with our academic objectives."

She was really bearing the brunt, with two small children and another on the way, as I put in extremely long hours at the laboratory and hospital. Her endorsement and support was enough. That ended the last temptation I ever had to enter pure private practice.

My surgical laboratories were in the same building as pathology and bacteriology, enabling me to create an intimate association with these scientists. I maintained much the same relationship with the physiologists and chemists, going to their conferences and seminars almost weekly. Basic scientists from the University of Mississippi's two-year medical school at Oxford would come for the physiology seminars at U.T. in Memphis. It was probably through this relationship that I was invited, in the late spring of 1952, to address the medical school faculty at Oxford. My subject was a general blend of experimental and clinical research having to do with the normal and abnormal physiology of the adrenal cortex, and with patients with Cushing's disease and related endocrine disorders.

Dr. David S. Pankratz, who was dean of the two-year medical school there, would drop by from time to time, since he and Harwell Wilson had both been at the University of Chicago and were long-time friends. Dean Pankratz was spearheading the development of the four-year medical school and hospital in Jackson, depending heavily on advice from officials at the University of Chicago. About this time Harwell Wilson had inquired whether I might be interested in being chief of surgery down at Jackson when the four-year medical school should be established.

Dean Pankratz invited me down to Oxford one afternoon to discuss possible clinical considerations for the new medical school, more as a consultant than anything else. After four hours of desultory conversation, largely about his experiences at the University of Chicago, he concluded the long afternoon by saying, "Well, Jim, we haven't discussed anything."

"That's certainly true, Dean Pankratz," I said, whereupon I departed for Memphis. I decided that he was an unusual person, to say the least.

On March 23, 1953, a tall gentleman entered my office and introduced himself as Coggeshall. "Tell me, Dr. Hardy, what are you doing and what are your future objectives?"

I described the various kinds of research I was doing, now with multiple grants and multiple technicians. He listened to all this and then said, "But what is your ultimate goal?"

Once again, as I had told Dr. Hyman originally, I said, "Dr. Coggeshall, I am going to work as hard as I can until I am forty-five years old. If I don't have a chair of surgery by then I am going into private practice, at least to a major extent."

"Dr. Hardy," he said, "there are many young surgeons in your position throughout the country, but only a few can ever become chairman of a department of surgery. Perhaps you should modify your ambitions somewhat."

I had not realized until we were well into our conversation that he was, in fact, the famous Lowell T. Coggeshall, head of the medical school at the University of Chicago, who was there to give the commencement address for the medical class that was graduating that evening.

About an hour later, in came Dean Pankratz, who was up from Oxford for the commencement. "Jim, the faculty down at Oxford has voted to offer you the chairmanship of surgery in our new four-year medical school in Jackson."

I accepted at once. What timing.

That evening I walked into the house, embraced Weezie, and said, "We've got a chair!"

PART IV

Jackson
1955–

CHAPTER 13

A New Medical School Is Established in Jackson

David S. Pankratz had been born in a sod house in Oklahoma in 1898. He had taken a Ph.D. in anatomy at Kansas University School of Medicine in 1929, and thereafter had begun teaching at the University of Tennessee College of Medicine in Memphis. Meanwhile he had studied medicine during summers at the University of Chicago and was awarded the M.D. degree in 1938. This was a remarkable achievement. He never served an internship, however, and this lack of in-hospital, clinical hands-on experience became a substantial handicap when he—often naive about political problems and special requirements in the clinical arena—began to organize clinical leadership for the new school in Jackson. The preclinical faculty had long been in place in the two-year program at Oxford, which would now be moved. In fact, the two-year school at the parent university campus had been founded in 1903. Dr. Pankratz had joined the Department of Anatomy there in 1939 and was appointed dean in 1946. Mild of manner, tall, and lanky, with almost a lope of a walk, he clearly wished everyone well, was anxious to please all. These qualities of kindness, while attractive, often rendered it difficult for him to make a clean decision and then see it through.

My first personal objective was, to the extent possible from Memphis, to try to make certain that we got chairmen in the other clinical departments who were as good as we could attract, physicians with a genuine background and interest not only in teaching but also in research. It can be assumed that most physicians can treat patients reasonably well, and that most of them can teach at least fairly well, though there is a wide range in the qualities of both these activities. However, it is rare that the physician who is truly effective at both can then include the third and fourth dimensions, those of research and administration. And yet, without good colleagues, I

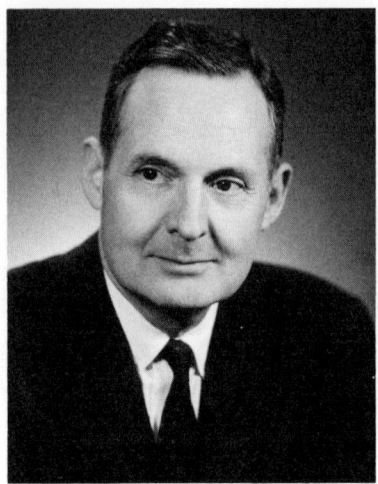
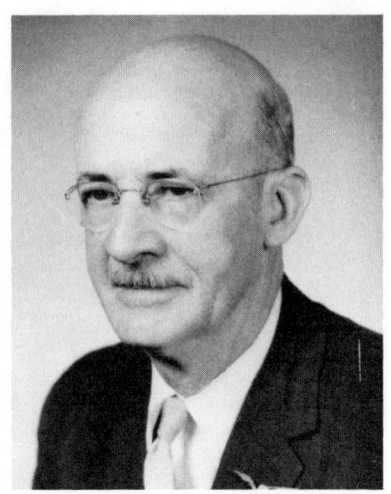

John D. Williams, Chancellor,
University of Mississippi

David S. Pankratz, Dean, University
of Mississippi School of Medicine

well knew that the Department of Surgery that would be my responsibility certainly would not thrive as well as it might.

My greatest ally was Arthur C. Guyton, chairman of physiology at Oxford. He was an enormously impressive person. Suddenly struck with massive poliomyelitis while he was in a surgical residency at Massachusetts General Hospital after graduation from Harvard, he surmounted his physical limitations and went on to become an internationally respected physiologist. His textbook spread throughout the world.

Dr. Guyton and Dr. Louis Sulya, the head of biochemistry, whom I had met at a meeting of the American Physiological Society in Chicago, chuckled when they asked me if I knew where the space assigned to surgery was to be located in the new complex at Jackson. The fact was, the two-year school at Oxford had been so cloistered that most of its faculty had assumed that surgeons spent most of their time either operating on patients or taking care of them in the hospital. Little serious thought had been given to their laboratory and office space. However, to an academician, space ranks only slightly below the other two requirements of the academic trilogy, faculty rank and salary.

There followed extensive negotiations between me, Dr. Sulya, and Dr. William Hare, head of pathology, whose departments were on the same floors where the operating rooms and surgery patient

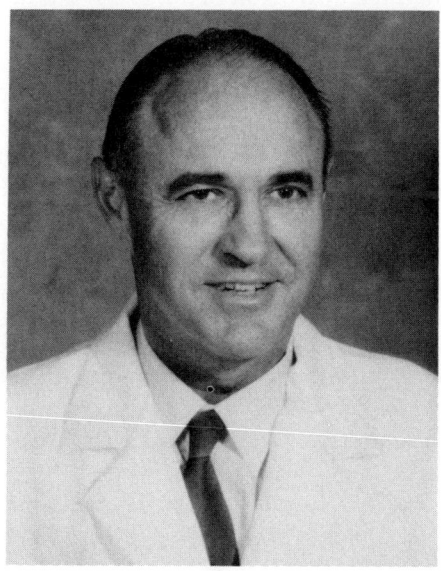
Arthur C. Guyton

wings would be located. They were generous, and we ended up with adequate space.

THE OTHER CLINICAL DEPARTMENTS
Hospital clinical laboratories

With the space problem settled, hiring the rest of the clinical staff assumed priority. I had been the first clinician appointed. Not long afterward, Dr. Warren Bell, a Canadian previously at the University of Pennsylvania, was appointed chairman of the Division of Hematology and Clinical Laboratories. He was a most pleasant, young, and able man, whose resilient personality was well suited to the flexibility so needed in the traditionally difficult job of running the hospital clinical laboratories. He also ran hematology, the blood bank, and chemotherapy for malignancies. The principal remaining appointments were those of the chairmen of the Departments of Medicine, Pediatrics, Obstetrics and Gynecology, and Radiology.

Department of Obstetrics and Gynecology

I was apprehensive regarding the recruitment of additional clinical faculty. Dean Pankratz had such an indirect and puzzling approach that I was concerned lest he fill these posts in such a way as to impair the possible future of the Department of Surgery. And my concerns were not idle ones. Obstetrics and gynecology, for example, is a specialty in which a lot of surgery is involved, and territorial conflict can arise. Imagine my surprise when one day Vice-Chancellor Hyman at Memphis called me from his office over in the administration building and said, "Hardy, I'm calling to congratulate you on your new chairman of obstetrics and gynecology."

"Who on earth could that be, Dr. Hyman? I don't believe anyone has been seriously considered as yet."

"Oh, yes," said Dr. Hyman, and he told me that a man had been just appointed by Dean Pankratz.

I was amazed. The man had been finally eased out of the University of Tennessee about a year before, after months of absence due to a chemical dependency problem, in addition to other problems. It was simply incredible that Dean Pankratz could have appointed him.

"Better call Pankratz, Hardy." Recall that Dr. Hyman knew Dr. Pankratz well, for he had also begun his teaching career in anatomy at Tennessee.

"You bet I will, Dr. Hyman, and thank you very much."

"Dr. Pankratz, how on earth could you appoint Dr. X?" I asked. "Everybody in Memphis knows what the problem was here. We will be the laughing stock of the area, if not the specialty generally. How did you happen to appoint him?"

"To tell the truth, he simply called me and said he wanted the job."

"Dean Pankratz, with Dr. X as head of obstetrics and gynecology, I really feel very depressed about our whole enterprise."

"Don't worry, Jim. I'll just call him up and tell him he can't have the job."

I could only imagine what the people at Vanderbilt were going to say about that turn of events, but under the circumstances, I thought it would be better to have consternation in Nashville than to have him actually in the chair in Jackson. True to his word, Dean Pankratz called and told Dr. X that he could not have the chair after all.

This episode was not the only occasion when Dr. Hyman showed informed interest and tried to prepare the way in Jackson. Early on he had told me, "Hardy, you'll do all right in Jackson, but they'll get at you through your family." I wondered if he spoke from personal experience.

In due course Michael Newton, my colleague at the University of Pennsylvania, accepted the position. He had graduated from the

University of Cambridge in England, then the University of Pennsylvania Medical School, and had trained first in general surgery and then in obstetrics and gynecology at Penn. Furthermore, he had in place an active research program and was an excellent speaker and teacher. His wife was a noted psychologist.

Department of Radiology

Another example. One day Dean Pankratz called me from Oxford and asked me to see a young man from Macon, Mississippi, who wanted to be chairman of the Department of Radiology. "Dean Pankratz," I said, "it is not my prerogative or responsibility to choose a person for the Department of Radiology. I would of course be happy to work with you and with any search committee you might wish to appoint."

"Well, Jim," he said, "look him over, and if you think he would do, we may offer him the job." I appreciated his confidence, but I did not want quite so much responsibility.

I found that the candidate had only just finished his residency at the Confederate Memorial Hospital at Shreveport, Louisiana, which was not then a university hospital, nor was there a medical school. Clearly, the doctor could not possibly have been exposed significantly to research and the teaching of medical students, even if he had had enough experience in the actual practice of radiology. However, he was a pleasant enough young man. After some general conversation I said, "Dr. X, what would you propose to do with the Department of Radiology down in Jackson in the new four-year medical school?"

"I would take X-rays."

"Yes, I am confident you would do that, but what else would you consider to be the responsibilities of the chairman of radiology in a modern medical school? You haven't mentioned administration of a large department, the teaching of medical students, technicians, and residents, and finally, research and the writing of papers. Have you ever written a paper that was published in a national journal?"

No, he hadn't.

After a few moments, he suddenly said to me, "I don't believe I am qualified to be head of the Department of Radiology."

"Dr. X," I replied, "why don't you consider the possibility of joining the Department of Radiology down in Jackson and then, after you have learned the various other responsibilities which a chairman has, in addition to the actual taking and interpreting of X-rays, then you will be ready to be chairman."

In time, Dr. Robert D. Sloan, then in the military service at Scott Field near St. Louis but recently trained at Johns Hopkins Medical School and Hospital, accepted the chairmanship of the Department of Radiology. He was definitely an introvert, but he conducted a solid Department of Radiology, so crucial to all the clinical services, and he himself was one of the best clinical radiologists of my experience. He won student awards for excellence in teaching.

After this second experience, I drove down to Oxford and urged Dean Pankratz to appoint a search committee which would include preclinical faculty, especially Arthur Guyton, to search carefully across the entire United States and thus try to recruit the very best possible person for each of the posts we had to offer. To come to a new medical school in Jackson, Mississippi, was perhaps not the most enticing academic opportunity on the horizon, but there was a definite attraction and challenge in the opportunity to begin a new department in a new medical school, which comes to very few academicians.

I talked with Arthur Guyton and with Dr. David B. Wilson, long since chosen to be head of the hospital, about getting together a more formal committee to search for recruits. Dr. Pankratz was depending on Dr. Wilson to get the hospital established, a large enterprise which he did quite well. But this was not Dean Pankratz's way, and we were not able to do much about it. Fortunately, and to give Dr. Pankratz due credit, he eventually secured good people in the remaining departments.

Department of Medicine

An excellent young academic internist at Cornell, who was from Tennessee, was very interested in the post of Chief of the Department of Medicine and made a splendid impression when he presented some of his research to the faculty at Oxford. He called me in Memphis several times to get news, since other chairs were available to him. Finally, exasperated, he remained in New York and rapidly rose to the top there.

Meanwhile, Robert Snavely at Tulane had been suggested as a candidate to Dr. Pankratz. I had not known him, so I looked in the *Cumulated Index Medicus* for his publications. He had very few publications, and none indicated an established field of scientific research. Moreover, this impression was soon confirmed by the chairman of medicine at Tulane, who stated in a recommendation that the candidate had failed to conduct original investigation. He was, though, a popular teacher and a good clinician. Arthur Guyton and I had hoped that the chairman of medicine, especially, would have more interest in research. However, it developed that the post had already been offered, and Chancellor J. D. Williams, who also had not been informed of the decision, felt that the university must stand by the offer.

Department of Pediatrics

The chair in pediatrics was filled quite late, though this need not have been so. In one instance, the candidate arrived in Jackson only to find Dean Pankratz was in the northwest; Dr. Pankratz had filed the correspondence in the top drawer of his desk, and his secretary, Mrs. Lallah White, knew nothing of the appointment. (This candidate later became dean and then vice-chancellor at Vanderbilt.) Another candidate took exception to the fact that, after having spoken before and submitted to a full inspection by the faculty at Oxford, he was then asked by Dr. Pankratz to go to Jackson and try to get the approval of the practicing pediatricians there. (He became dean at the University of Cincinnati.) In the end, Blair Batson, a solid academic pediatrician trained at Vanderbilt but currently at Johns Hopkins, was appointed.

Thus, the most pressing needs for chairmen of clinical departments, who would each recruit his own respective personnel, had been met. The psychiatry post would be filled later. Incidentally, the story was told of one psychiatrist who had already visited. After having been wined and dined, he was asked what he thought of our proposition, that we looked upon ourselves as pioneers. He was said to have replied, "You're not pioneers, you're missionaries!"

Arthur Guyton and I continued to push for the appointment of people who had a track record in published research; if the chairman does not do research and writing himself, the people below him will all too often reflect this same attitude. There are no great medical school departments that do not have effective research in progress.

Meanwhile, many of my friends cautioned me not to go to Mississippi, not only because it was a new school, with all the attendant problems and hazards for any chairman, but also, since politics was so hopelessly interwoven into education in Mississippi, I would always be at the mercy of the next governor elected. (Professor Ben Eiseman, who went to the new University of Kentucky Medical School as chairman, later declared that his next move would be to a *new* house and an *old* school.)

But Dr. Ravdin was in favor of the move. "Jim," he wrote, "I suggest that you take the job and show what you can do. The salary they are offering is really very low by national standards, but when you do a good job things have a way of getting better. Not many people get a chance to run a department of surgery at your age." It was unclear whether I would automatically be accorded tenure on becoming full professor and chairman at Jackson. But Dr. Ravdin said it made little difference, that they could always get rid of you if they wanted to by cutting your salary, taking your space, stopping promotions, assigning onerous duties, and all the rest.

The administration of the University of Tennessee was generous in allowing me to go back and forth to Jackson, a distance of 213 miles, when necessary. There was no point in a surgeon's going to a hospital that had not yet been built, where he certainly could do no operating. Meanwhile, the medical politics in Jackson had heated progressively until it represented such formidable opposition that it became doubtful whether the school could be established on a truly effective basis, and indeed whether I would want to be a part of it.

THE TOWN-GOWN CONFLICT

There is a "town-gown" problem in any city where there is a medical school, but it reaches its greatest intensity when a new medical school is going to be established in a relatively small city, especially if the new faculty are to treat private patients. Basically, it has to do with income. Though at first quite happy over my appointment, I became more and more apprehensive that my position was going to be somewhat tenuous at best. Practicing politics, Dean Pankratz would suggest one set of financial arrangements but then, after another salvo from organized medicine in Jackson, would ask me if I would accept different arrangements. Meanwhile, I was appreciated more and more in Memphis, as my research support had enlarged and my publications, including two additional books, established a national reputation. I conveyed my dismay to David Wilson, and he wrote as follows:

With reference to Dr. Pankratz and the changes that he makes with reference to financial arrangements with individuals. The best statement that I can make about Dr. Pankratz is one which Dr. Arthur C. Bachmeyer (at the University of Chicago) made to me about three years ago. He told me at that time that when I first began to know Dr. Pankratz that I would have some misgivings. He assured me though that as time went on Dr. Pankratz would "grow on me." May I assure you that this is exactly what has happened. I have come to know Dr. Pankratz well and to admire him. I have a great deal of respect for him and he has "grown on me." At times he does appear to change. I think that is because he has the qualification of certain strictly teacher types. I mean by that that sometimes he does not take some of the practical things in life too seriously. I believe, however, that you will find that he is loyal and will do everything he possibly can for your own good. I merely make these statements in generalities to give you a general assurance that I think you really have little to worry about even though it appears that he has changed from time to time.

One sticky point was whether or not any private patients would be treated in the University Hospital. If the practicing physicians in Jackson could prevent the treatment of private patients in the University Hospital, then they would of course have effectively quarantined the full-time members of the faculty. Again, Dean Pankratz,

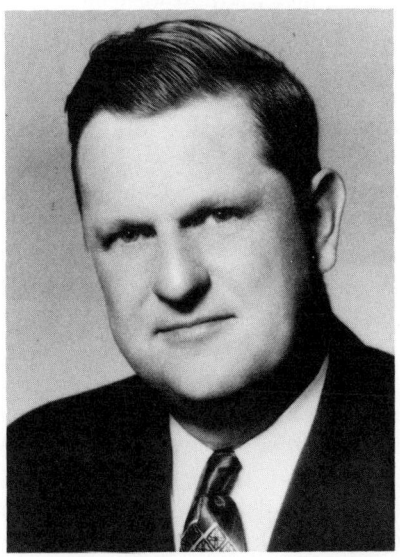

David B. Wilson

having been cloistered in Oxford for so many years as a professor of anatomy and part-time dean, and having never had any in-hospital experience as an intern or resident, really did not understand the dimensions of a town-gown problem, as I noted previously.

Curtis Caine, an anesthesiologist and the representative of a group in Jackson, came to see me in Memphis and, right there in my office, said bluntly to me, "Dr. Hardy, if you insist on seeing private patients, we are not going to have you in Jackson."

This certainly put the matter squarely. I decided that the time had finally come for someone to face and to state facts.

"You will realize I mean nothing personal, Dr. Caine," I replied, "for you and I have just met. But let me say this: We could put that medical school on a Pacific atoll if somebody wanted to pay for it. And the Mississippi legislature has already voted the money."

He departed and remained a rival thereafter.

After the emissary had reported back to his colleagues in Jackson, Dean Pankratz called and asked if I would meet with a group of physicians in Jackson at a dinner. Dean Pankratz said that he and Dr. David B. Wilson, the hospital director, would also be present to meet with these other physicians, virtually all of them surgeons, though some had had limited training.

Because my flight was delayed, the assembled thirty or so physicians and surgeons were well along with their meal when I arrived. I sat in the only vacant chair, at the foot of the table, and ate quickly. The meeting was being chaired by Harvey Johnston, Jr., a very able surgeon who had the orientation of having trained at Charity Hospital in New Orleans, which had no private patients. Further, he was well aware how the support of Charity Hospital had been utilized, albeit indirectly, in the establishment of the Ochsner Clinic. Some preliminary talk about policies of medical school practice followed, and then Dr. Johnston, at the head of the table, got right to the point. He said that he had a signed list of all the surgeons in Jackson; they would serve the University Medical Center without pay, but none of them would assist the university in any way if Dr. Hardy (and presumably the rest of the full-time school faculty) were allowed to see private patients. He looked down at me and said, "Dr. Hardy, do you think you could influence me with five thousand dollars?" (I had insisted on budget funds to pay for part-time help.)

"No, Dr. Johnston, I don't think I could influence you with five thousand dollars. I'm told that you have the best practice in Jackson and probably the best in the whole state of Mississippi. However, there would be some well-trained young surgeon who'd just come to Jackson, who badly needed five thousand dollars, and who would start in that position the following morning."

"Maybe you'd like to see this list of surgeons' signatures," he said, and passed it down along the table. I looked carefully for one particular name, one I knew would not be on the list, and it was not there.

"The list is incomplete," I said.

"Then maybe this will help you, Dr. Hardy." He then passed down a single sheet of white paper bearing a single signature. I was deeply disappointed over this particular signature. True, this doctor was in private practice and depended on good peer relationships for patient referrals; yet, at the same time, he was the only plastic surgeon in Jackson and probably the only one in Mississippi. But the list was now complete.

"Dr. Hardy, now what is your position?"

"Absolutely unchanged, Dr. Johnston."

Dean Pankratz had sat there, immobilized by this exchange. It was a Mexican standoff, it seemed to me. The hazard of losing such a battle is that, while the town practitioner can withdraw to the privileged sanctuary of his private practice to fight another day, the full-time man, having little practice, must move.* I returned to Memphis full of doubts, and began to voice serious misgivings about the chances for success down in Jackson.

That brought a call from Dr. Billy Guyton, the father of Arthur Guyton. He was a leading ophthalmologist, practicing in Oxford, and a former dean of the existing two-year medical school. I had met him earlier, at a men's service luncheon, where I had said that I would not want our daughters to be doctors. He had taken exception, which proved to be prophetic, "Why not? First, they'd be assured of interesting and rewarding work, and second, they'd be surrounded by intelligent and eligible men to marry."

"What's all this I hear that you may pull out?" he said. "Could you see me tomorrow afternoon about three o'clock?"

"Certainly, Dr. Billy."

The next afternoon his chauffeur drove him up from Oxford and was told to get coffee and come back in about forty-five minutes.

Dr. Guyton and I discussed all the problems, the political maneu-

---

*Once policies had been settled, Dr. Johnston and his qualified colleagues served the university faithfully and well.

vering, and the fact that Dean Pankratz had repeatedly suggested different arrangements for my contract to placate some new demand from the opposition in Jackson.

"Jim, I'm surprised that you've never met Chancellor J. D. Williams. Promise me you won't do anything radical. You'll hear from him very soon."

Chancellor Williams called the next day and set up an appointment in the lobby of the Peabody Hotel (often called the capitol of the Mississippi delta). We selected two overstuffed chairs near the duck pond. "I want to hear how you see the situation in Jackson, from one end to the other," he said.

He must have listened for almost an hour, asking an occasional question. I discussed the financing of a modern medical school, and tried to convey that some private practice was essential to recruiting and keeping clinical staff and for political influence, that high standards were essential, that the inevitable town-gown conflict must be faced, and that definite and long-range policies should be set and then steadfastly adhered to. He agreed to limited private practice, but he was reluctant to accept the proposition that all surgeons operating in the University Hospital be either board certified or at least board qualified. This was political dynamite.

As we closed he said, "Dr. Hardy, I'm confident you are the man we want to head up our surgery department. But before I leave I want to tell you a story. A farmer had a prize bull, very expensive. One day, as the farmer talked with a drummer along the barbed wire fence, a freight train was seen coming right through the pasture. The bull ran and planted himself in the middle of the track, pawed the ground, and prepared to charge the onrushing locomotive. 'Quick,' yelled the drummer. 'Aren't you going to save the bull?'

"'Magnificent animal,' said the farmer. 'Such courage.'

"'Yes, I don't question his courage,' said the drummer, 'but I wonder about his intelligence!'"

Several weeks later Chancellor Williams called and invited Weezie and me to Oxford for a luncheon, at which I would sign a contract as the first clinician appointed. "Chancellor Williams," I said carefully, "I really would like to come but I must decline, with thanks, for we've not yet settled the issue of just who will have surgical privileges in the University Hospital."

But he would not take no for an answer, so I finally agreed to come. Driving down to Oxford that Saturday morning, June 26, 1954, Weezie said, "Jim, do you want the job in Jackson?"

"Yes, I'd like to try my hand at running a department of surgery."

"Then what if the chancellor insists on an open staff? After all, he has compromised on everything else, including the return to the Department of Surgery of a part of the money you earn from private patients but aren't allowed to keep yourself." (A part of my income was to be earned from private practice but with a fixed upper limit of salary plus practice receipts.)

"Weezie," I replied, "Chancellor Williams is an experienced man. He's hired many a person. He's giving this luncheon for an important out-of-state academician. You can rest assured that he has a position to fall back on if I'm not bluffing—and I'm not bluffing, for without high standards the Department of Surgery could not be a national competitor."

"All right," Weezie said, "but you may be sorry."

We arrived at the chancellor's home, and after a splendid luncheon, Chancellor Williams asked me, Dean Pankratz, and Provost W. Alton Bryant to accompany him over to his office to sign the contract. I felt very awkward, since we had discussed the point of the requirement for board qualification no further.

As we gathered around the table, Chancellor Williams said, "Dr. Hardy, why don't you just let the board qualification ride. Perhaps we could activate it in a year or so. It would make things much easier all the way around."

I had been thinking for months about just how best to have Chancellor Williams fully comprehend the situation.

"Chancellor Williams," I asked, "who teaches Ph.D. candidates?"

"Ph.D.'s, of course," answered Chancellor Williams.

I said, "How do you think a general practitioner can teach a fifth-year surgical resident to do major surgery? It is precisely the same situation as having simple graduates try to develop Ph.D. candidates."

"Dr. Hardy, you've made your point. Why don't you and Dean Pankratz go into the next room and write a contract. Do you have your thoughts arranged?"

Reaching into my inside coat pocket, I said, "I just happen to have a few notes here."

He laughed and said, "I just knew you would have, Dr. Hardy, which is one of the reasons we want you!"

And thus the final and formal contract was signed, and I knew that it would have the backing of the chancellor, and with him the Board of Trustees. Regardless of what problems we might have in Jackson, as long as we were firmly supported by the chancellor and the nonpolitical Board of Trustees, we would succeed.

By way of an epilogue, within a few years after the University Hospital had instituted the requirement of board qualification, the other leading hospitals in Jackson gradually adopted the same requirement. And, to varying degrees, the requirements for operating privileges were eventually strengthened in most hospitals throughout the state of Mississippi. Thus, the University Hospital had already begun to fulfill the mission of any university hospital: to establish and maintain the highest standards possible in its geographical area.

My appointment as chairman at Mississippi certainly did not impair my credentials for membership in various surgical organizations. I was soon elected to membership in the Southern Surgical Association, the American Surgical Association, the Society of Clinical Surgery, and the Surgical Forum Committee of the American College of Surgeons, and was elected secretary of the Society of University Surgeons, a post that almost automatically led to the presidency if one did a good job.

Preparing to Leave Memphis

I asked Dr. Wilson and Vice-President Hyman what they wanted me to leave behind in the way of special laboratory equipment purchased on my grants. I then requested permission from the National Institutes of Health and the army to duplicate all the research equipment that we were currently using and to move it intact to Jackson. Furthermore, the three technicians in Memphis—Mrs. Anne Cole Bass (who had just become Mrs. Turner), Miss Virginia Ward, and Miss Thelma Carter—also moved to Jackson, along with Dr. M. Don Turner (who had recently married Mrs. Bass). Thus we were able to continue our research immediately in Jackson. In addition, Dr. Wilson agreed I might take one surgical resident with me. I chose William A. Neely, a Harvard Medical School graduate and a Mississippian who had worked with me in the laboratory for a year. Four rotating interns came along, as did John H. Dickson, a masterful photographer and movie producer. Dr. Jorğe A. Rodriguez, a trained surgeon from Mexico who gained further experience with us, came and provided excellent medical illustrations.

During the last days in Memphis in 1955, Dean Roberts asked me if I would give the honor address to Alpha Omega Alpha, the national scholarship society of medical schools. (He had told me to

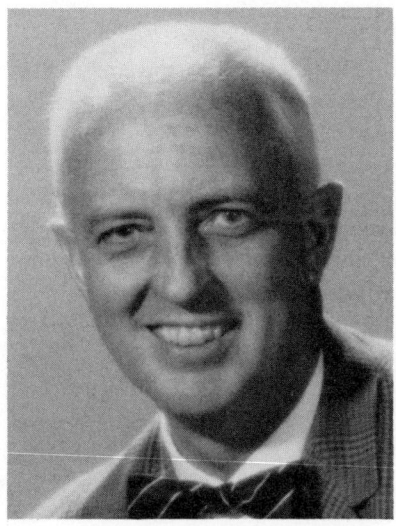

William A. Neely

come back to U.T. if I were forced to retreat northward from Jackson.)

"Dr. Roberts," I said, "I accept with pleasure, on the condition that I can say exactly what I think needs to be done around here."

Dr. Roberts was a little taken aback. He grinned and said he would have to ask the boss (Vice-Chancellor Hyman).

He called the next day and said, "Hardy, go ahead, but let me tell you that you are strictly on your own!"

Dr. Hyman was seated beside me at the head table on the night of the AOA banquet at the Memphis Country Club, with the student president of the society on the other side. "I would like to state at the outset that the opinions to be expressed are not necessarily those of the management," I began. The audience roared, for Dr. Hyman really ran that school with an iron hand.

I went on to say that the University of Tennessee sorely needed more full-time faculty. Remember, I was the only full-time surgeon that the school had ever had. There were not more than one or possibly two full-time people in the Department of Medicine.

The main points of my address were duly published in the *Memphis Commercial Appeal* the following morning. Incidentally, in the years following, the University of Tennessee gradually developed a full-time system in virtually every clinical department.

Our move from Memphis to Jackson was with four young daughters, ranging from a few weeks to five years in age. Bettie had been born in 1953 and Katherine in 1955.

The Divisions of the Department

The overall progress of the clinical years of the medical school was now well under way, with the appointments of the chairmen of the various clinical departments. The recruiting of the personnel for the Department of Surgery moved front and center. Actually, I had been holding back, to some extent, until I, myself, had been assured of a specific salary ($15,000), a limited practice income, the return to the Department of Surgery of 60 percent of the money I made from practice but was not allowed to keep (the other 40 percent went to the Dean for discretionary use), and the requirement that all surgeons operating in the University Hospital be either certified by the American Board of Surgery or at least board qualified. Of those not on published lists of certified specialists but who claimed to be board qualified by residency training, a letter to this effect was required from the office of the American Board in Philadelphia. Some proved to be qualified, others not. In case of the "nots," lasting hard feelings were generated, but it was pointed out that nothing was being subtracted from previous hospital staff privileges, since *no one* had ever operated in the University Hospital before. Actually, there was a second reason for the "board qualified" regulation: residents just finishing their training would not be able to take their boards for quite some months thereafter.

Regarding the subdivisions to be recognized in the Department of Surgery, Dean Pankratz wrote me on December 23, 1954, as follows:

> Dear Jim:
>
> You may remember that I said Dr. Jobe [Executive Secretary, Board of Trustees of Institutions of Higher Learning] felt that it would be helpful if I could have a list of the subdivisions in the Department of Surgery. And if you cared to make any statements about the use of local men, names would not have to be used. I believe this would not be "out of line." You and I have frequently discussed the various divisions that we plan to have.

The subdivisions were to include anesthesiology, orthopaedic surgery, urological surgery, plastic surgery, ophthalmology, general and cardiothoracic surgery, otolaryngology, oral surgery (including the dental section), neurosurgery, and later, pediatric surgery.

The chair in neurosurgery was to be filled by Orlando Andy, who had graduated from the University of Rochester School of Medicine. I had first met him at the University of Tennessee when he was

A New Medical School in Jackson 199

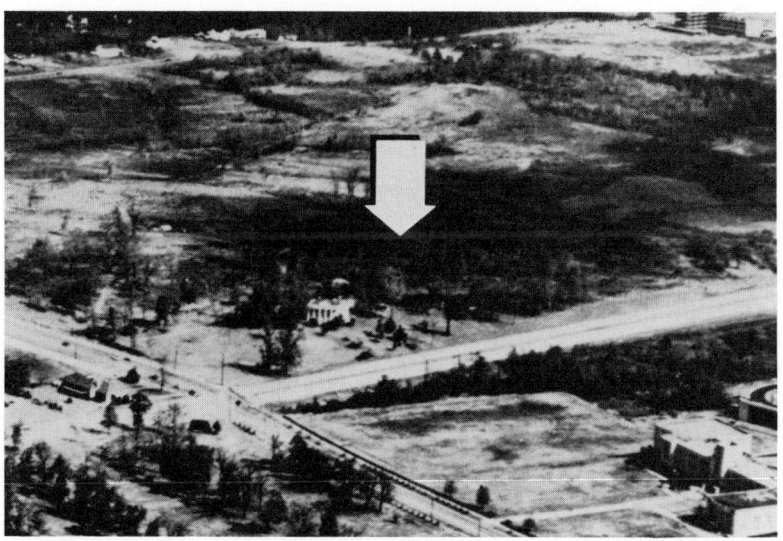

Hole in ground, future University Medical Center, 1952

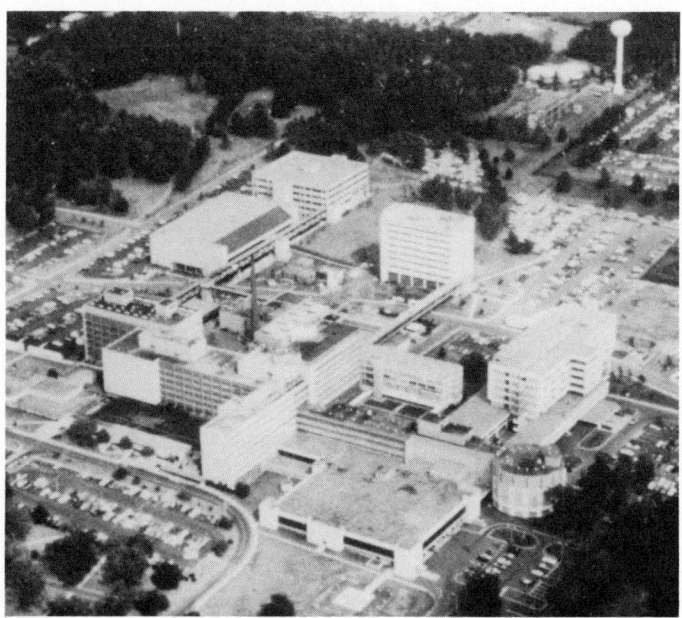

University Medical Center, 1985 (Veterans Administration Hospital, not visible, located to right)

a resident in neurosurgery there, but for the past several years he had been at Johns Hopkins getting advanced training, especially in research. At that time there was only one well-trained neurosurgeon in the state of Mississippi, Charles L. Neill, a very competent man trained originally at Cornell University. Dr. Neill could have filled the clinical and teaching responsibilities handsomely, but his large private practice was thought to preclude the possibility of his doing laboratory research. Hence we chose Dr. Andy, but I was forever grateful to Dr. Neill for his generous acceptance of the situation, since he certainly could have rightfully expected to head the Division of Neurosurgery. He remained loyal, and the rich experience of his large clinical practice strengthened the university over the years.

The members of the Semmes neurosurgical group in Memphis, who were in charge of the residency, reported that Dr. Andy was very bright, though one or two of them alluded obliquely to his at times less-than-rigid adherence to carrying through on clinical duties.

The chair in anesthesiology was always a hard post to fill. Relatively few medical students entered this specialty, and those who did were not often inclined to accept for long the salary and other strictures involved in accepting an academic position. However, we were able to locate G. B. Bittenbender, chief of anesthesiology at the Veterans Administration Hospital at Baylor University Medical Center at Houston. I decided to go to Houston and meet Dr. Bittenbender on his home ground, so that I could talk not only with him but also with my surgical colleagues at Baylor. The cooperation between the surgeon and the anesthesiologist is so continual, and at times of such a delicate nature, that personal qualities can prove a major consideration. Dr. Bittenbender was said to be a competent anesthesiologist who had been trained at Charity Hospital in New Orleans. He would also be able to bring a number of trained graduate nurse anesthetists with him. He was said to be crusty and perhaps a bit cynical, but in general easy enough to get along with. We were concerned, however, that about a year before, in the course of operating for a tubercular focus, Drs. Michael DeBakey and Oscar Creech had noted a small nodule on the surface of Dr. Bittenbender's lung. Microscopic examination of this nodule had revealed cancer, and that entire lung was then taken out. DeBakey and Creech felt that if anyone had ever been cured of lung cancer, Bittenbender should have been cured, so small was his lesion out at the periphery of the lung, but there did remain the possibility that in the future he might have a recurrence of this tumor. Even so, all things considered, and in view of the dearth of academic anesthesiologists who were willing to come to Mississippi to a new medical center, Bittenbender was offered the chairmanship of the Division of Anesthesiology and he accepted.

Thus, the two specialties that none of the general surgeons could cover in any respect, neurosurgery and anesthesiology, were filled. It would be the responsibility of the head of each surgical division to recruit and recommend his subordinates.

Orthopaedics was to be run by attending orthopaedic surgeons in practice in the city, and Dr. Thomas H. Blake, the veritable dean of that specialty in Mississippi, was clearly the appropriate person. (So pervasive was his reputation that some said many Mississippians could not distinguish between the two words, Blake and break.) Unfortunately, within months it became apparent that the practitioners could not devote sufficient time to the effort and that a full-time person must be found. Accordingly, Dr. William F. Enneking was recruited from the University of Chicago, where he was just completing his residency.

As with orthopaedics, urology was represented in Mississippi by a strong local practitioner, Dr. Temple Ainsworth, and he was the natural choice. He was already prominent nationally, and he went on to become President of the American Urological Association. Of all the various divisions, urology manned by Dr. Ainsworth and his staff was the most stable and clinically solid, and was a greatly appreciated support to the Department of Surgery.

Plastic surgery was covered quite faithfully and effectively by Dr. James Hendrix and the staff he later developed. Actually, I had delayed this particular appointment for a thoughtful period.

The local practitioners of otolaryngology did not wish to select from among themselves a head of the Division of Otolaryngology in the University Medical Center, lest this give someone's private practice an advantage over their own. Therefore, they requested that Dr. Edley Jones in Vicksburg, who did have a national political reputation in ENT circles, be appointed. To his credit, Dr. Jones put in a lot of time driving the 40 miles from Vicksburg to conduct the ENT affairs and, later, get a residency approved. Meanwhile, the ENT practitioners in town were of much assistance, especially Dr. Eugene Hesdorffer. This arrangement was of course makeshift, and ultimately it became desirable to bring in a full-time head.

Ophthalmology presented the most thorny appointment politically. In Jackson there were a number of richly experienced ophthalmologists who had been there for years. In this one instance, however, Dean Pankratz was very anxious to have a hand in the decision, and he wished to have Dr. Samuel B. Johnson appointed. Dr. Johnson had completed his training at Tulane University two years before, in 1953, and had then opened his office in Jackson. Dean Pankratz put forward two particular considerations in favor of Dr. Johnson. First, he had just recently completed his ophthalmology residency training in a well-known medical center and would be current with academic affairs and problems. Second, he was the son-in-law of Dr. Henry Boswell, one of the major political medical leaders in the state of Mississippi at the time. Dr. Boswell had for many years been head of the Mississippi Tuberculosis Sanitorium. He had not only a large leadership role in Mississippi, including influence with the legislature, he also had a well-earned national reputation as well. The other major leader in Mississippi was Dr. J. D. Underwood, head of the state Public Health Service, who likewise enjoyed a national and indeed international reputation for the public health work that he had fostered in the state.

I knew none of the ophthalmologists in Jackson, including Dr. Johnson. I was well aware that to appoint so young a man, competing in practice, when the leading ophthalmologists had been there for years, would not sit well with his older colleagues. But in this one instance, having no strong feeling about the situation other than my concern over the political ramifications of this appointment, I agreed when Dr. Pankratz asked that this appointment be made. Actually, in retrospect Dr. Johnson was a good choice anyway, since he did have recent and continuing academic ties with Tulane, and he served well. Probably predictably, however, virtually all the other Jackson ophthalmologists declined to serve with him.

Oral surgery was conducted by Dr. Walton Shannon, who worked with the dental faculty members. I must confess that I offered little nurturing to the dentists: they had been placed, administratively, under the Department of Surgery, but I did not know them individually and their needs were foreign to me. The dental school was far in the future.

In general surgery we were fortunate to recruit Curtis P. Artz, trained at Ohio State University, who had already had a brief but fruitful army research career. He was peerless in the treatment of burns, and he later directed the first Shriner's Burn Hospital, at the University of Texas, Galveston. Watts R. Webb, a Johns Hopkins graduate, had trained in surgery at Washington University and

First full-time faculty, Department of Surgery

Barnes Hospital in St. Louis, with particular specialization in thoracic surgery. He was an excellent technician and was primarily responsible for getting the pump-oxygenator set up for open-heart surgery, in which he and I collaborated.

Dr. Artz later became professor and chairman of the Department of Surgery at the Medical University of South Carolina in Charleston, and Dr. Webb, after a series of upward moves, became chairman of the Department of Surgery at Tulane University. These able men were most effective in accepting responsibility and in generating competent leadership in clinical surgery, teaching, research, and administration in our department.

One other group of departmental appointments should be mentioned. These were the nonpaid teaching staff members in private practice.

To my surprise, I found that the two-year school at Oxford already had a chief or chairman of surgery. I was reminded of the classic title "grand admiral of the Swiss navy." Actually, it was then still a common practice to pad the faculty catalogue with clinical appointments that were all too often honorary and required no service; unfortunately, to the uninformed or naive these appointments were indistinguishable from the hard core, hard won, meaningful academic ranks. I wrote Dean Pankratz on August 12, 1954:

> Just exactly what is Dr. Parson's title supposed to be? He suddenly confronted me with this subject, saying that he had been led to understand first one thing and then another. Certainly he expects more than we can give him without disrupting our "scale" of titles. For example, he thought "Professor of Surgery, Part Time" would be appropriate. I said nothing, but he does not deserve such a title. Actually, he is probably asking for more than he expects to receive. Yet, we do want his enthusiastic cooperation if we can obtain it on reasonable terms. What would you think of Assistant Professor of Clinical Surgery? This would give us the opportunity eventually to raise the title to Associate Professor if he finds time to give to teaching. I am opposed to full professorships as "honorary" titles, such as Dr. R. L. Sanders has here—he never teaches anything.

Dr. Willard H. Parsons served loyally and was progressively promoted in due course.

The general outlines and overall policies for the establishment of the University Medical Center in Jackson had become fairly firm by April of 1955. The original philosophies at Oxford had been slowly but substantially modified. In the beginning, Dean Pankratz and his advisors, who had worked long and hard for the establishment of a four-year medical school in Jackson, had envisioned a fairly low-cost operation. Their plan had been to have a full-time chairman of each major clinical department, and thereafter to use volunteer assistants from the physicians already in Jackson. However, for many reasons including political skirmishing, it had become apparent that additional full-time help would be required in each department.

We had agreed to have only one new medical school class a year, instead of one every six months, as was the case at Oxford at that time, or four per year, as in Memphis. Also, the faculty would be allowed very limited private practice. The policy of what to do with that portion of funds from private practice which the clinical teachers would generate but could not keep personally had also been settled. In a codicil to my original contract, it had been agreed that 60 percent of the "overage" earned from practice would revert to the department that had earned it, and 40 percent would go to the dean's office for discretionary distribution.

I had a very clear idea of what I hoped to do with the Department of Surgery. Teaching, patient care, and research would all be given strong emphasis in our surgical effort in Jackson. All decisions would be made solely on the basis of what was good for the Department of Surgery and the Medical Center. In Memphis, I had had an opportunity to compare the full-time system in Philadelphia with the private practice system at the University of Tennessee. Inevitably, some of the administrative decisions Harwell Wilson had made were subtly, to varying degrees, influenced by the fact that he received only a nominal stipend from the university and depended on patient referrals from friends who might take exception to some necessary decision.

We planned to provide the students and residents with a broad spectrum of learning and experience that would enable them to be whatever they wished to be: a full-time private practitioner (which most would inevitably be, anyway), a private practitioner closely associated with a university medical teaching center, or a full-time career academic surgeon. To achieve these objectives, we obviously had to have not only good patient care but effective and ongoing research. Above all, I and my colleagues in surgery were dedicated to ensuring that our residents would be able to operate and take care of patients effectively when they completed their training.

The difficulties involved in recruiting staff and residents from numerous universities, at various levels of training, were substantial.

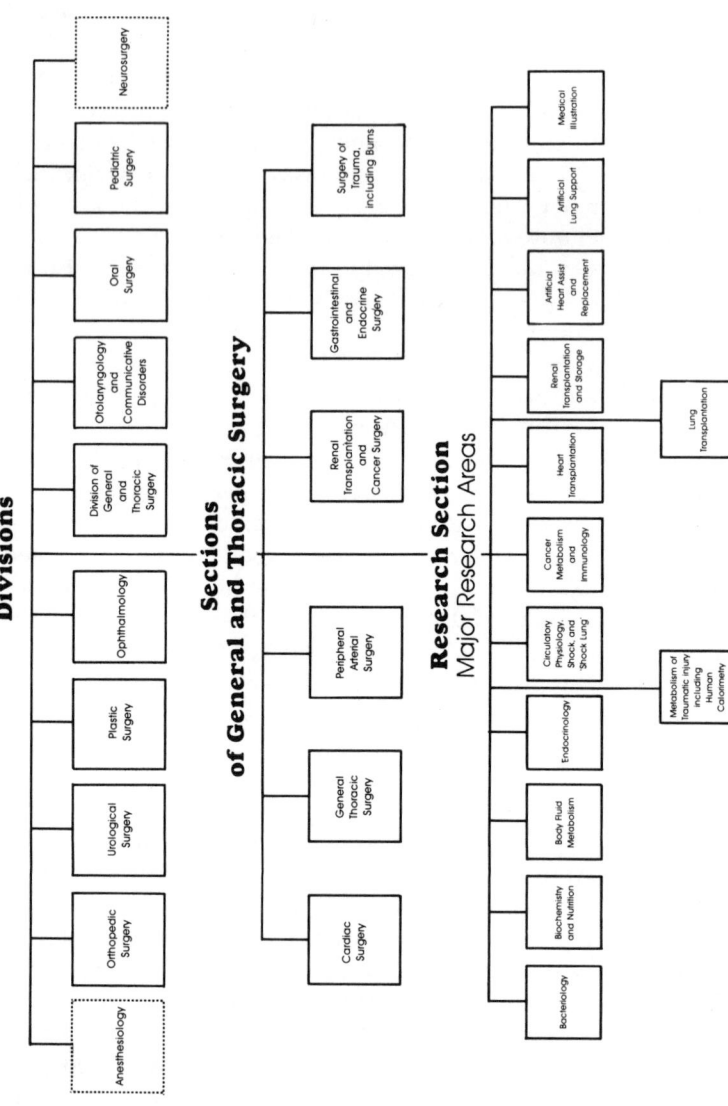

Administrative organization, Department of Surgery

Nonetheless, it was my hope that we could achieve some reasonable consensus at the beginning, and then gradually develop our own traditions over the months and years. At both the University of Pennsylvania and the University of Tennessee, most members of the surgical staff had been alumni, and the majority of the surgical residents at Tennessee had gone to the University of Tennessee Medical College. But even with my awareness of the different views and backgrounds that would exist among the people we were able to recruit, I still did not fully appreciate the concerns which would ultimately be my lot from this particular source. Thirteen different medical schools were represented by the initial resident cadre—five from the University of Tennessee, three from Tulane, three from Harvard, and the rest from all over the country, including California.

The Department of Surgery was most fortunate, over the years, in having capable women who came to work, often just out of college, and remained for many years. Four key persons were with me for a total of 104 years, affording invaluable continuity in the overall effort. Mrs. Virginia Keith, chemistry technician and later editorial assistant, had moved with me from Memphis. Mrs. Hazel M. Mattox was engaged as departmental secretary, later was administrative assistant, and still later became executive assistant. Among her many contributions to the progress of the Department of Surgery was her ability to modulate tactfully her telephone response to the position and personality of the caller. Jane Peters took over when Mrs. Mattox retired. Mrs. Mary Ruth Ruffin has now been my private secretary for twenty-five years.

With the looming obligation of daily participation in operative surgery, teaching, research, and the heavy administrative tasks of recruiting and developing a department of surgery in a new medical school–hospital complex—with all this and a growing family—clearly I had to alter my work habits. I lived only five minutes from the hospital, so travel time was for me at an absolute minimum. Also, we began operating at eight o'clock in the morning, and later at seven o'clock, earlier than I had in Memphis. There I had been a night owl, working commonly until midnight and still getting my six hours of sleep. In Jackson, however, there had to be a change, especially if I was to complete the book *Pathophysiology in Surgery* for the Williams & Wilkins Publishing Company.

Therefore, on reaching Jackson I began to go to bed after the children about 9 P.M., setting the alarm for 3 A.M. In the morning hours

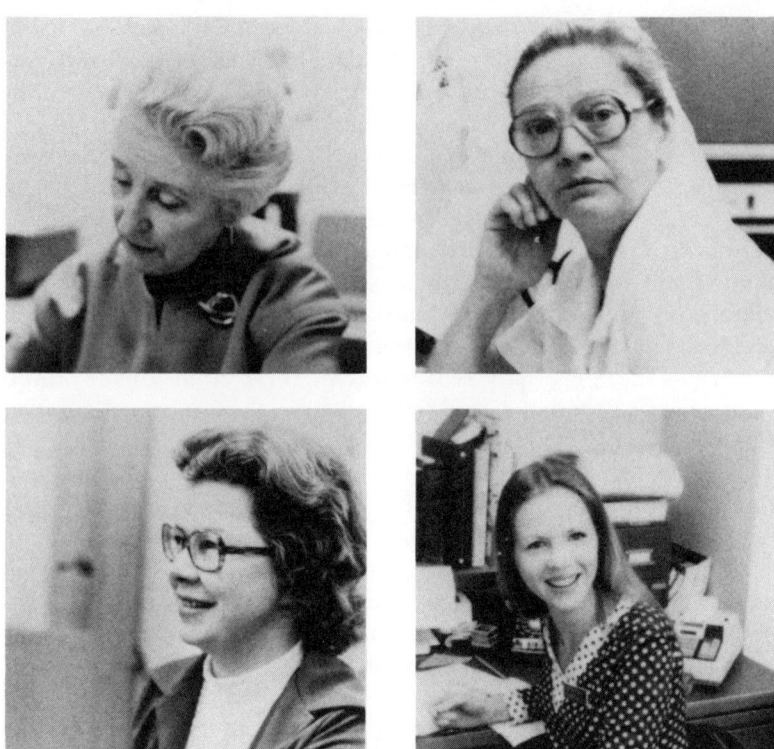

Top left: *Hazel M. Mattox;* top right: *Virginia W. Keith;*
bottom left: *Mary Ruth Ruffin;* bottom right: *Jane E. Peters*

there was absolute quiet. Peace. Mind absolutely clear. I would plug in the coffee pot while shaving, drink a cup in the darkness lit only by the streetlight outside while thinking through the operations to come that day, then list objectives for the rest of the day, and finally begin either handwriting or dictating on the book. Just before leaving for the hospital for the first operation, I would have a quick breakfast with Weezie and the children, another cup of coffee, and scan the *Jackson Clarion Ledger* for news. So heavily engrossed was I in getting things started in Jackson, that I fear I did not fully realize just how much Weezie had on her hands, with getting a new house filled and occupied and nurturing four small daughters.

This general practice of early to bed and early to rise was to remain in effect throughout my professional career, over which span some seventeen books were authored, edited, or co-edited, and several hundred papers published in medical journals. I tried to adhere to Sir William Osler's advice to live in "day-tight compartments." Or, as "Farmer Jim" Neal would say on the car radio as I drove to the hospital: "Wake up, ever'body. It's a brand new day. Ain't never been used yet." However, if I had a critically ill patient, like most surgeons I was rarely able to put him or her completely out of my mind. Sometimes the urge to call about the patient at 3 A.M. would get the better of me, but knowing my detachment would be lost if I did, I was usually able to assume that the condition was at least no worse or the resident would have called me during the night. The resident on duty always called me at 9 P.M. with a complete rundown on all the patients on our service.

Occasionally, I simply rented a room at a motel for the day, in order to get the detachment and isolation necessary to finish some manuscript or grant request. The only way I could then be reached was through the hospital switchboard on my pager.

University Hospital Opens

The University Hospital was scheduled to open on July 1, receiving twenty-three chronic patients from the old Charity Hospital in downtown Jackson. These patients represented mostly the "three B's": breaks (fractures), burns, and bladders (prostatic obstruction patients who were usually wearing a urinary catheter). In no way could they be considered acutely ill or a heavy load to take. However, at an emergency meeting called on June 30, the nursing service urged that this transfer be delayed because the hospital simply was not yet ready to receive patients. This proposed delay seemed to the clinicians unnecessary. It was pointed out that in Germany our 81st Field Hospital had admitted well over one hundred patients to tents in a single day. The clinicians' insistence prevailed and the patients were moved on July 1.

But we had a surprise. An hour after the opening, we received a call from the emergency room saying that a patient was there who had a groin hernia which had caused intestinal obstruction and that he must be operated upon immediately. We rallied to the cause. Several members of the surgical staff scrubbed, came into the operating room, and placed or tied one stitch each in the repair of the hernia, this being the historic first patient ever operated on in the University Hospital.

During July and August the principal focus was on getting the hospital procedures and policies fully in order. For example, when a patient had a venous pressure measurement done, he was likely to have a chilly sensation. We first suspected that the solution used to fill the pressure manometer was somehow contaminated by bacteria, but we found that the person assigned to prepare the material was using distilled water instead of normal salt solution. The distilled water caused destruction of red blood cells.

There were difficult experiences with infections. Later, an expert from Boston pointed out that infections were more likely to occur in a brand new hospital than in an old and well-established hospital. This was due, he said, to the fact that the personnel and procedures had been well developed and in consistent use in the established hospital.

Another problem was the blood bank. We were chronically short of blood donors, and members of the state legislature frequently sought to find out whether we kept the "white" blood and the "black" blood segregated. (We never did, but some fancy verbal brokenfield running was at times required to avoid telling an outright lie.)

We also had our first brushes with potential political interference. In one case, I had instructed the chief resident, Dr. Robert Caldwell, to accept no more burn patients, since chronic burn patients were being dumped on us from hospitals all over the state. Therefore, when the next burn patient came to the emergency room, Dr. Caldwell made certain that the patient was in stable condition and getting the proper fluids, and then referred the child to a hospital in Vicksburg. The patient arrived there in stable condition but later died. This resulted in an investigation by the Mississippi state legislature to learn why their new state university hospital had not accepted this burn patient, who had died. I refused to disclose to the legislative investigating committee the name of our chief resident, which caused them much agitation but which was finally accepted, though with newspaper comment all along the line. One of the three newspapers—which had a number of stockholders in town, the other two papers being owned by the Hederman family—regularly seemed to publish articles attacking the University Medical Center. A crisis was reached after a woman had rushed into the emergency room with her husband, saying he'd had a heart attack. The nurse told them to sit down and wait, that the doctor was at lunch. Desperate, the woman scooped up her husband and rushed to another hospital, where the husband died on the doorstep. At an emergency session of our staff, held to try to prevent such disasters in the future, one exasperated chief exclaimed, "That was a put-up job if I ever saw one." "Well," someone rejoined dryly, "One thing's for sure: they're going to run out of volunteers."

In another instance, I had been named to a committee with Bob Snavely and Dave Wilson for drawing up the specifications for intravenous fluids to be used in the University Hospital. This choice contract had been put out on bid, and some firm other than Baxter Laboratories had come in with the low bid. However, Baxter Laboratories had been brought to Mississippi by then governor Hugh White. The governor called Chancellor Williams in Oxford, and the chancellor called Dean Pankratz. The specifications were revised; not surprisingly, Baxter Laboratories was found to have the low bid according to the new specifications. Incidentally, when I told this story to my brother John, of the Alabama building construction firm of Jones and Hardy, he had a story of his own. He said that Jones and Hardy had bid on jobs in Mississippi for some years, but always unsuccessfully. Then one day, at the opening of bids in Jackson, Governor White, an elderly father figure, had drawn John aside and said, "Son, I hate to see you keep wasting your money to work up bids on Mississippi construction projects. Frankly, only Mississippi contractors are going to get these jobs."

There were, naturally, a host of problems and procedures to be worked out in opening such a large institution, and Michael Newton's very orderly mind added much to establishing clear and coherent policies.

The residency training program

Initially, all the surgical specialties were to be covered by the residents in general surgery, with the exception of a single resident in neurosurgery and one in urology. We had been advised by surgeons in whom I had confidence that it would not be wise to try to develop independent residency programs in each of the surgical divisions, with the limited number of surgical beds that we had in the 350-bed hospital. Nonetheless, I knew that if we got full-time chairmen in the various other divisions of the department, it would be necessary to offer them the opportunity to develop their own residency training programs with their own assigned quota of beds.

Accordingly, we set up a solid training program in general surgery patterned after that at Penn. Since the residents were at various levels and had come from so many different places, it was hard to know just what they knew, how much experience each had had, and what surgical judgment and surgical conscience they had developed—in other words, how far the leadership and clinical discipline of each could be trusted.

Some residents develop sound surgical judgment very early, but others may cause concern and require close supervision almost to the end of their training program. Therefore, we established a modified pyramidal residency so that those without genuine surgical aptitude could be released early—though most of those released found further surgical training elsewhere if they were determined to have a surgical career. To be sure, the reader might ask, if the resident was not good enough to continue at Mississippi, would it be moral for him to finish elsewhere and then foist himself on the public? I can offer three answers. First, the resident might have been a good surgeon but did not exhibit the overall leadership qualities needed to run the teaching service in a university hospital, as compared with others allowed to continue. Second, as in the medical school class, some students are better than others, but all who pass graduate. Third, all residents must eventually pass the American Board of Surgery examinations before they are certified.

As required by the national Joint Commission on Accreditation of Hospitals, a Tissue Committee was promptly established, and all tissue removed at an operation was submitted to pathology for periodic monitoring of a surgeon's results.

We established a searching Mortality and Morbidity Conference, which was held at first monthly but later weekly. The reason for greater frequency was that the case of the patient who had died, or the complication that had occurred, was much more vivid one week later than one month later. The M & M Conference gradually proved to be useful in discouraging an occasional board qualified surgeon who was automatically allowed to practice in the University Hospital but who was not in step with modern surgery. Such a person might feel embarrassed by the fact that the surgical residents knew more than he did. In fact, one surgeon came into my office and frankly said that the kind of surgery we were doing had moved beyond him, and that he would like to be allowed to drop out quietly, which he did. I admired him for this.

Complications in special types of surgery, particularly in the new vascular surgery, were discussed so openly, and criticized so objectively where justified, that this policy gradually caused surgeons unqualified for specific procedures to transfer their private patients to other hospitals in Jackson, which did not have rigid mortality and morbidity reviews. In all this, we sought to develop in the residents a strong surgical conscience. Early on, we kept the name and hospital number of each patient so considered, but later, when malpractice suits became commonplace and paid informers for lawyers were said to be present in most hospitals, we no longer used the patient's name but simply an index number. Otherwise, the naked appraisal of circumstances went unchanged. In fact, a British research fellow from Liverpool who spent a year with us said on departing, "Never will I forget that barbarous exercise you folks call the Mortality Conference!"

The mere fact that each complication and death is going to be presented to his colleagues tends to have a bracing effect on the individual surgeon's constant pursuit of excellence in the care of his patients. We also conducted a Chest-Heart Conference, Gastrointestinal Conference, Tumor Conference, and grand rounds. In addition, obviously, there were daily rounds on all patients—morning, evening, and in between. All resident operating was closely supervised, first, because we did not know what the residents at various levels had been allowed to do at their previous hospitals, and second, because we wanted to build the reputation that the University Hospital provided surgical care at the highest level. The patient's welfare always had to come first.

Gynecologic surgery required special consideration because, while the ob-gyn service required these procedures for their teaching, most of the general surgeons in Jackson did hysterectomies. This problem was solved by an agreement that, first, we would do no gynecologic surgery if Dr. Newton's group did no breast surgery (a quid pro quo) and, second, I would ask general surgical members of my staff to do their gynecological surgery at other hospitals in the city.

Hospital affiliations

The hospital affiliated with our residency program in general surgery and other divisions was the Veterans Hospital, supervised professionally by the University Dean's Committee. This facility, with which we always had the most harmonious relations, was an invaluable resource in patients for housestaff, students, and staff. Certain financial support was also available. Varden Cockrell was initially Chief of Surgery, but later relinquished this post to Harold Conn when he moved up to chief of professional services.

The thoracic residents rotated through the Mississippi State Sanatorium until the tuberculosis surgery dwindled. We had had continual difficulties with the financing of staff and anesthesia coverage of the residents for operations at the sanatorium, and we had asked on numerous occasions if at least some of the patients were not covered by insurance policies which would provide additional income. The business officers there steadfastly insisted that no insurance coverage was available, but this was to be proven untrue. Sadly, the State Auditor eventually exposed embezzlement, unknown to the superintendent, extending back for years—resulting in tragic subsequent events.

Two attempts were made to establish resident rotations at the Baptist Hospital, but this rotation was never very successful. Initially, the problem was inadequate supervision and little resident responsibility. The second time, the residents just got tired of the continually expressed animosity against the university (a classic town-gown conflict) and asked that this elective rotation be discontinued.

Medical student teaching

One hundred thirty-eight medical students were enrolled in September 1955. Thirty were juniors, down from Oxford, and would be the first doctors of medicine graduated in Mississippi for over forty-five years. The members of the clinical faculty had agreed on a classical curriculum for student teaching, at least at the outset. There were lectures, conferences, and patient rounds. We did a lot of spoon-feeding, and for our students this type of instruction proved to be effective over the years. In surgery we emphasized shock and cardiac arrest, infections, fluid and electrolyte problems, wound healing, trauma, intestinal obstruction, and neoplasia. Classes were small, we knew each student personally, and the Socratic method of teaching was applicable and much used.

Patients

The ward or charity patients would of course come as they might, referred by physicians not only in Jackson but from all over the state. However, our means by which to attract private patients were limited. Certainly we would receive virtually no private patients from physicians in the city of Jackson because of the town-gown controversy, which had continued to build slowly.

Few referrals could be expected from other physicians in the University Hospital, since they had very few private patients themselves. Moreover, if one were to vote against some pet project of a clinical colleague at the executive faculty meeting, referrals from that source were apt to be limited for some time.

Clearly, the only way to improve the situation was to do precisely what Dr. Ravdin had always told his staff in Philadelphia: "Gentlemen, we must get our patients from outside Philadelphia." Thus, I accepted any invitation to speak anywhere in the state of Mississippi and nearby states, especially if I could get back in time to operate the next morning. In this way, I gradually built up a referral pattern that made me largely independent of the internal rivalries, which are always a part of any medical center and, indeed, of any other human endeavor.

Research

Inasmuch as we moved our research effort from Memphis to Jackson virtually intact, getting started was easy and immediate. However, we could not do a lot of clinical research with the limited number of patients admitted to the University Hospital, so animal work would be important, fitting in with research in open-heart surgery and organ transplantation. I had sent one of our future residents to the University of Minnesota almost a year before, supported by the Mississippi Heart Association, to observe the open-heart surgery that had just been initiated there and to bring to Jackson, for use in the animal laboratory, the equipment necessary to assemble a heart-lung machine for open-heart surgery. We began this work immediately in our animal laboratory. Experimenting teams in Boston and Paris were vigorously pursuing kidney transplantation, and this appeared to me to be a field where we could begin with the pioneers. Clearly, though, we were going to be far behind Minnesota and other centers in open-heart surgery by the time we could get our program established.

Meanwhile, there was the problem of refinancing our research program, for only part of its support could be transferred from Memphis to Jackson. This time, however, in contrast to the situation I encountered when I arrived in Memphis, our team had a proven track record. Research applications to the National Institutes of Health were promising, and committees assigned to inspect project sites were dispatched to Jackson to see what we had by way of personnel, laboratories, and equipment. In general, they were impressed with the fact that we had an ongoing program, actually transferred intact from Memphis. Research support was soon ample.

One episode concerning a research application is worth recounting. The world-famous cardiologist Paul Dudley White led a team of project-site visitors to review our situation, in response to our request for a broad heart grant. After looking over the hospital and our laboratories, the entourage had got all the way down to the basement. Suddenly noting a men's room on the left, just across from the hospital record room, Dr. White indicated that he and I were to enter the men's room while the other members of the group remained outside. After taking a quick look around, Dr. White turned back to me and said, "Dr. Hardy, now tell me exactly how much money you need." What a situation! I was afraid that if I asked for too much I would appear greedy, and it would militate against our getting the grant. On the other hand, I certainly did not want to ask for a penny less than we might otherwise get.

Looking at him carefully, to see whether he flinched or not, I replied, "Dr. White, we need a great deal of support here to get under way. Would thirty thousand dollars per year be excessive?"

"If that's what you need," he told me, "that's what you'll get." And that was precisely what we got.

We were equally fortunate in getting support from other agencies. Dr. Webb, a superb surgical technician, interested himself in transplantation of the heart and heart-lung, and was able to show a movie at the American College of Surgeons about a year later of a living dog walking around the laboratory postoperatively. Dr. Artz, who had been director of the Brooke Army Medical Research Center and who placed a major emphasis on burns, had his team of research fellows and residents working on metabolic problems. Our research program was off to a good start.

In November 1956, Dr. Ravdin had me invited to a large committee meeting at the NIH of perhaps fifty surgeons from around the country to plan a large-scale chemotherapeutic attack on solid malignant tumors not amenable to surgical excision or radiation. The internists and pediatricians were working with drugs for leukemia. Thus, once I had definitely left Philadelphia, the Professor was very attentive in seeing that useful opportunities were sent my way.

Each surgical resident was required to spend a few months on a research project, following which he could spend additional time in the laboratory if he had found some problem he wished to pursue further, or he could return to the clinical rotations. The objectives were to have the resident learn how to derive statistically valid data, and how to write a paper for publication and present the work at some national meeting. The experimental laboratory work was facilitated by the assistance of thoroughly experienced surgical assistants. I believed then, and still do, that such laboratory experience enriches the physician's critical approach to the physiologic management of his patient, and this program was, on the whole, very successful. However, it was not without surprises. At the annual business meeting of the Southern Society for Clinical Research in New Orleans in 1959, I had urged that the moderator of each scientific session be *instructed* to ask a question or so of each speaker in order to stimulate audience participation during the discussion period. Well, at the 1960 session, one of our residents had read his ten-minute paper well, and I was very pleased. Then the moderator, as instructed, began with, "Doctor, what was the error of your blood volume method?" Our man, rattled, said he didn't know, although he actually did. After a pause, the moderator then asked if he had tried another blood volume method, for comparison. No, he hadn't. Then,

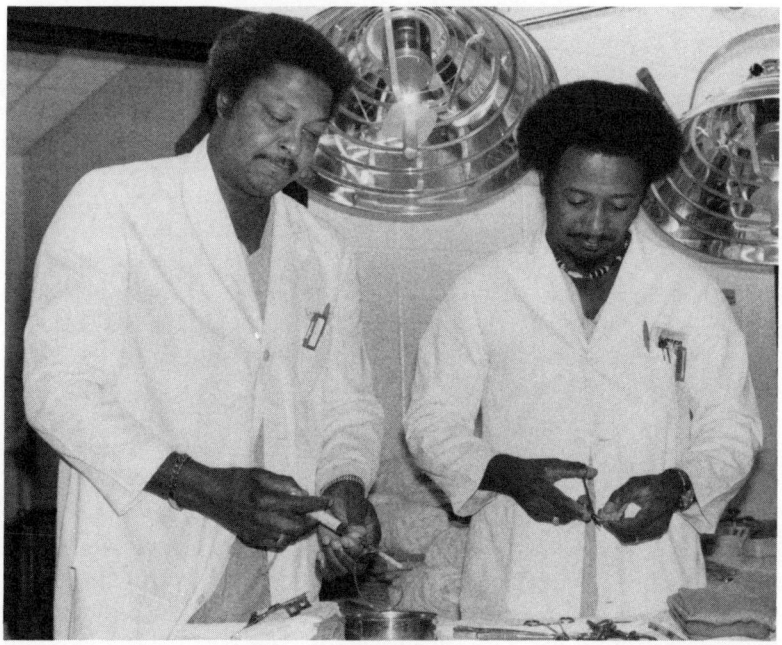

Lynch Evans, Jr. (left) *and Cleveland S. Owens* (right), *experimental laboratory surgical assistants, 28 and 24 years of service, respectively*

as the moderator was trying to think of some question the essayist *could* answer and thus relieve the increasingly awkward situation, our resident faced the moderator and said, "Frankly, Doctor, I never thought much of this work myself!"

Electrical anesthesia

During some metabolic studies that involved stimulating the brain with electrodes, we suspected that such stimulation minimized or abolished pain sensation in the animal. These observations, plus reports from elsewhere, suggested that a carefully controlled electrical current could be used as a general anesthetic (psychiatrists had used electroshock therapy for many years).

After studies in a great many animals, the technique was extended first to minor biopsies in patients, and later to other operations in several patients with far advanced tumors who were willing to give permission to use this anesthetic modality. Extensive psychological and psychiatric tests were conducted, and various other parameters carefully monitored, throughout the operations. There appeared to be no significant aftereffects from the current. The patients felt a tugging but no pain at the site of the incision. They remained awake and were able to repeat precisely anything that might have been said during the course of the operation.

We were not able to raise electrical anesthesia to a level of dependability that could seriously challenge ether anesthesia or other drugs available for this purpose. Our studies halted abruptly when our engineer was hired by a private corporation, for without him I did not feel safe in using the electrical equipment. It has since been shown that electrical stimulation of the brain causes the release of endorphins, the morphinelike substances produced by the body itself.

Laboratory fraud

Every research scientist with a large program risks the publication of imperfect data. My first experience with fraud involved a research technician who had not received the training in chemistry she had recorded on her résumé. She claimed to have graduated in chemistry from a midwestern university, but when she was found absolutely ignorant of what she had been doing for several months, a careful check of her college experience (which should have been done before employment) showed that she had started in chemistry but had dropped out.

The most distressing development, however, involved one of our otherwise satisfactory residents who was caught in flagrant fraud in a research project. Feeling hard pressed to complete some research work amidst his other responsibilities, he had delivered for chemical analysis specimens purported to have come from animals that had undergone a special type of operation, when in fact he had drawn the specimens at random from normal animals. Fortunately, my chief chemical technician routinely reviewed raw data before going over the data with me. She brought in the analyses derived from the specimens delivered to her chemistry laboratory and said, "Dr. Hardy, these results don't make sense and I question their validity." The facts were soon exposed.

Fortunately, we had been spared publication of incorrect data in the national literature. Fraud or simple incompetence in laboratory experiments has seriously impaired the reputations of some of this country's most outstanding scientists and universities. It is an ever-present hazard where many people are conducting experiments without adequate monitoring by an experienced scientist.

Departmental finances

The basic medical school salaries were not adequate to attract and retain clinical faculty for long without supplementary income from private patients, and most of our patients were indigent. This was still ten years before the advent of Medicare and Medicaid, and in Mississippi, the money paid by the latter would never be comparable to that paid in most other states. Therefore, other sources of income were sought; the most helpful in this regard were the Vocational Rehabilitation Service and the Veterans Hospitals. The Vocational Rehabilitation Service, while not paying to the university physicians the full rates paid to surgeons elsewhere in the state, was nonetheless a strong supporter of the University Medical Center.

Eventually the Crippled Children's Service was helpful, but early on it was not to the extent it should have been. The CCS was, to me, the quintessential example of what I came to know as the "Mississippi medical inferiority complex"—that is, the belief that almost any operation could be done better in Memphis, New Orleans, Birmingham, Houston, or the Mayo Clinic than it could be done in Jackson. For example, for years the Mississippi CCS had manned a whole office suite in the Le Bonheur (Children's) Hospital in Memphis to handle all its referrals to doctors in that city, while its own University Hospital in Jackson went begging for patients. Of course, the CCS replied that the patients were sent to other states because either the families or the doctor, often for pure convenience, wanted the "client" sent there. But one suspected that somewhere along the line the welfare and progress of medical growth in Mississippi could have been better served. After some years, the flow of patients toward Jackson did increase measurably and, of course, the state of Mississippi has long since gained confidence and pride in a *variety* of areas.

Departmental financial controls

Before leaving the subject of departmental financial support, the crucial importance of internal monitoring and auditing should be acknowledged. Many an academic administrator's career has been destroyed through embezzlement by a trusted assistant. Therefore, from the beginning, I *made* time to keep up with the monies from all sources and their expenditure, and gave particular attention to the considerable sums the department received from third-party vendors, prior to depositing these funds in university accounts. It was time-consuming, yes, but it represented very economical job insurance. Of course, the best protection is to have honest and highly moral office assistants, with whom I was richly blessed.

Town-gown showdown

The town-gown controversy had continued to build slowly until it reached its high-water mark in a dramatic confrontation on the evening of April 3, 1956. The medical center had proved a much more expensive enterprise than the state legislature had expected. Hence, the university administration was anxious to announce publicly the considerable amounts of grant money brought in by members of the faculty. Our six-county Central Medical Society, however, had a regulation that the appearance of the name of any practicing physician in a newspaper represented unethical competition. After various unsuccessful attempts to reach a compromise, Dean Pankratz and Chancellor Williams decided to release a single announcement to the newspaper, but one that contained the names of all grant recipients and the dollar amounts of their grants; this was to avoid piecemeal releases involving single recipients, who then could be picked off individually by the opposition. Feelings ran high. Each of us on the list received a letter from the secretary of the Central Medical Society, dated March 12:

Dear Dr. Hardy:

According to the Constitution and By-Laws when the Censors Committee receives a complaint against any of the Society's members, they notify the member of the complaint; and the Censors Committee request an explanation from the accused member.

As Secretary of the Censors Committee, I am writing you in regard to the complaint received by the Censors Committee, and the charges which are as follows:

"Your attention is called to two clippings, one each from the Clarion-Ledger, Jackson, Mississippi, dated Feb. 23, 1956 under the title of "U. Medical Center has over $200,000 in Research Funds," in which the names of individuals who are members of the Central Medical Society are used in the announcement. A clipping in the Jackson Daily News of the afternoon of Thursday, Feb. 23, 1956, under the heading "Medical Center is Helped by Grants-in-Aid" which also mentioned names of members of the Central Medical Society. . . ."

As a member of our Society, you have violated the provisions set-up in the policies and recommendations regarding newspaper releases passed by this Society on January 3, 1956. A copy of this policy was distributed to the Directors of the various Hospitals embraced in our Society. In the case of the University Medical Center, a copy was handed to Dr. David Wilson on December 8, 1955 by me, as Secretary of the Society.

The Censors Committee expects an explanation from you to clarify this complaint at your earliest convenience.

Sincerely yours,

Wm. E. Lotterhos, M.D.
Secretary

I answered Dr. Lotterhos, relating the facts as they stood.

The Central Medical Society's Censors Committee called on all of us on the afternoon of April 3 and voted that we be censured at the society's meeting that night. It was of course an embarrassment, and could possibly lead to expulsion from the medical society and the opprobrium resulting therefrom. That night we all went down to be "executed" at perhaps the best-attended meeting ever. But between the meeting in the afternoon and the one in the evening, the Executive Committee had changed the recommendation to censure of only Dean Pankratz (as representative of the medical school), preferring not to attempt to get a positive vote against each individual faculty member. (As is recorded in the archives of the medical society, this decision to censure the dean alone was made by the Executive Committee at 5:30 P.M., before the evening full meeting, but no one at the university was made aware of it.)

We were stunned. Everyone knew that Dean Pankratz did not practice and could not have profited financially from the newspaper announcement. At this point, Orlando Andy leaned across the table and said, "Did you hear that? Only Dean Pankratz!" It was instantly clear they'd made a huge tactical blunder. Everyone knew the dean wouldn't hurt a flea, and a vote to censure him was unlikely to pass. Meanwhile, it gave me the splendid strategic position of defending not myself—their primary target—but my leader, the dean. I decided on the spot to make the most of it. Asking for the podium, I said all the things that should have been said over the past three years by those charged with organizing the medical school. I minced no words, letting the chips fall where they might, and closed with the ringing declamation, "I cannot believe that medical statesmanship is dead in this town, and I want a vote!" The vote was taken, and of perhaps one hundred or more doctors present, only one or possibly two stood up, neither one the ringleader. That night at home I got a number of telephone calls from town physicians, congratulating me and affirming their support.

The minutes of that meeting were recorded in the archives as follows:

> Dr. James Hardy expressed his convictions in defense of Dean Pankratz by saying the University Medical Center was going to be a first class Medical School and this was the main goal of Dean Pankratz. In order to be a first class Medical School and have first class students, Research Funds were necessary, and publicity of such funds were necessary to impress students and grantors of the work that the University Medical Center was doing. Research is one of the prime objectives of the University Medical Center.

Dr. Arthur Guyton spoke in behalf of the Dean and the Medical School, of the necessity of Research Funds and asked for the committee that Dean Pankratz suggested to be formed to "iron out" the differences in publicity of the Medical School and the Society.

Dr. Thomas Marland defended the Dean, but asked that the Committee be formed as the Board of Higher Learning were not members of the Society and could not make the rules for the Society's member.

The motion to censure Dean Pankratz was defeated overwhelmingly. Following this face-to-face encounter, there was a standoff in which both sides drew back and let the years reduce this inevitable competition to a permanently sustained but tolerable level. (Now, in 1985, the majority of the members and officers of the Central Medical Society are graduates of this school, to my great pride and satisfaction. In fact, the Executive Committee has granted my request to be allowed to bring Weezie, the only nonphysician, to each dinner meeting, so that I do not leave her to dine alone now that the children are all gone.)

Medical school policies

It became increasingly apparent, indeed urgent, that committees be established to regulate the admission and also the promotion of medical students. James Rice, head of pharmacology, and I began to push for a permanent Student Promotions Committee, with membership rotating among the faculty. This was to protect the dean from pressure to reinstate individuals who had flunked out or had been dropped "for reasons other than academic." Curiously, some departmental chairmen were strongly opposed to such a committee, for reasons that were a mystery to me.

I recall one student who had spent six years in three medical schools but had never made it through the third-year class. Now, out of kindness, Dean Pankratz had let him come to Jackson and had admitted him in our third-year class. Some of us were astonished by this. After some very vigorous and even acerbic discussions at a faculty meeting, I stated that my investigations disclosed that for the past eleven years not a single medical student had been dropped from the two-year medical school at Oxford for academic failure; the students had been allowed to keep repeating until they finally got out and transferred to other schools for the third year. Dean Pankratz challenged this statement, but Mrs. Lallah White, registrar, on cue promptly confirmed it. Mrs. White had herself long deplored the reinstatement of inadequate students.

In another case, the executive faculty had dropped a student for academic failure as well as for character deficiencies. To our surprise, however, he showed up again the following fall, having prevailed upon Dean Pankratz, who was a long-time friend of the family. Here again, the dean was so sympathetic that he simply could not turn down a request.

Finally, the faculty managed to pass the motion that a formal Student Promotions Committee be established. So close was the vote that when two of us were out of town this decision was reversed. However, it was later reversed again, and a lasting promotions committee was established. The dean retained the ultimate prerogative of overriding the promotions committee, but one suspects that he was relieved to be freed from continuing pressure from outside. Incidentally, the advent of a formal Student Promotions Committee put an end, at a single draconian stroke, to the old policy of allowing inadequate students to keep repeating until they finally graduated. This, not surprisingly, thinned the ranks of the student body considerably, for a time. In fact, the national medical school accreditation authorities cited our school for an excessive withdrawal rate. However, research showed that while our drop-out rate of 12 percent was higher than many other schools in the nation, it was equalled or exceeded by twenty-five of the approximately eighty-five schools.

Another need was the creation of a Faculty Promotions Committee. Some department chairmen automatically put up their members for promotion by the dean, whether they deserved it or not. Other chairmen, especially those involved in research and publication, felt that clinical faculty members should demonstrate some academic pursuit other than treating patients and giving occasional conferences and lectures. While the well-worn motto "publish or perish" has often been ridiculed, it still remains a major objective criterion by which promotions may be evaluated. If no one in the department publishes, the department will itself perish on the national scene.

Ultimately, we were able to establish a promotions committee, which was advisory to the executive faculty and ultimately to the dean, though the dean usually went along with the recommendations. This was true of all seven deans or administrative officers who were to serve during my tenure.

There were weaknesses in the promotion system. By the time the committee was fully active, many promotions had already been made which were patently undeserved and which tended to diminish the stature of the associate-professor and full-professor ranks. Also, sometimes it became necessary to promote a clearly undeserving individual simply to maintain clinical coverage in a given specialty. To be fair, I must acknowledge that before the Faculty Promotions Committee was established I had promoted freely also, so as not to penalize surgery faculty members.

A Faculty Search Committee mechanism, for the recruitment of department chairmen, was also established.

When the national Liaison Committee on Medical Education Representing the American Medical Association and the Association of Medical Colleges came to inspect the medical school, it was fully accredited without limitations.

By the end of 1956–57, the general policies and procedures in all phases of the Department of Surgery's activities were in place and the department was moving steadily forward.

An operation

During his campaign, Governor James Plemon Coleman had repeatedly had indigestion following political dinners. He had attributed his symptoms to the rubbery chicken and pasty peas of the campaign circuit, but after he was in office the symptoms continued. His longtime good friend, Dr. Verner Holmes, whom he had appointed as the medical member of the Board of Trustees of Institutions of Higher Learning, persuaded him to be admitted to the University Hospital for a complete checkup. Dr. Snavely and I were asked to examine the governor. After each of us had done a very careful history and physical examination, we withdrew to a conference room across the hall, sat down, and looked at each other.

"What do you think is wrong with him?" Snavely asked.

"If he weren't the governor, I'd say he has gallstones."

"That's exactly what I think," Bob said.

Appropriate X-ray studies disclosed that he did have gallstones.

After we had discussed the situation with Governor Coleman and Dr. Holmes, the governor's retinue, accompanied by highway patrol cars, sped out from the University Hospital and spirited him back to the Governor's Mansion. We thought this was the last we would hear from the governor. We suspected he would not come to the new University Hospital and its young staff for the gallbladder operation which he needed, but a few days later he returned and announced that he was there to have his operation. He said we had done the most careful physical examination he had ever had.

Bob Snavely urged me to get surgeons from the city to scrub with me. However, it was only a gallbladder, a relatively minor operation in my opinion. The only thing major about it was that it was on the governor. Therefore I insisted that my assistants would be my two chief residents, in whom I had every confidence. Snavely was considerably perturbed over this. The operation was set for September 18, 1957. After I had scrubbed and was about to back through the swinging door into the operating room to perform the operation, I turned to Bob Snavely, who was pacing the floor in the hall, and said, "Well, Coach, any last words?"

He fixed me with a baleful stare and said, "Look, Buster, this had better be good."

It was good enough, and the governor made an uneventful recovery. He became a devoted supporter of the University Hospital throughout his term of office and in the years afterward when he was a federal judge with the Fifth Circuit Court of Appeals in New Orleans. As he left the hospital, he hinted that the medical school's biennial budget would have no problems when the legislature met the following January. Had the medical center been denied all access to private patients, this fortunate medical admission to the University Hospital could not have occurred. I hoped that this fact had not escaped Chancellor Williams up in Oxford.

The question then arose at higher levels as to whether or not the governor should be sent a bill. Dean Pankratz and Chancellor Williams decided that he should be sent a bill, though it need not be excessive.

Accomplishments and mistakes

By 1957 the research and teaching programs were effective, and we were beginning to get more patients, though the University Hospital was still far from full most of the time. Good-natured hassles with Dr. David Wilson, hospital director, concerning various policies and needs continued, and Dean Pankratz remained a lovable but indecisive administrator.

The mistakes I made were, in retrospect, avoidable—at least to a considerable extent. My concern was that we must push forward, as hard and as fast as possible, while affairs were still fluid and subject to influence. I knew that things could easily settle into a comfortable mediocrity, because Dean Pankratz did not have the same academic aspirations for the school that I did. Perhaps he was right, since his main objective was to place more doctors in Mississippi, whereas my objective was to produce doctors from a nationally and hopefully even internationally recognized department of surgery. It would be impossible for surgery to achieve its full potential unless the other departments of the medical school likewise aspired to academic excellence.

Certainly I wrote too many letters. Reading the file copies of those letters now, I realize that they were often too firm—though factual, they were sometimes less than diplomatic. Even so, I had long since learned the value of a letter as a record, as opposed to a telephone call which might or might not be answered or considered carefully. I knew that happy and welcome letters, such as those of admiration or congratulation, were treasured, kept, and read again and again; the alternative—a simple phone call—is far easier but also evanescent. On the other hand, I may not have been quite so fully aware that unwelcome letters can likewise be filed and read again and again.

Administration has to be learned. For example, I was perhaps too short in giving directions without asking for comments. A certain amount of seniority (and, in the army, often physical stature) is helpful in commanding, but most of us were approximately the same age.

Another of my mistakes probably was failure to hold enough staff meetings or to consult my colleagues often enough. Actually, I was not unaware of this, but I hesitated to ask for advice that I might not take. Despite many opinions from many people of different medical backgrounds, only one policy could be adopted and it had to accord with the overall objectives of the department. It had become abundantly clear to me that some colleagues viewed the request for consultation as a definitive "How should I treat my patient?" or, "How should I handle this situation?" If that advice went unheeded, the consultant might be acutely offended. In my view, a consultant was one who gave advice, which could then be taken or ignored as the original physician deemed appropriate. Certainly I had pushed everyone hard, as indeed I had pushed myself.

During that first year I was sometimes guilty of failing to get all the facts from various sources before making decisions, especially in interpersonal disputes. I learned to sleep on important administrative decisions rather than make them when I was tired. Moreover, new as I was in handling responsibility for a large enterprise, I initially found it difficult to delegate authority and then allow that designee to carry out the mission. For example, once when I had asked Dr. Artz to perform a particular function, some of the residents promptly came to me to complain about what he was doing. They seemed to have a point, and I asked Dr. Artz if he would be willing to modify his approach accordingly. To this, Curt, a master organizer, replied, "Jim, if you want me to do something I will do it, but please don't undercut me when I try." He was right. In another instance, Dr. Harold Conn, chief of surgery at the Veterans Administration Hospital, said much the same thing. "Jim," he said, "this loyalty business works both ways. Your troops have got to know that you support them, if you expect them to support you." I got the point and did not forget it.

And, last, I am sure I appeared truculent to some. But I was afraid to leave important decisions to protection by the dean's office, because of unsettling administrative experiences in the past.

Departmental unrest

Some unpleasant departmental problems began to surface, with the struggle of the chairmen of the divisions of anesthesiology, neurosurgery, and orthopaedics to become separate departments in the medical school. This was a national struggle as well.

As his cancer recurred, Bittenbender began campaigning to make anesthesiology a separate department, believing this would be required to entice anyone else to take his position in the future. To my dismay, Dr. Wilson had apparently joined Dr. Bittenbender in writing letters to numerous centers in the United States stating that anesthesiology had in fact been made a separate department. This was not true, and as much as I liked "Bit" personally, I did not believe that the wishes of any individual should so profoundly alter stated and published medical school policy. I still don't. Therefore, I opposed this at the executive faculty meeting and requested a secret ballot to protect those who did not wish to vote openly against Dr. Bittenbender; the executive faculty supported my position. Actually, I had been doubtful of the outcome. With regard to most prospective executive faculty meetings, I knew which third were with me, which third were against, and which members might not know much about the subject and thus would not have a firm conviction—and which of these might be persuaded by a firm and eloquent presentation. Incidentally, in my experience, I have found it is best to speak last, taking into consideration the points made by the previous speakers. (With nominations, however, it is often preferable to nominate first, for this may discourage further entries.)

During Dr. Bittenbender's terminal illness, we had been searching for a new chairman of anesthesiology and had attracted a good man from Western Reserve University. He was to bring a young assistant with him. Literally the week before he was to have moved to Jackson, he called, in genuine embarrassment, and regretted to say that, at the last minute, he could not come. He thought he had cleared the matter of female tubal ligations with his church in Cleveland, but this decision had been reversed, even though we had assured him that he need never have any association with sterilizations in our University Hospital. The archbishop had ruled that he could work in no hospital where sterilizations were permitted, no matter what his arrangement might be.

The young deputy did come, however, and he did his best with the cadre of nurse anesthetists we had at the time. The responsibility was very stressful, in view of his relative youth and limited independent experience. Some months later he was found dead on a sandbar in the Mississippi River, with his boat pulled well up onto the gravel.

Thus, the anesthesiology search had to begin once again. Throughout my tenure, personnel recruiting remained a most time-consuming activity, as it was so often fruitless for long periods. Moreover, it now became clear that the ground had been pretty well cut out from under my position that anesthesiology should be part of surgery. Under the circumstances, I suggested that Dean Pankratz do what he thought best in this matter, and he did grant anesthesiology departmental status. Dr. Ravdin later told me that here I had made a major mistake, but he did not know the circumstances firsthand. I really had no other choice. Parenthetically, the national shortage of academic anesthesiologists persisted and presented problems intermittently throughout the entire thirty years of my tenure.

Meanwhile, as noted previously, it had become clear that we could not expect sufficient orthopaedic coverage from local surgeons in practice. After all, they were fully engaged already. We had tried to attract a full-time head of the Division of Orthopaedics, and we had been considering a young surgeon who was just completing his residency at the University of Chicago, Dr. William F. Enneking.

He clearly was an able individual who had a good academic record. On the other hand, there were those who suggested that he was difficult to get along with, and in fact, one of Dean Pankratz's friends told him we would rue the day if Enneking were invited to come to Jackson. But we were in a weak position, and we decided to take a chance on his firm personality in order to get his competence in orthopaedics. We offered him the title of associate professor of surgery (orthopaedics), though he was just completing his residency. He accepted with the clear understanding that orthopaedics was not a separate department and that there were no plans to make it so. But hardly had he arrived, proving surgically able as had been reported, than he began to agitate. He pushed first for a full professorship and, soon after that was granted, for a separate Department of Orthopaedics. When he threatened to resign unless he got a separate department, however, Dean Pankratz, to my surprise, accepted his resignation.

Diminished political capital

Dean Pankratz, to his great credit, at times invited Chancellor Williams to sit down for private interviews with heads of departments at the medical school. To my best memory, Dr. Pankratz was the only one of the seven administrative officers who presided during my tenure—David S. Pankratz (1954–60), W. Alton Bryant (1960–64), Robert Q. Marston (1961–66), John A. Gronvall (1966–67), Robert E. Carter (1967–70), Robert E. Blount (1970–73), and Norman C. Nelson (1973–)—who did this, though each served earnestly, according to his basic personality. It seemed to me a generous and courageous thing for Dean Pankratz to do, and it showed that he was not concerned about having different views expressed to his superior.

Chancellor Williams asked me how things seemed to be going, and perhaps I told him my views a bit too forcefully. He listened for a time and then said abruptly, "Dr. Hardy, do you play golf?"

"No, Chancellor Williams, I almost never play golf, some tennis."

"Do you cook steaks in the backyard?"

"No, Chancellor, I don't."

"Well, thank you very much." It was clear that the interview was at an end.

I did not have to be clairvoyant to perceive that my stock with

Chancellor Williams had been sadly depleted by the skirmishes with anesthesiology, orthopaedics, and neurosurgery, not to mention my prodding of Dean Pankratz to take actions to assume what I saw as the proper posture for a medical school that aspired to greatness. One has various political strengths with almost every individual in one's orbit. I judged mine with Chancellor Williams not more than five on a scale of one to ten. It was obvious that I had done about all I could to influence medical school policy. Therefore, it was no great surprise to me when neurosurgery, in addition to anesthesiology, was declared a separate department, without prior consultation with me, in early 1960. Actually, it was apparent that this decision had been made for some time, but the announcement simply delayed. I was distressed, for it appeared that the chairman had been rewarded for consistently ignoring administrative and resident supervision duties, though he was a prodigious worker in the laboratory. Future events were to vindicate my perception.

My judgment that Chancellor Williams saw me as a disturbing element, if not a downright troublemaker, was soon confirmed. During our interview, I had complained that the medical center had no clear sense of direction, that there was a desperate need for some type of planning so that we wouldn't simply stumble or drift from day to day. Whether as a result of my remarks or not, several weeks later there came down from Oxford the directive that a Long-Range Planning Committee be established. Somewhat conspicuously, I thought, my name was not listed among those invited to become members of this large and important committee. My reaction was mixed. The directive confirmed my judgment that I had pretty well played out my hand with Chancellor Williams and could expect no more support there, at least for the time being. On the other hand, I shuddered at the thought of the interminable hours spent in the meetings of such committees, and on that score at least I was gratified.

What nettled me most was that I had accepted the chairmanship with the firm understanding, approved by the Board of Trustees and definitely a part of my agreement, that all the three restive divisions would be a part of the Department of Surgery.

Dean Pankratz had announced his resignation shortly after having made neurosurgery a separate department. He went to Memphis as a resident in psychiatry at age 62. No other individual had labored as long and successfully to establish the solid four-year medical school. He left the state of Mississippi forever in his debt.

Robert Q. Marston was recruited as dean and soon became vice-chancellor. Thereafter I never had to expend time and energy wastefully to maintain the integrity of the Department of Surgery.

Drug addiction

The problem of drug addiction in patients is common to all hospitals. Surgeons are alert for patients who return to the emergency room repeatedly, complaining of abdominal pain and even asking for still another operation, just to get shots of morphine or Demerol. Practicing physicians, too, are at risk of drug dependence because of strain and fatigue, and because the relief of the opiate is so readily available through professional sources.

I was completely unprepared, however, for my first confrontation with the addiction of a surgical resident. This young physician had been a medical student at Mississippi, had interned elsewhere, and had begun his residency July 1. He called me at home on the fourth of July and said he had to see me at once. Surprised, I told him to come to my home.

He expressed much agitation, as we sat on a bench on the lawn, away from the children. "I just can't face the responsibility," he said.

"What responsibility do you mean?"

"The responsibility for patients' lives. I'm constantly afraid I'll do something wrong and kill somebody."

"You must not feel that way. Your job now is simply to see the patient and then call your immediate superior—pass the buck. After all, you've been on the job only four days. Why don't you keep trying for a while? If at mid-year or next summer you still feel the same way, you can resign gracefully without prejudicing your future."

A year or so later a very responsible resident came and told me he thought he had seen R., through the crack at the hinges of a partially open door, injecting himself with something about three o'clock in the morning. He and another resident had then gone to R.'s room and found highly suspicious paraphernalia and a tourniquet.

Confronted, R. adamantly denied taking any drug whatsoever, not even a barbiturate. Dean Marston thought we had better call the director of the state Department of Health. We did, and the director told us that not more than five percent of such addicts were ever completely cured. As Dean Marston and I were not trained to catch an offender, he offered to send over their narcotics investigator, a former FBI man. Within thirty minutes the officer brought

R. back to my office in tears and told him, "Drop your pants!" There, on his thighs, were perhaps as many as fifty needle marks. He had been volunteering to help the nurses by taking narcotic syringes to the patients. He would then pop into an empty room or closet and shoot himself right through the cloth of his pants pocket. Patients, whom he then injected with salt solution, had complained they got no relief from pain. The outcome was that he took the cure several times but eventually died of an overdose elsewhere.

We were equally oblivious to the development of addiction in another resident, who was caught promptly at his first job as he stole narcotics from the medical bags of his colleagues. Here again, we should have been more suspicious of the marked change in personality that he had exhibited.

The pressure of clinical responsibility, or perhaps the burden of selfblame for a patient's death, has broken many a young physician.

First open-heart surgery in Mississippi

We began working in the animal laboratory with the heart-lung machine in 1956, but it was not until 1959 that we operated on our first patient. The nurses from the operating room and anesthesia had joined Watts Webb and me in the animal laboratory to practice before doing the first human case. The difficulties had been substantial. To begin with, the University Hospital did not have the finances to buy a new heart-lung machine, and we had to bring the equipment from the experimental laboratory to the hospital operating room for the operation. The blood bank was a perennial problem, with even routine surgery cases frequently canceled for lack of blood. Heart cases had far greater transfusion needs. (At that time we had to depend substantially on blood drawn by our residents from donating inmates at the state penitentiary about 170 miles away.) There was no intensive care unit and only a modest recovery room. The anesthesia available was limited. Twenty-four-hour laboratory support was restricted because of a need for equipment to perform arterial blood gas analyses promptly.

Therefore, it was with much satisfaction that Watts Webb and I did our first open-heart operation on a five-year-old child under hypothermia on January 27, 1959. It required opening the patient's stenotic pulmonary valve leading out of the right ventricle, a simple procedure as open-heart operations go. This went well, so we operated on another boy for the same heart lesion ten days later, but this time we used the heart-lung machine. We were thus launched, and though progress was not as rapid as we would have liked it to be, we were ultimately successful in making the open-heart program stable. We were not surprised that the pump oxygenator had functioned satisfactorily, but in those days the almost laboratory-built heart-lung machines were associated with many hazards, the worst being the constant risk of air being pumped into the patient through the arterial blood return line. This could have a devastating effect on the brain as well as on the muscle of the heart itself.

"The Closed Society"

The political forces in Mississippi, by an intricate series of maneuvers, had managed virtually to ignore the United States Supreme Court decision in 1955 in favor of public school integration. Increasingly, Mississippi was indeed the "closed society."* Almost all public news sources rigidly maintained the hard segregationist line, whether from actual belief or from social and economic coercion. Almost every village and town developed its white Citizens Council with the avowed purpose of maintaining segregation, ostensibly under law. Economic boycott and social ostracism were commonly the lot of those who exhibited even the slightest evidence of moderation on racial relations. Private schools, almost nonexistent before, sprang up like mushrooms. Public swimming pools were closed, denying a generation of children the chance to learn to swim. (I recalled how many soldiers on our ship during the war had been afraid of the water when depth bombs were exploding or during abandon-ship drills. They could not swim.)

The one voice of moderation that could be heard publicly was that of the *Jackson State Times*. Editor Oliver Emmerich wrote editorials from time to time which took at least a moderate tone in acquainting his readers with the facts of life, i.e., that federal law ultimately was going to have to be obeyed. Personally, I had become increasingly concerned over the direction in which our political and economic establishment was taking us; especially, that it was becoming increasingly hazardous even to discuss dissenting views. Accordingly, I had written Mr. Emmerich about one of his editorials, that "strikes a blow against the type of thought control which has been creeping upon us steadily for the last several years."

"I was cheered by your editorial concerning censorship in Jack-

---

*James W. Silver, *Mississippi: The Closed Society* (New York: Harcourt, Brace & World, 1963, 1964).

son," I wrote. "I know nothing whatever about the movie *I Passed for White*, but I deeply disapprove self-appointed censorship by any group not duly elected to serve this purpose. Furthermore, except for the protection of children, I find no need for censorship of any type except where the national security is at stake, or where individual personal rights might be violated by public disclosure of certain types of information.

"I am sure you know that your editorials have had a far reaching effect upon a great many thinking people in this state. I can say for all of them that we hope you will continue, and that gradually the general intellectual climate which has begun to constrict us will be dissipated by the naked truth, courageously delivered from your pages."

That night, in September of 1960, I had a number of telephone calls congratulating me on my courage. This was the first I knew that Mr. Emmerich had published my letter. Naive as I was, it had not occurred to me that he would publish the private letter, and I felt that the congratulatory telephone calls were perhaps misplaced. Nonetheless, I did want the black people to get a fair shake, if only to unburden my own conscience—as Martin Luther King had often said would be the white man's reward.

The University Medical Center, as Mississippians at large saw us, represented an island of moderates in a sea of reactionary arch-conservatives. True, most of the senior faculty at the University Medical Center were from other states, or at least had received extensive medical training in the North. It was a sad time for Mississippi. The University Medical Center, located about 175 miles south of the university proper at Oxford, led a charmed life with respect to direct political interference in its daily affairs. But obviously it suffered the same fate as all other Mississippi educational institutions with respect to the rapidly increasing difficulty in recruiting and retaining teachers and trainees.

During this period I began to get offers from other universities, but conditions were still tolerable and we all kept hoping that integration would come to pass without too much more damage to our medical school.

> Listen, please listen, a distant voice chanted:
> Stay, just stay, and bloom where you're planted.
> —Gilbert S. Campbell

Integration comes to Mississippi

Ross Barnett was elected governor in 1960. He was an ultraconservative in racial matters, a damage suit lawyer in private life. He had around him the leaders of the white Citizens Councils and doubtless a considerable representation of the Ku Klux Klan. He had run on a "segregation forever" platform in this, his third try for the office. In my judgment, his administration represented the most difficult period for the University of Mississippi that occurred during the entire thirty years of my association with the institution. Some of the public pronouncements he made and the things he did, in open and flagrant defiance of federal law, were so exasperating that one day I asked his distant cousin and my faculty colleague, Dr. William O. Barnett, "Bill, who on earth is advising Ross Barnett?"

"Nobody is advising him. He believes exactly what he says."

Up until 1962, the political system had succeeded in preventing the entrance of any black student to the white universities, including the University of Mississippi. James Meredith, a military veteran, had applied in 1961, but his admission had been blocked, often by long, drawn out court procedures. By the fall of 1962, however, all legal maneuvers available to the state had been exhausted, and on October 1, 1962, the United States Supreme Court refused to review the decision of the Fifth Circuit Court of Appeals that had directed, in effect, that Meredith be admitted to "Ole Miss."

Riots ensued in which the federal marshals accompanying Meredith were overwhelmed and required reinforcements. The radios and one television station were constantly breathing defiance, even inciting to arms for defense at Oxford. One person, and one alone to my knowledge, a young executive with the Lamar Life Insurance Company, came on the company's television station and agonizingly declared the folly of resisting federal marshals and troops. He was William H. Mounger. If there is no risk, there is no courage. At great risk of corporate retaliation, he performed possibly the most courageous act I recall witnessing in Jackson. Ultimately, by the U.S. Army troops, Meredith was matriculated.

Even now, it is impossible for me to convey to the reader the hold that Ross Barnett had on ordinary Mississippians. Indoctrinated by tradition in the first place, they had heard virtually nothing but racial propaganda from their leaders and public media for years, some since their childhood. I came to fully comprehend this Mississippi mindset at a football game which became a political microcosm. The game was planned by Dr. Jorğe A. Rodriguez, a member of our staff who also was an outstanding medical illustrator. He had arranged a football game between a Mexican team and a local college team from Jackson in the municipal football stadium on the night of September 15, 1962. My wife and I attended, and there was a large crowd present, considering the relative obscurity of the two teams that were playing. Just before the game was to begin, the floodlights were directed to a gate at the end of the stadium and in came Governor Ross Barnett and his entourage. Stepping to a microphone, he intoned his standard call to arms, "*I love Mississippi!*" Instantly, the crowd was on its feet, cheering with a frenzy that could hardly have been exceeded by that at a Nuremberg Congress. It was almost frightening in its intensity, underscoring the fanaticism of the average citizen and reflecting the momentous inner struggle that would have to occur before Mississippi could emerge into the mainstream of the United States. My wife and I refused to stand, but we were actually afraid of physical violence to our persons by those surrounding us. It was not a happy time. At halftime, a message from President John F. Kennedy was read, since this was an international event to foster good will between our country and Mexico on the anniversary of Mexico's independence from Spain. The president's message was roundly booed.

These kinds of events had pervasive and devastating effects on the University Medical Center. For years after the Oxford riots, we received virtually no applications for surgical training in our department from senior medical students outside the state of Mississippi. Not unexpectedly, many faculty members quietly found posts elsewhere, and the replacement of these able people proved enormously difficult. Even when a doctor could be induced to look with favor upon coming to our Department of Surgery, the spouse would absolutely refuse to go to Mississippi, no matter what the attractiveness of the position itself.

Finally, before letting the matter rest, the disaster (or fiasco) at Oxford crucially blunted the reputation for increasing excellence that Chancellor J. D. Williams had achieved at the University of Mississippi, his administration having been the longest in the history of the school. He was criticized by some for not defying Ross Barnett and the state government, but such critics simply did not know the situation. No lesser force than the U.S. military could have had any effect on the state government, the white Citizens Councils, or the Ku Klux Klan at that time. President Kennedy came on television on the Sunday afternoon before the Oxford riots. Using both argument and flattery, he pleaded eloquently with the state to admit Meredith in accordance with federal law. There was much speculation that Governor Barnett had already agreed privately but had later reneged under pressure from his fanatical henchmen. The army then installed Meredith at Oxford, using troops and tanks, and the rest is history.

Months later, Chancellor Williams invited Dean Robert Marston and me to go fishing with him at Sardis Lake, a few miles outside of Oxford. He had brought along the university chef, who set up tents. That evening, at a table with white linen, illuminated by candlelight amidst the whispering pines under a starlit sky, the chancellor told us quietly—he said for the first time—just what his personal thoughts had been during the Oxford crisis. Its destructive impact upon this proud and able academician was all too clear. He had always taken pride in his long administration, in the fact that there had never been political interference—only to end in such a shambles. Of the many humiliations and embarrassments he had suffered, he said one of the most wryly cynical was an article in the *New York Times*. It had described him (as I recall now) as "a man who over the years has developed protective coloring—dark suits, dark ties, timid statements. . . ." I fully realized, for the first time, the staggering assault that the chancellor had sustained.

The federal government, affirmative action programs, and full compliance

The federal government seemed to single out Mississippi, and in particular the Hospital of the University of Mississippi, as the strategic battleground to integrate hospital services. While the University Hospital had presented no problem for several years, focus turned to a nearby private hospital; it did not receive federal funds directly, making it impossible to force integration there. There was a loophole in the Medicare law that permitted payment to noncompliant hospitals for emergencies—it was said that the largest private hospital in Jackson had the largest number of emergency admissions in the entire South. I doubt this, but there can be no question that many patients were admitted to noncompliance hospitals who were not in fact emergencies, but for whom the federal government continued to pay. The federal teams from Atlanta utilized every possible means to harass and gain leverage over hospitals. One day I received written instructions that I must at once cease allowing residents to go to the Baptist Hospital. Otherwise, there was the threat, always hanging over us, that *all* University Medical Center funding from the federal government would be cut off abruptly. This would be disastrous.

We had residents in plastic surgery who went to observe special surgery at Baptist Hospital, but who were not paid by that hospital, nor did they have any organic connection with it. The federal monitors sought to halt even these visits, using the argument that the University Medical Center, though in full compliance itself, was indirectly assisting a hospital that was not in compliance. The solution to the problem was obvious: If the government would simply cut off Medicare payments to noncompliant hospitals, the situation would change immediately. Medicare and Medicaid had now come to represent a substantial segment of the financial support of most major hospitals in the United States. This situation dragged on for a period of time, but ultimately the government appeared to stop payments to noncompliant hospitals, and general compliance was achieved.

We had our own experiences with affirmative action in the University Medical Center. One day Mrs. Maurine Twiss, Director of Public Information, was making a television tape for in-house projection, depicting the early days of the University Medical Center. She first interviewed me and then turned to a large, black, uniformed and armed policewoman, for both of us had been present from the founding of the hospital.

"Officer Kelly," Mrs. Twiss began, with her best television smile, "you first had a career in our laundry. Would you please tell our viewers just what influenced you to shift from your laundry career to assume your present career in law enforcement?"

"Well, Miz Twiss, it wuz like this. Chief Wilson, he done come up to me and said, 'Look, the feds say we got to have two women on the force, one white and one black. You want the job?'"

CHAPTER 14
Human Organ Transplantation

The possibility of replacing worn-out individual organs has challenged human imagination throughout the ages. Consider the imagery of the Greek Chimera, the Minotaur, and the wings of Daedalus and Icarus. And now this dream is at hand.

It would be hard to impart to beginners, at this late date, the huge excitement and challenge the pioneers of transplantation felt in the 1950s and 1960s. I will explain how transplantation has come about, first in a general discussion and then in sections dealing with specific organs.

GENERAL CONSIDERATIONS
History

The skin was the first organ transplanted. It is recorded that the ancient Hindus and possibly the Egyptians treated destruction of the nose by transplanting a pedicle of full-thickness skin from the cheek. However, it was G. Baronio, in Italy, who demonstrated at the beginning of the nineteenth century that while full-thickness skin autografts (from one site to another on same subject) persisted indefinitely, allografts (from an unrelated donor, also called homografts) sloughed in a few days. However, the significance of this observed difference was not understood, and the problem was not examined carefully again until a century later.

The monumental studies conducted by Charles Darwin and Gregor Mendel, in the middle of the nineteenth century, led to discoveries which ultimately provided much of the foundation on which modern transplantation biology has been established. Darwin gathered his specimens and data, on which his *Origin of Species* was based, while on several years of exploration voyages on H.M.S. *Beagle*. His theories implied basic biological differences between species. Father Mendel, an Austrian monk, worked out the classic

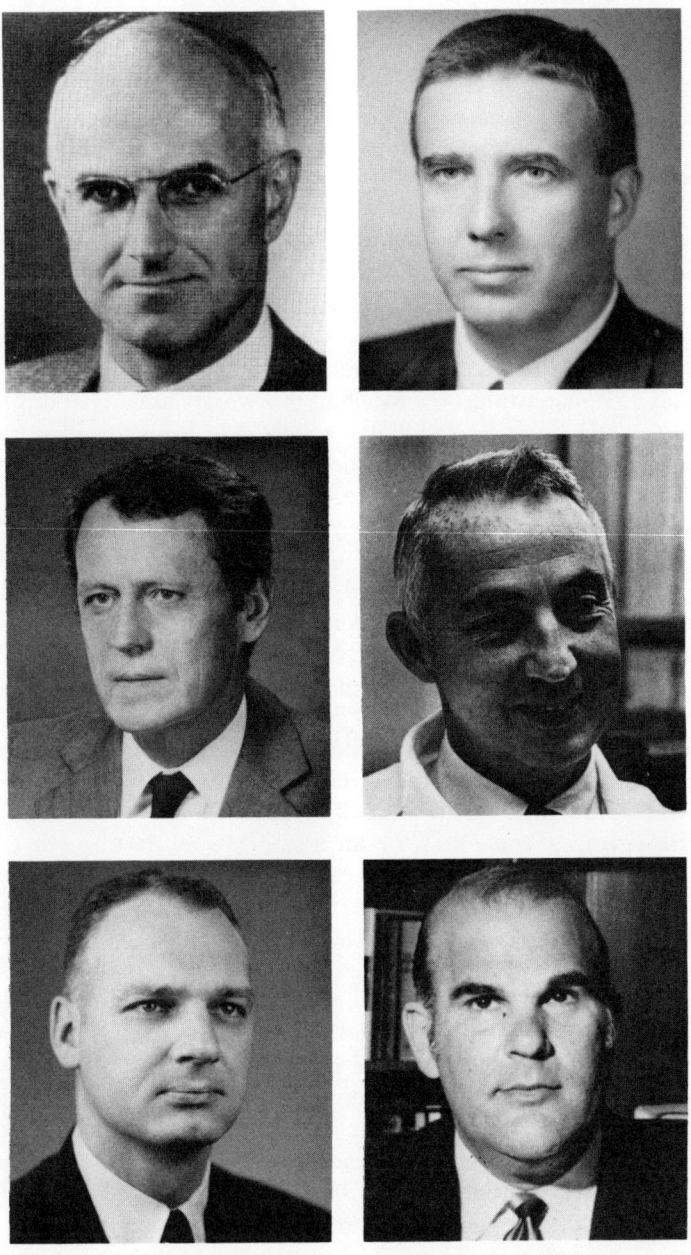

Some American pioneers in organ transplantation: Joseph E. Murray (top left); *David M. Hume* (top right); *Thomas E. Starzl* (middle left); *Norman E. Shumway* (middle right); *Keith Reemtsma* (bottom left); *John S. Najarian* (bottom right)

Mendelian laws of genetic inheritance by patiently observing the results of crossing peas of different strains in his garden. As was to be clearly demonstrated almost a century later, the degree of genetic difference determines the degree of immunological difference. That is, the greater the genetic difference between the donor of an organ and the recipient who receives it, the greater will be the reaction of the recipient's body to reject this allograft.

For many decades the laws governing biological differences went largely unused, but at the beginning of the twentieth century investigators began extensive exploration of organ transplantation using blood vessel anastomoses. Much of this work was carried out by Alexis Carrel at the Rockefeller Institute. He used the blood vessel anastomosis technique established with Charles C. Guthrie at the University of Chicago, after the method of J. Dorfler in Germany. Carrel transplanted both kidneys in a cat, with prompt function of these allografts and survival of the animal for three weeks. He showed that autografts survived, that allografts were rejected, and that xenografts (also called heterografts—from a different species) were rejected even more rapidly. For this and related work, Carrel was awarded the Nobel Prize in 1912. Arteries and veins were transplanted extensively in animals, but blood vessels were not to be transplanted clinically until Robert E. Gross reported replacement of a coarcted segment of the aorta with a human allograft in 1948. In 1906 Eduard K. Zirm successfully grafted a cornea.

However, it remained for Sir Peter Medawar, through experiments performed during the 1940s, to present lucidly a theory of actively acquired immunity. He showed, in both man and the rabbit, that second-set allografts (i.e., transplants made to an unrelated recipient that had received one or more transplants from the same donor on a previous occasion) survived for a much shorter time than did the original transplants. Medawar also showed that the period of survival of skin allografts in the rabbit was reduced if the recipient had previously received intradermal injections of a suspension of leucocytes from the prospective donor. He postulated that the skin and the leucocytes shared common antigens (and chromosomes, the genes and subcomponents), and that the prior injection of the leucocytes produced active immunity (antibodies) against the subsequently grafted skin. Thus, the recipient could distinguish self from nonself.

For this work Medawar shared the Nobel Prize with Sir Macfarlane Burnet of Australia in 1960. As it happened, I had visited him only two days before he was awarded the prize. It came about in this way. The American College of Surgeons had needed ten speakers to assist in putting on a program in London, and Dr. Ravdin had engineered my participation. Before going over, however, I had secured a letter of introduction to Medawar. On arrival in his office-laboratory, I asked to see Dr. Medawar. "I'm very sorry," said his secretary, "but the professor is frightfully busy. He won't be able to see you."

Rising to leave, I happened to say, "I'm sorry, too. I had this letter."

"Oh, you have a letter?"

"Yes," and I offered it.

"Just a moment, please." She disappeared around a screen and I could hear whispering. Just then the tall, handsome scientist strode swiftly around and pumped my hand. He spent an embarrassing amount of time with me, as we discussed transplant science and the morality of human kidney transplants. He felt that clinical transplants were perhaps premature, but I pointed out that many if not most of these patients would not have access to chronic renal dialysis and would thus die otherwise. Each time I tried to comment on his superb research he would say, "Oh, no, my dear fellow, I must enter an immediate disclaimer; we've done nothing here."

He recommended that I visit the British Museum and the National Gallery. At the latter I fell under the spell of the French Impressionists—my favorite was Monet—from which I never recovered.

I spoke the next day at the meeting at the Royal College of Surgeons.

Passing through the Atlanta airport in the early morning hours on my return, I saw on the front page of a newspaper "Medawar wins Nobel Prize." It was indeed Peter Medawar. I immediately sent him a telegram: "Magnificent lifetime prize. No further disclaimers accepted here!" I received a handwritten note from him a week or so later. He had received no warning before a Swedish reporter arrived and began beating on his door.

Genetics, immunology, tissue typing, and immunosuppressive therapy

The basic immunological barrier to allografting having been defined, it remained to search for ways in which to abrogate this barrier. Clearly, since the greater the genetical disparity, the greater

UNIVERSITY COLLEGE LONDON
DEPARTMENT OF ZOOLOGY

Telephone: EUSton 7050
Professor P. B. Medawar

GOWER STREET WC1

28 Oct.

Dear Dr. Hardy,

I was delighted to get your generous and kindly message. One has no idea that these prizes are going (the awarder, I'm not sure) till one's name is under consideration — my first news was from a Reuters reporter at 11 a.m. on the 20th. You can imagine the turmoil that ensued — I'm so very glad you weren't visiting just then! Many thanks again for writing —

Yours sincerely,
P.B. Medawar.

Note from Peter Medawar, 1960. Reproduced with permission.

the allograft reaction, it was advisable to obtain the donor tissue from a close relative who shared many chromosomes-genes-antigens with the prospective recipient. However, since a close and willing relative would often not be available, it became desirable to develop tissue typing—similar to ordinary blood typing but infinitely more complex—so that an unrelated donor whose tissue was reasonably compatible with that of the recipient might be found.

Meanwhile, the previously unknown function of the thymus gland was discovered: the thymus (with its thymic lymphocytes, T-cells) proved to be a major, if not *the* major, organ responsible for the development of the immunological capability of the individual, the capacity to distinguish self from nonself. For example, if the thymus is removed from a newborn rat, the rat can then accept skin from an unrelated rat. Indeed, it can accept a malignant tumor from a hamster, a xenograft. This led to the realization that the science of transplantation would shed light on malignant tumor genesis. In fact, one of the complications of immunosuppressed human kidney or heart recipients has been the development of spontaneous malignancies. Parenthetically, the intimate relationship between different branches of science is well illustrated by the discovery of the function of the thymus. Its probable nature was indicated by Bruce Glick of Mississippi State University in his studies of the bursa fabricius in the chicken, which corresponds to the thymus in mammals. However, since he published in a poultry journal, his important observations were not immediately discovered by the human transplant scientists.

In addition to tissue typing, however, drug therapy became the mainstay of preventing graft rejection in human recipients, with selected use of antilymphocyte serum prepared in the rabbit (or the horse) and on occasion radiation to the kidney allograft site. The drugs used were principally azathioprine and prednisone. A major complication of their use has been infection, since they not only suppress the allograft rejection reaction but also the ability of the host to combat bacterial invasion. Recently, cyclosporine has come on the market as an especially useful immunosuppressive agent, since it offers essentially equal protection from rejection of the transplant, while causing less impairment of immunological defenses against bacteria and viruses.

For some time, splenectomy was done in the recipient, since the spleen represented a large mass of lymphocytes already immunologically activated by the thymus and thus presumably available for producing antibodies against the foreign nonself tissue, the allograft. Now few transplant surgeons remove the spleen.

Organ procurement and storage

A vast amount of work has been done to develop methods for long-term storage of organs and tissues. However, the cold storage of the cornea and bone, and to a far lesser extent the skin and parathyroid tissue, are the principal successes so far. At present, complex organs such as the kidney, liver, or heart can be safely stored in ice only a matter of hours: the kidney for twenty-four to seventy-two hours, the liver perhaps less than ten hours, and the heart only four hours or so. Obviously, air transport is vital when the donor organs must be shipped long distances. These times will surely be extended by developments in the future. Already, our group has shipped two kidneys to Great Britain and one to Turkey. Every effort is made to coordinate the harvesting of permitted organs from the donor and matching with the most suitable recipients: the heart may go to New York, the liver to Pittsburgh, one kidney to Minnesota, and the other kidney to San Francisco. The current general acceptance of brain death in the donor with a still-beating heart has enormously advanced the success of harvesting organs while they are still capable of functioning adequately in the new host.

Early on, few relatives were willing to sign permission for use of an organ of the deceased for transplantation. It seemed macabre, ghoulish, foreign to anything most people had ever been asked to consider, and some religions were opposed to it. However, as time passed and kidney transplants became more successful, the idea of donating an organ became more familiar and hence more readily accepted. In time, the public acceptance of organ donation steadily increased, for which the public media—print, radio, and especially television—must be given much credit.

Ethical and moral questions

Organ transplantation was beset by ethical and moral questions from its inception, in contrast to skin allografting in treatment of burns, which had been used for decades. These considerations arose from the reluctance of relatives to give a part of the deceased patient for transplantation, from the reluctance of the prospective recipient to accept a part of the deceased body, from the high risk of

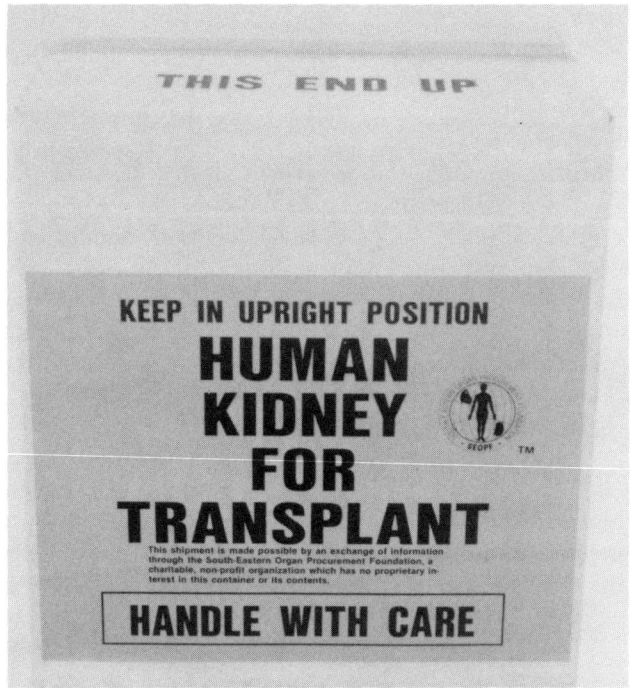

Container for cold preservation of kidney during shipment

failure of transplant in the early years of this clinical science, and because some religious leaders, and indeed society in general, were affronted by the whole concept of swapping organs from one person to another. However, there were usually two persons willing to try: one was the patient, facing early death unless some new form of treatment could prove successful; the other was the physician, who had the responsibility for preserving the life of the patient. In other words, those most vigorous in criticizing the early transplants were those farthest removed from the desperate clinical situation. Moreover, as the transplants slowly became more successful, they were perceived as less unethical or immoral. All radical new treatments must begin *somewhere*.

Nonetheless, transplanters were acutely aware of the ethical and moral dimensions of these exquisitely sensitive considerations, and I believe these intellectual and emotional reservations were generally handled with perception and humanity.

The high-water mark of criticism was probably reached in 1964, when we transplanted a chimpanzee heart into a dying man. Physicians, and the public in general, had begun cautiously to look upon kidney transplants with restrained interest and a degree of acceptance. However, few were aware of the extensive experience with heart transplantation in a number of laboratories. The mere fact that a *heart* had been transplanted, not to mention a lower primate heart (but one genetically very close to man), fell like a bombshell on the world. The resulting clamor was enormous.

At this point, as will be told again later in connection with the description of this first heart transplantation in man, I proposed to our dean and vice-chancellor, Dr. Robert Marston (later director of the National Institutes of Health), that he appoint a widely representative Human Investigation Committee of members from both the University Medical Center and the community—physicians, other scientists, clergy, and legal representation. Any new projects would be proposed first to this committee. This mechanism would serve to protect the patient, the public, the transplant team, and the University Medical Center. Soon the National Institutes of Health required such review on all research receiving financial sup-

Are Transplants Morally Wrong?

THE COMMERCIAL APPEAL, MEMPHIS.

SUNDAY MORNING, MARCH 15, 1964

Title of a discussion of transplant ethics and morality.
Education of the public was a vital element in the progress and acceptance of organ transplantation.

port from that source. And thereafter, the Helsinki Declaration of guidelines for human investigation was accepted internationally.

Even so, I had considerable confidence that transplants would be accepted as the public became more familiar with the concepts and the need; the public media did much to further this acceptance, if in no other way than simply to keep transplantation in the spotlight. People generally accept a new idea once they get used to it.

I find that my general position was expressed in my reply to Mr. Byron Scott of the *Journal of the American Medical Association* in 1967:

December 4, 1967

Dear Mr. Scott:

Thank you so much for sending me a copy of the recent legislation passed by the Italian Chamber of Deputies and Senate. It is of special interest to me in view of the legal uncertainties surrounding human kidney transplantation which I found when I visited Italy several years ago. The general medico-legal situation in Italy appears to be somewhat different from that in the United States, as it doubtless varies somewhat in all countries.

The essential features of the Italian legislation that are particularly pertinent in the United States are the requirement of a medical board which would certify the results of the histocompatibility testing and other factors involved in the given transplant experience. This special appreciation and cognizance of the importance of histocompatibility testing may well have been stimulated by the outstanding work of Professor R. Cepellini in the Institute of Medical Genetics at the University of Turin. In fact, this university was host to an international conference and workshop on histocompatibility testing last June. The conclusions of this conference were reported at the First International Meeting of the Transplantation Society in Paris a few days later. This report formalized the fact that histocompatibility testing had advanced to a point where it promises to be a useful adjunct to human transplantation in the prediction of probabilities of long-term success in the given case. Of course, a great many other factors also influence the ultimate success of the given transplant.

I personally have sound faith in the moral integrity of physicians. Almost all physicians engaged in clinical investigation are acutely aware of the many obvious and the many more subtle hazards involved in the total effort to improve the ultimate health of mankind through investigation. In fact, these physicians are usually far more intimately involved with these problems than many of those less involved could appreciate. The restraints implicit within a profession such as medicine are ancient, far reaching and comprehensive. I fully believe that the ultimate scientific and moral progress of the medical profession in the United States would be better left to regulation within the profession rather than by Federal Law. It is often extremely difficult to decide upon a course of action which may or may not prove successful. It is impossible to cover all the considerations, which go into the making of such a decision, in a legal document. In conclusion, one feels that the ultimate health needs of the population will be best served by not restricting the initiative of qualified centers. On the other hand, the fact that we do enjoy substantial freedom, within the self-imposed ethics of the medical profession, obligates each of us to employ the most advanced and responsible information and techniques available.

Sincerely yours,

James D. Hardy, M.D.
Professor and Chairman

Meanwhile, the international Transplantation Society had been established, and I had been elected a member of the Executive Committee. Professor Jean Dausset of Paris, also of this group, was named chairman of the Ethics Committee and I was named a member of this subsection. Thus, the transplant community was very much aware of, and active in, the moral problems surrounding human transplantation. Incidentally, Professor Dausset was to share the Nobel Prize only a few years later; it was awarded for his discoveries related, generally, to tissue typing.

There have been legal problems with transplantation, in some instances. Lawsuits have followed the harvesting of an organ from a donor, when some member or members of the family claimed not to have been fully informed and appropriate consent was not obtained. In the case of one murder trial, the lawyer for the defense apparently claimed that the transplant surgeon, not the lawyer's client, had killed the decedent when he removed the still beating heart. And there is always the possibility of litigation when a high-risk operation is not successful in the recipient.

Today, twenty years after the first heart transplant, hearts are transplanted daily around the world.

In the broad sweep of medical history, there come moments when it is possible to perceive the end of one era and the start of a new one. For example, with the advent in the early 1970s of widespread coronary bypass for coronary artery disease, it became clear that the remaining thrust of cardiac reparative surgery would be directed mainly toward the refinement of existing modalities and the development of corrective procedures for lesions of lesser general importance. Such a historical milestone or watershed is now clearly discernible with respect to clinical organ transplantation. The uncertain experimental years are largely behind us. Organ transplantation is accepted as standard treatment. Like open-heart surgery, but even more so, clinical organ transplantation requires a *team*—surgeon, internists, pediatricians if needed, pathologists, tissue typing immunologists, radiologists, and an organ procurement organization.

The United States Congress has recognized the clinical arrival of organ transplantation and is processing legislation to make available sufficient funding to render donated organs available nationwide, hopefully without respect to the financial resources of the prospective recipient.

KIDNEY TRANSPLANTATION

The kidney has served as the prototype for the transplantation of other organs. The reason for this has been the clear need in uremia, the relative simplicity of inserting the kidney into the pelvis, and the availability of artificial kidney dialysis should the transplant be rejected—support not effectively available for liver, heart, or lung transplant failure. The artificial kidney had been developed by Willem Kolff in Holland during the German occupation of World War II. (He also developed the immediate prototype of the currently used artificial heart.) At the present time there are approximately fifty thousand patients on chronic dialysis in the United States, at a cost of from nine thousand dollars (at home) to forty thousand dollars (in hospital) per year for each.

Sporadic attempts had been made to transplant the kidney, after vascular anastomosis was developed at the turn of this century, but these had been unsuccessful. The modern approach to renal transplantation was begun in 1947 at the Peter Bent Brigham Hospital in Boston. At the suggestion of George Thorn, surgeons Charles Hufnagel, David Hume, and Ernst Landsteiner transplanted a cadaver kidney to the antecubital fossa, anastomosing the renal vessels to the brachial artery and a large adjacent vein. The organ functioned immediately, and by the next day the patient was much better. After two days the transplant was functioning less, but by that time the patient's own kidneys were functioning again and she recovered.

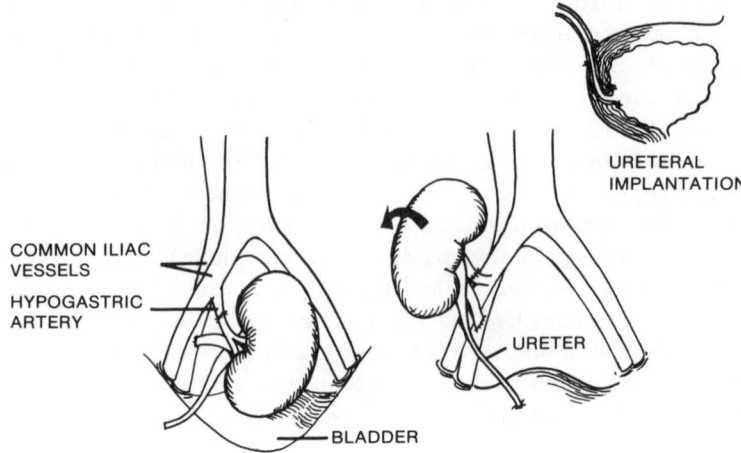

Vascular and ureteral anastomoses in renal transplantation. From Hardy, J. D.; Timmis, H. H.; Weems, W. L.; et al., "Kidney Transplantation in Man: Analysis of Eleven Cases," Annals of Surgery 165 (1967): 933.

Many others began investigating renal transplantation, but the absolute feasibility of this new modality of treatment for uremia was proven by Joseph Murray, John Merrill, and their associates in 1954, in a transplant between identical twins. There existed no genetical difference, and hence no immunological barrier; the kidney donated by one twin to the other survived permanently. Clearly, only the immunological barrier hindered routinely successful renal transplantation, and this obstacle was to give way slowly before massive research. Thousands of kidneys have now been transplanted throughout the world. The one-year survival rate of kidneys harvested from cadaver donors is now approximately 85 percent, and rejection rates fall off rapidly after one year. So good is the success achieved with cadaver kidneys that many transplant groups now consider it inappropriate to accept living donors, no matter how good the tissue match. Major leaders in achieving this goal included David Hume, Roy Calne (Cambridge University), Jean Hamburger (Paris), Thomas Starzl, and John Najarian.

Kidney autotransplantation for high ureteral injury

Our group at the University of Mississippi Medical Center began kidney transplantation in animals in the late 1950s and in man in the

1960s. Except in one instance, however, we mainly followed the lead of our colleagues in the vanguard.

A contribution for which we were given gratifying credit was generated, as is often the case, by a specific clinical need. In certain types of abdominal surgery and in traumatic injuries, the ureter may be injured. When only a short length of normal ureter remained attached to the kidney, the urologist often considered the situation irretrievable and removed that kidney if the opposite kidney exhibited adequate function.

On a number of occasions we had suggested that the kidney with an injured ureter need not be sacrificed, that it could be transplanted down to the pelvis. The remaining short segment of ureter could then be anastomosed to the bladder, and the renal artery and vein could be anastomosed to the adjacent iliac vessels. The kidney does not need extrinsic nerve supply. The ureter has its own *intrinsic* nerve circuit which permits muscular peristalsis to propel the urine along toward the bladder.

Eventually, an appropriate case became available in 1962, and we readily transplanted the involved kidney successfully and without event. (Pasteur's dictum: Fortune favors the prepared mind.) This operation led to "bench surgery" (surgery outside the body) on the cooled kidney to remove large stones, or a tumor or cyst, following which the organ might be returned to its normal location, though it was usually placed in the pelvis, as we had done before. Still later, a technique was developed by others which permitted operation on the cold kidney *in situ*, without removing it from its normal attachments. I presented our work before the American Urological Association.

Three kidney transplant vignettes

Examples of the vast range of scientific, ethical, and moral problems and surprises that confronted the early transplanters are illustrated by three cases. The first patient had received a kidney from an unrelated living donor (actually a prisoner volunteer—this was allowed back in those days). The transplant had functioned well from the start. Some months later he had come by on Christmas Eve, just to say hello, as he came to the hospital for his routine checkup. I said, "Bobby, you are of course taking your pills daily?"

"Doc, you've been so nice to me, I'm going to level with you. I haven't taken those pills for months, and I'm doing just fine."

This was absolutely astonishing. He had continued to live in happy coexistence (symbiosis) with the unrelated transplant without taking the drugs to prevent rejection of the kidney. He went on to say that he had picked up the pills regularly to please us. He was not stupid; he and his wife were dairy farmers who ran their own enterprise.

My first reaction was to scold him and tell him that he must take the pills. Nonetheless, here was a truly remarkable experiment, which the patient had performed on himself. I called several transplant centers and consulted them as to what we had best do with this "experiment." Some advised that the drugs be restarted at once. Others felt that he could be followed closely, with blood and urine studies and the annual biopsy of his transplanted kidney. If evidence of rejection developed, the drug treatment could be reinstituted. He went for almost a year before he began to exhibit definite evidence of rejection, and the drugs were then restarted, successfully.

Another patient was a young housewife. She had received a cadaver kidney transplant many months previously. About three o'clock one morning I received an excited telephone call from Laurel, Mississippi, about one hundred miles away, informing me that Irma had had a baby!

"Why, that's impossible," I said. "We've been seeing her regularly, and she is not pregnant."

"Well, we've got the baby right here."

Irma had developed the round face and obesity (Cushing's syndrome) caused by the prednisone she was taking to prevent rejection of her transplant. Since she had had somewhat the appearance of a pregnant woman already, and since such steroid therapy can cause cessation of the menstrual periods, we were caught completely by surprise. She was not the first transplant patient who had had a baby, but all of us were pleased that the baby, a boy, was completely normal. The patient is still living, eighteen years after losing her own kidneys, but she is currently on dialysis.

The third patient was a fourteen-year-old boy who was stabbed in the chest with something like an ice pick in a Jackson school hall amidst a group of other boys. He initially felt little, but on going downstairs to his locker he saw that there was blood on his shirt over his heart. He suddenly collapsed on the floor, and by the time he was finally brought to the University Hospital emergency room, he appeared to be dead. Although he was resuscitated, with a beating heart and functioning kidneys, there was no evidence of brain function. What had happened was that he had been stabbed in the heart. The blood released into the pericardial sac around the heart had compressed the heart so that it had virtually stopped. It was a simple matter to operate on him and repair the heart injury, but unfortunately, the lack of oxygen to the brain had already produced irreversible brain damage, as documented by the neurologists and neurosurgeons. He was brain dead, as this state later came to be called in clinical and legal terms. We discussed the situation with the parents and cautiously asked whether they would be willing to have the kidneys used for transplantation, should he not live (and we knew he would not).

"No, Doctor, we are opposed to having his kidneys used."

"Well, I certainly do understand that, for the situation is tragic enough as it is," I agreed.

The boy went gradually downhill, and on what appeared to be his final night of survival, I told his mother and father, who were educated people—school teachers I think—that this appeared to be his last night and that we had done all we could, inadequate though it was.

About four o'clock in the morning the hospital called and said that the parents wanted me to come down. I remonstrated mildly, since I already had done everything possible and had explained the situation to them, but when they insisted, I got up and went down.

"Doctor," the father said, "we want to give our boy's kidneys for transplantation."

"That's certainly generous of you," I said. They went through the formality of signing consent forms.

As I was about to walk away, the father said, "Dr. Hardy, don't you want to know why we changed our minds about giving the kidneys?"

"Why, yes, I do."

"Doctor, his mother and I were afraid you wouldn't work quite as hard with our boy if you were waiting to get his kidneys."

LIVER TRANSPLANTATION

Early workers in the field of experimental liver transplantation included Stuart Welch and Francis Moore. However, it has been Roy Calne of Cambridge University and, preeminently, Thomas Starzl, formerly of the University of Colorado but now of the University of Pittsburgh, who have, through prodigious effort, rendered liver transplantation an increasingly feasible and successful form of treatment.

Many efforts have been made to transplant an auxiliary liver to a more accessible site, such as the lower abdomen, with vascular anastomoses to the iliac artery and vein. But these heterotopic (to an abnormal site) grafts have generally failed. Orthotopic transplantation of the liver (to the site from which the patient's own liver is removed) has now been accepted universally as the operation of choice.

The liver is a fragile organ, more so than the kidney or even the heart, and its functions in the overall preservation of life are complex indeed, whereas the heart is only a pump (though a magnificent one). On the other hand, the major problems encountered in liver transplantation have been associated less with rejection than with management of the structures to be anastomosed, especially the common bile duct and the gallbladder. Bile leakage has been a frequent source of infection.

Transplanted organs reflect rejection through evidence of impaired function: the liver by the appearance of jaundice, the kidney by decreasing urine output, the heart by decreasing cardiac output.

At present, the one-year survival of liver transplants in the most experienced centers is approximately 70 percent, though of course many patients are alive years after receiving their transplants. Human liver transplants now number in the hundreds.

Starzl's group originally selected principally recipients who had a malignant tumor of the liver, but the long-term cure rate was disappointing. They have long since moved to accept patients suffering from hepatic failure due to such various causes as cirrhosis in adults, congenital biliary atresia in children, or severe disease caused by liver dysfunction. The need for liver transplants is great, and the need for donor organs has grown steadily as liver transplantation has been brought into routine therapy.

PANCREAS TRANSPLANTATION

There is also a great need for successful transplantation of the pancreas. Approximately five million people are known to have diabetes in the United States, and there may be as many as five million undiagnosed diabetics as well. More than half the blindness in the United States occurs as a complication of diabetes; other major complications include arterial atherosclerosis, renal failure, and peripheral neuropathy. Despite the increasing success of continuous infusion of insulin at a variable rate by subcutaneously implanted devices, these complications continue to develop. We know that the pancreas does much more than secrete insulin. If the complications of diabetes are transmitted on a gene separate from that causing hypoinsulinism, however, successful pancreatic transplantation may not prevent all the problems met in the diabetic patient. Fortunately, there is early evidence, derived from experimental transplantation in rodents and in several human patients, that successful transplantation of the pancreas does reverse certain complications of chronic diabetes.

Thus far, clinical transplantation of the pancreas, while contributing much information, has enjoyed limited success. The largest clinical experience is probably that of Najarian and his associates at the University of Minnesota, who recently published a report on one hundred patients. Some of the transplants maintained normal blood sugar levels for variable periods. Since early successes have been achieved, however, commonly successful transplantation of the pancreas for diabetes mellitus may be anticipated with considerable confidence.

Small Bowel Transplantation

Each year there occur in the United States accidents or disease that damage the small intestine, rendering its remaining absorptive surface inadequate to preserve the patient in nutritional health. Successful transplantation of the small bowel would solve this problem, and much experimental work has been done. The small bowel can be removed from the experimental animal, and then replaced in the same animal, with ready survival; or, in the human patient, a segment of small bowel can be transplanted to the neck to replace an esophageal defect with virtually routine success. However, human allotransplants, as by C. Olivier in France and Joseph G. Fortner in New York, have ultimately failed. The principal obstacle appears to be a combination of infection (for the bowel is inherently contaminated) and rejection. Research continues in many laboratories, including ours.

Certain problems are illustrated in the following case report on an intestinal transplant in man.

A child was brought to our hospital with severe abdominal pain. Operation disclosed gangrene of almost all the small bowel and the right part of the colon. The dead bowel was removed and the duodenum was anastomosed to the remaining colon. A length of only about four feet of the normal approximately twenty-two feet of small intestine is absolutely essential for adequate absorption of nutrients, especially if the colon remains to absorb water. Clearly, this patient would not survive without a transplant, though the as yet imperfect intravenous feeding would suffice for a time. A few bowel transplants had been performed in humans, but with limited success.

Our little patient's mother was a rather good tissue match. On June 12, 1969, we operated on her and the child in adjacent rooms, and transplanted three feet of her small intestine to her son, using vascular anastomoses. We did not insert this transplanted gut into his own alimentary canal at that time, since we wanted to observe the ends of the transplant, brought out through the abdominal wall, to be sure the graft had survived. The graft was not clearly rejected, but when a week later he perforated a duodenal ulcer, we decided that it would be wise to remove the transplant to avoid any further possibility of intraabdominal crises. Weeks later, he eventually died of infection and inanition.

Endocrine Tissue

Parathyroid transplantation

Allotransplantation of endocrine tissue has been conspicuously unsuccessful, but the survival of parathyroid tissue autotransplants to the forearm following excision of all four glands in the neck, as espoused by Samuel A. Wells, Jr., has provided a way to avoid permanent hypoparathyroidism, if all or most parathyroid tissue has been excised in the neck.

Adrenal autotransplantation in Cushing's disease in man

We became interested in the transplantation of slices of an adrenal gland into a muscle in the thigh, following total resection of the two adrenal glands in the abdomen for Cushing's disease. Total removal of the adrenal glands is of course fatal unless the patient takes replacement steroid hormone for life. We reasoned that if the adrenal tissue transplanted to the thigh survived (and here there was no genetic-immunological barrier, since this was self to self), the patient would be spared lifelong obligatory medication. On the other hand, if this transplanted adrenal tissue itself hypertrophied and produced recurrent excessive adrenal function, the surgeon could easily remove a portion of the transplant using local anesthesia.

In brief, the transplanted tissue did survive in most patients, but it was sometimes several years before maximal function was achieved. In two patients the transplants eventually functioned so well that they caused recurrent Cushing's syndrome and had to be removed.

For some time we believed that this first such clinical adrenal transplantation in the United States was also the first in the world. Later, however, we found in the literature a prior report from Sweden and one from New Zealand.

Utero-Ovarian Reimplantation

A gynecologist came to me with a specific request: Could we transplant a uterus and ovaries? He had a young woman who had had a hysterectomy. She had now remarried and her new husband badly wanted children. As always, I replied that what we might accomplish in the laboratory was not necessarily transferable to human patients, but that his request was an intriguing one worth exploring.

Sadan Eraslan and I found in dogs that it was possible to remove the uterus and ovaries *en bloc*, cool them for a period of time, and then replant them in the same animal using vascular anastomoses. (This did not cross a genetic barrier.) After establishing the technique, we found that seven of ten dogs later exhibited changes in the vaginal epithelium that reflected ovarian function; three of them had puppies. The work was not extended to allografting in dogs, and the technique was never applied to humans. Clearly, however, utero-ovarian transplantation in man is possible, as drugs for suppression of the allograft rejection reaction continue to improve. Of course, the mother would not be the genetic parent of a child unless she still had her own ovaries following the hysterectomy, though the father would be.

Unfortunately, our routine report to the NIH became public

knowledge. From one quarter there was outrage from the antivivisectionists, and from another quarter came queries from women who had the specific problem addressed in the research.

Lung Transplantation

Chronic respiratory disease causes more than forty thousand deaths in the United States each year. The majority of these deaths are due to emphysema from cigarette smoking. If the patient with terminal lung disease does not actually asphyxiate, the diseased lungs may harbor a fatal infection, or the resistance to blood flow through the lungs may cause the right side of the heart to fail. Chronic pulmonary failure is a massive public health problem.

In contrast to the effectiveness of the artificial kidney for the treatment of renal failure, efforts to develop an artificial lung for long-term support have been unsuccessful. Lung transplantation, or combined heart-lung transplantation, appears at present to offer the most promising modality for the management of otherwise fatal chronic respiratory insufficiency.

The modern experimental transplantation of the lung apparently began with V. P. Demikhov in Moscow in 1947, when he transplanted both the whole lung and separate lobes in dogs. Henri Metras, of France, suggested in 1950 the commonly used anastomosis of a cuff of the atrium (containing the inflowing pulmonary veins) to the atrium of the recipient, thus diminishing the incidence of thrombosis in the multiple separate pulmonary veins.

In the United States, significant work was reported by André A. Juvenelle, by Wilford B. Neptune and associates, by David A. Blumenstock, and by Creighton A. Hardin and C. Frederick Kittle, in which it was demonstrated clearly that the animal could survive on both the reimplanted lung and the allotransplanted lung.

The first lung transplant in man will be described in the next chapter.

Heart Transplantation

A number of groups began experimental heart transplantation in the 1950s. These included, in the United States, C. Rollins Hanlon, Vallee L. Willman, and Theodore Cooper at St. Louis University, Blumenstock at Cooperstown, New York, preeminently Norman E.

Shumway at Stanford University, and Watts R. Webb at the University of Mississippi Medical Center. Initially, hypothermia of both the donor organ and the recipient animal was used to slow the metabolism and thus reduce the oxygen requirements, and there were some early survivors. However, it was only after the pump-oxygenator became generally available, after 1954, that experimental heart transplantation flourished, and long-term survival of significant numbers of animals permitted long-term assessment of reimplanted and allotransplanted hearts.

In 1961, Richard R. Lower, Raymond C. Stofer, and Norman E. Shumway described a transplant technique that involved division through the atria, the pulmonary artery, and the aorta—thus avoiding the time-consuming suture of the vena cavae and the pulmonary veins and the greater risk of their thrombosis.

The immunosuppressive therapy employed in kidney transplantation was used, and it was found that the heart was no more likely to reject than the kidney, perhaps less so. Impending failure of the transplant was reflected in changes in the electrocardiogram, the cardiac output (when measured), and the general health of the animals. Much later, Shumway's group demonstrated that biopsy of the right ventricle, using cardiac catheterization, gave more secure information regarding the impending rejection of the cardiac allograft, as biopsy did for the kidney.

The first heart transplant in man will be discussed in a subsequent chapter. "It is sufficient to know in the large, that a thing may be possible and not to despair of it at first sight" (report attributed to a committee of the Royal Academy of Science, Paris, 1710, sent to investigate the claim of a successful colostomy).

Suffice it to say that at present the most experienced heart transplantation centers report 80 percent one-year survival, and many heart transplant patients have survived more than a decade. The improved results have come about through better selection of recipients, and improved management of the diagnosis and the treatment of allograft rejection. Importantly, the disease should affect solely the heart itself, without significant disease of other organs of the body. Recently, however, Shumway's group has reexamined the clinical transplantation of the heart and both lungs as a single unit, with 70 percent survival. This technique affords an approach to the management of congenital and acquired diseases that affect both the heart and the lungs.

The Mitchell Banks Lecture

The William Mitchell Banks Memorial Lecture in Liverpool was a landmark between our early transplants and what was to come. Professor Charles Wells, head of the Department of Surgery at the University of Liverpool in England, had written to me in mid-1962, inviting me to give the William Mitchell Banks Memorial Lecture of the University of Liverpool, in association with the 1963 annual meeting of the Association of Surgeons in Great Britain and Ireland. That fall, at the meeting of the American College of Surgeons in Atlantic City, he and I had stood on the boardwalk and discussed possible topics. He had waved off all my suggestions until the topic of transplantation of organs was mentioned. "That's it, Hardy," he said.

Meanwhile, the segregation fight raged on, with condemnation of Mississippi in the press throughout the world. When I arrived in England, this struggle was prominent in the newspapers and general conversation. Imagine my position and that of Professor Wells. Here he was, having invited an unknown surgeon from the United States to give what was to his department the centerpiece: The William Mitchell Banks Memorial Lecture. Disastrously, the Oxford fiasco had continued to reverberate around the globe. Mississippi, to the British, was just about the worst place that the William Mitchell Banks speaker could have come from. The tension was obvious, and Charles Wells was grim and silent. I saw that this was going to be a very long day, as I would discuss another speaker's paper in the morning and then give my formal lecture at five o'clock. I had been informed by letter that my discussion that morning had to be spoken, not read. Nervous anyway, and still far from over the jet lag, I had slept little the night before.

When the morning speaker had given the vascular work that I was to discuss, the chairman announced that Professor James D. Hardy, of Jackson, Mississippi, would now comment on the paper. There was absolute, stony silence. Clearing my throat, I walked to the podium and said: "First, I want to say how much I appreciate being invited to be with the British Association on this occasion." Steely stares. "Next, I bring to you the best wishes of our faculty at the University of Mississippi Medical Center." (Pause.) "I bring you also the best wishes of our dean." (Pause.) "I likewise bring you the best wishes of the chancellor of the university." (A longer pause.) "Lastly, I would like to have brought you the best wishes of our governor—but relations are strained."

At this the audience roared and rapped on their armrests as they often do in Great Britain instead of clapping. I then went on to discuss the paper on atherosclerotic arterial disease in the legs.

As I sat down beside Professor Wells, he was no longer grim—he was all smiles. "My God, Hardy," he said, "that was brilliant!" The ice had been broken and we were on our way.

Principals marched in to the lecture that afternoon in academic regalia. The mortarboard slipped on my head as I looked up to find the auditorium packed to the very last, upper circular rows. It was late in the afternoon, after a long day and many talks. The room was warm and dark, with only the light of the lectern and the lantern slides. The audience was drifting and the lecture threatened to be a miserable failure. Something radically different had to be done. Reading to the end of the paragraph (reading was permitted at the Banks Lecture), I then emphatically closed the folder with my two hands and placed it down on the podium. I turned to the screen and began to talk, just as if I were speaking to our Department of Surgery at home. Released from the manuscript, I soon warmed to the subject in which we had invested so much thought and energy over the past seven years. The excited interest of that distinguished audience was fully recaptured. The slides finished, the formal lecture was closed with the movie showing that lung and heart transplantation could be performed in animals. Asking for the lights, I concluded with, "Gentlemen, these transplantations will be performed in man in the very near future."

CHAPTER 15

The First Lung Transplant in Man

My prediction in Liverpool that lungs would soon be transplanted in man had not been an idle one. In early 1963, Watts Webb and I went to Dean and Vice-Chancellor Robert Marston and reviewed with him our results in several hundred animals over the past seven years. We said that we now planned to transplant a lung from a cadaver to a patient in terminal respiratory insufficiency, should the appropriate clinical and ethical circumstances arise. No lung had ever been transplanted in man. Our criteria were as follows. First, the patient must have a probably fatal disease so that, in the event of untoward results, his life would not have been materially shortened. Second, it must be a reasonable possibility that the patient would benefit from the lung transplant. Third, the removal of the patient's own diseased lung must not result in the sacrifice of a significant amount of his own functioning lung tissue. And fourth, since transplantation of the left lung was technically easier than that of the right lung, because of its longer unbranched portions of the pulmonary artery and main bronchus, we preferred to perform the first human lung transplant on the left side. It was clear that considerable time might elapse before a morally acceptable recipient was admitted, for many patients with apparently terminal respiratory failure can be improved by vigorous medical measures to increase lung function.

A number of possible lung recipients were considered and carefully studied over the months, but it was not until June that an acceptable patient presented. As it happened, he was a prisoner from the state penitentiary—the University Hospital cared for all prisoners who could not be managed at the prison infirmary. The fifty-eight-year-old white man, a heavy smoker, had respiratory distress even at bed rest. His collapsed and infected left lung contained a large cancer which we had diagnosed with bronchoscopic biopsy. No distant metastases were demonstrated. There was minimal function in the left lung. Antibiotics had failed to cure the infection behind the cancer. There was the possibility that his respiration could be improved by a lung transplant.

He also exhibited evidence of right heart failure, probably due to chronic pulmonary emphysema. He had chronic kidney disease, but thus far his renal function had proved marginally adequate.

Our two surgical teams were in tense readiness the first week of June. One team would remove the left lung of a cadaver donor in one operating room. In an adjacent room my team would remove the patient's left lung and prepare to insert the homotransplant.

Days went by while no prospective donor materialized. At about 7:30 P.M. on June 11, however, a patient entered our emergency room in shock from a massive heart attack and died almost immediately. His family agreed to lung donation.

Waiting expectantly at home, I received an excited telephone call from the thoracic resident, Martin Dalton: "Come on, Dr. Hardy, we've got a donor!"

Both surgical teams performed admirably. Both the donor and the recipient protocols were followed meticulously. We collected all the data we had hoped for and the donor lung was transplanted effectively. The four necessary anatomical structures—the two pulmonary veins, the pulmonary artery, and the main bronchus—were anastomosed. We did encounter two unanticipated problems. The cancer and surrounding infection were even more extensive than we had expected, and there was some difficulty in removing the patient's chronically collapsed left lung. Next, since this lung had been collapsed and the size of the chest space on that side had shrunk accordingly, we were at first concerned that we would not be able to transplant the large donor lung and then close the chest over it. We even began to consider removing one of the two lobes of the transplant. With adjustments, however, a satisfactory result was achieved. The prompt function of the transplant as an organ of respiration was documented immediately, using blood gas analyses. The patient had withstood the operation in stable condition. We walked out of the operating room thoroughly pleased with our effort.

On reaching the front desk of the operating suite we found much excitement, but the excitement was not for us. Medgar Evers, the black civil rights leader, had just been brought into our emergency room with a gunshot wound of the chest and had died on arrival. Resuscitation efforts were unsuccessful. The injury could have been

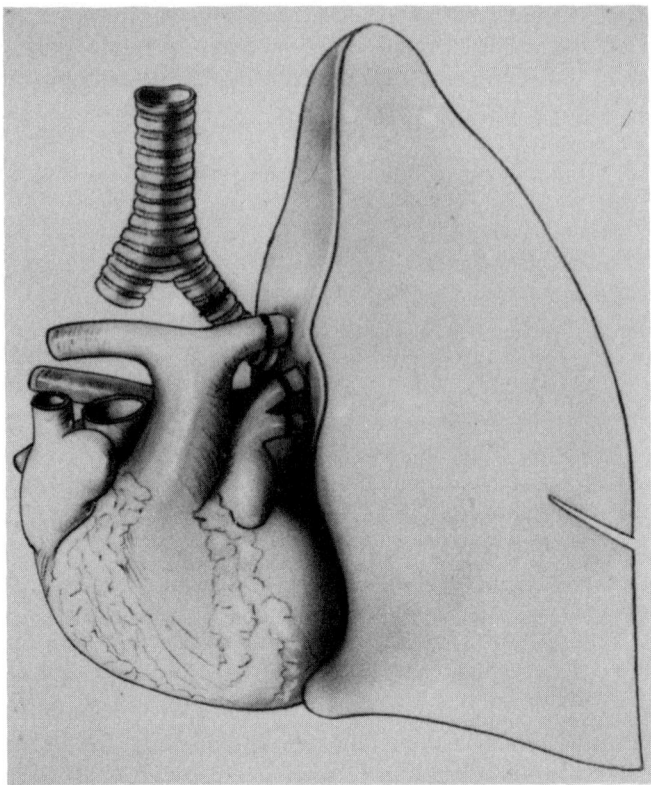

Operative technique used for first lung transplantation in man. From Hardy, J. D., "The Transplantation of Organs," Surgery 56 (1964): 685.

readily repaired had there not been delay in bringing him to the hospital. But racial conflict was intense, and ambulance drivers had been afraid to enter the area of his home.

Our patient did well from the lung transplant itself, but he slid into renal failure from his chronic kidney disease and eventually died three weeks later. The immunosuppressive therapy had consisted of azathioprine and prednisone. Radiation therapy to the thymus gland was given daily for a five-day period, beginning on the first postoperative day. At autopsy the lung did not appear rejected, and this was confirmed by microscopic studies.

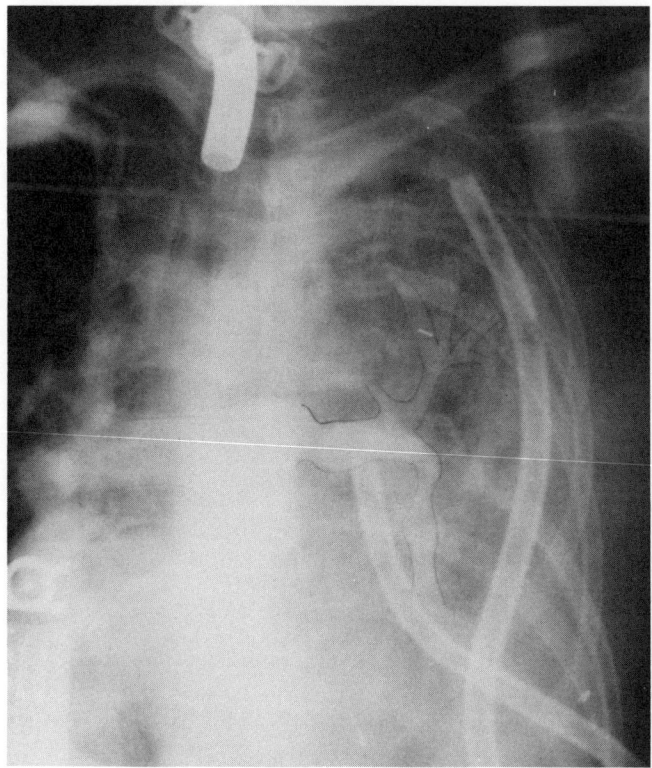

Pulmonary arteriogram on first postoperative day following first human lung transplant. The branches of the pulmonary artery of the transplanted lung are outlined. From Hardy, J. D.; Webb, W. R.; Dalton, M. L., Jr.; et al., "Lung Homotransplantation in Man: Report of the Initial Case," Journal of the American Medical Association 186 (1963): 1065, copyright 1963, American Medical Association.

The technical feasibility and functional validity of lung transplantation in man, using techniques developed in the laboratory, had been established.* The Smithsonian Institution in Washington requested the transplanted organ, and some years later we formally donated the preserved lung, which had been mounted in transparent plastic.

*J. D. Hardy; W. R. Webb; M. L. Dalton, Jr.; and G. R. Walker, Jr., "Lung Homotransplantation in Man: Report of the Initial Case," *Journal of the American Medical Association* 186 (1963): 1065.

The management of public interest posed a problem almost equal to that of transplantation of the lung itself, though in an entirely different sphere. The degree of acceptance of the operation varied with almost every individual. Some considered the transplantation unethical or even immoral, while others agreed with us that the effort was morally acceptable if all appropriate conditions of need had been observed and if informed consent had been obtained. Of course, when a startling new treatment proves successful, its ethical problems are immediately abolished. Had our lung transplant patient lived for a year or more, in comfortable health, criticism relative to an unethical procedure would have been muted. Actually, criticism of this first lung transplant was not even comparable to that which was to attend the first heart transplant in man the following year. Moreover, by this time Dr. Webb and I had become fairly well adjusted to critical situations in the course of open-heart surgery, as had every other cardiothoracic surgeon operating during those early days of this developing field.

The results of single lung transplantation in man may be expected to improve slowly.

CHAPTER 16

The First Heart Transplant in Man

Heart transplantation research was begun in our laboratories by Watts Webb and his associates in 1956. They achieved short-term animal survival the following year. Not only was heart transplantation investigated, but cold heart storage and heart metabolism were also studied.

On the basis of several hundred heart transplants in animals, and encouraged by the success of our first human lung transplant, Webb and I again met with Vice-Chancellor Marston. He agreed to a careful and cautious approach to heart transplantation in man.

To prepare for the eventual human heart transplant, we set up two teams in the animal laboratory. One team operated on the donor animal to ready the donor heart for excision, then to quickly cool it in iced salt solution, and to have it promptly available for transplantation into the recipient. The other team put the recipient animal on the heart-lung machine ("the pump") and excised the heart.

We were well aware of possible criticism. At that time the heart still carried strong emotional overtones: "I love you with my heart and soul," or "heartfelt," or "no heart for it," or "heartsick," or "fainthearted." How would one lover feel, for instance, if within the other's breast beat the heart of a stranger? On various occasions among social groups, we broached the matter of heart transplantation obliquely and listened to what was said and assessed attitudes.

We evaluated a number of possible candidates for heart transplantation, but none was acceptable—they were either too far gone, or they surprisingly got better. Originally, we thought it would be relatively easy to get a donor who died at the same time as a possible heart recipient went into final shock from heart disease. It became evident, however, that it was going to be extremely unlikely that both the donor and the recipient would die at the same time. At that time it was not accepted in the United States to remove the still beating heart; the concept of brain death was not accepted generally, and certainly it would not be accepted in Jackson.

Our plan was to gain permission for the donation and then to insert cannulas into one femoral artery and both femoral veins so that, the moment the prospective donor heart stopped, the heparinized body could be cooled immediately with the heart-lung machine to preserve the heart until it could be removed. As time passed and we gained more insight through our open-heart work in patients, we came to believe that the donor heart should be preserved during insertion not only by cooling but also by perfusing its coronary arteries with cold oxygenated blood while it was being transplanted into the new host.

Our greatest concern, as we approached the first heart transplant in man, was that the new heart might not start up and beat at all, after the patient's own heart had been removed. This haunting worry stimulated us to do heart transplants in calves, where the coronary arteries were much larger and the catheters for their perfusion with blood were more quickly secured in place than in dogs. In time, we had this aspect of the transplantation technique securely established.

Meanwhile, we continued to sample what the reaction by both physicians and laymen to a human heart transplant might be. Even kidney transplantation had barely begun to receive emotional acceptance. When asked, an audience might raise hands to indicate that, yes, they would accept a kidney transplant; yes, they would accept a liver transplant; yes, they would at least consider a lung transplant; but no, most would not even consider a heart transplant. The probable reaction of university personnel was sampled at my Alpha Omega Alpha Lecture at Columbia University in New York. There was much ambivalence.

Some religious leaders opposed transplantation altogether. Actually, transplantation of organs was so new that many practicing physicians knew only what they had read in the newspapers—certainly they did not read the arcane medical journals where transplantation research was usually published. The heart transplant was to hit them like a bombshell.

Chimpanzee kidney transplants in humans

It had become ever more apparent that, in the absence of general acceptance of the concept of brain death, the odds of having a dying heart patient and a dying brain injury donor die at precisely the same time were small. Meanwhile, unable to obtain human kidney donors at a time when few relatives of the deceased were willing even to listen to the need for donation, we had become very interested in some research at Tulane University in New Orleans. Recognizing that the chimpanzee, of all subhuman primates, has probably the greatest genetic compatibility with humans, Keith Reemtsma and his associates had transplanted chimpanzee kidneys into a number of patients when no human donor could be found. I had visited Tulane and had been much impressed by the early success and the laboratory data of the two such patients who were in Charity Hospital at that time.

Accordingly, since we also had a severe problem getting donor kidneys, I had purchased four large chimpanzees. It occurred to me that the largest of these, a male weighing over one hundred pounds, might conceivably serve as a heart donor under dire circumstances. We tranquilized him and measured his cardiac output per minute asleep. It was over four liters, equal to that of a fairly small human adult.

Meanwhile, our surgical team suffered a setback. Dr. Webb was induced to accept the chair of cardiothoracic surgery at Southwestern Medical School of the University of Texas in Dallas. Dr. Carlos M. Chavez advanced into his place and we pressed on.

The first heart transplant in man

The year 1964 was to have a profound influence on my life and career. Dr. Chavez and I, with our teams, transplanted hearts as often as we could, subjecting ourselves to criticism that we were spending too much time in the animal laboratory and neglecting our clinical and teaching responsibilities. This was true. As Harvey Cushing had remarked, when one is driving toward some specific goal, something else must go by the board.

On January 11 we had a dry run, which served the useful purpose of bringing nurses, anesthesiologists, and both surgical teams to full readiness in anticipation of a possible heart transplant. We had been working together in the animal laboratory for some time, but the prospect of the first human transplant posed infinitely larger problems of all kinds.

A thirty-six-year-old man who had sustained a knife wound to the left ventricle was referred to University Hospital. Clots had formed in his heart and had embolized to occlude multiple major arteries in his body. He had had a right-sided stroke caused by these clots shooting out from his heart to arteries in the brain. There was severe impairment of mental function and incontinence of urine and feces. Later, another clot caused gangrene of the left leg which necessitated amputation. A month later, an additional clot eventuated in amputation of the right leg for gangrene. The patient was referred to us for surgery on the heart to prevent still further clot embolization. Could the patient survive an operation for removal of the clots, presumably from his left ventricle? Both transplant teams were in readiness, with the thought that a heart transplant might be a possibility—and a patient with a massive head injury who was being kept alive solely with a respirator in the recovery room was a possible donor. The largest chimpanzee available as a donor weighed around 100 pounds. The patient, legless, weighed 73 pounds.

During the operation for removal of the clots, which was performed on January 18, we found that the patient did have the suspected traumatic left ventricular aneurysm, which doubtless had been the source of the clots. However, the heart promptly restored blood pressure once the heart-lung machine had been discontinued, and there was no acceptable reason for a cardiac transplant. The patient improved and was sent back to his local hospital.

Even though we performed no transplant this time, our entire large team had been brought to a high state of mental preparedness, and it was apparent that everything would function smoothly when we actually did have the opportunity to perform a clinical heart transplantation.

The first heart transplant in man: report of a case

On January 22, 1964, a sixty-four-year-old man was referred to the surgical service with gangrene of the lower portion of his left leg. He had a long history of hypertension and multiple heart attacks, for which he had been taking digitalis and diuretics. He had been admitted to his community hospital in a comatose state and with no detectable blood pressure. Rapid atrial fibrillation had been recorded there, and drugs had been given in high doses to elevate the blood pressure and assist in resuscitation. The following morning it was possible to maintain his blood pressure level with minimal vasopressor drug therapy. His sensorium had cleared slightly. Whether this impaired mental state was secondary to the previous shock, with the resulting hypoxia imposed upon already atherosclerotic

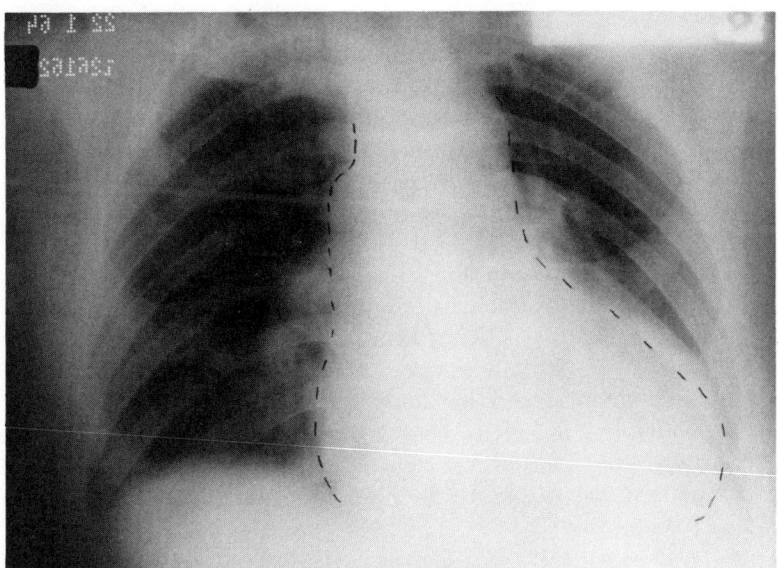

Huge decompensated heart of prospective recipient.
From Hardy, J. D.; Chavez, C. M., "The First Heart Transplant in Man: Historical Reexamination of the 1964 Case in Light of Current Clinical Experience," Transplantation Proceedings *1 (1969): 717.*

brain arteries, or to intracranial hemorrhage, or to a blood pressure level that remained abnormally low for this previously hypertensive patient was not determined. He was able to move all four extremities, but this motion was limited.

Further details were later recorded extensively in the previously cited report published in the *Journal of the American Medical Association* and need not be repeated here. In brief, the conclusions of Thaddeus D. Labecki, cardiologist, were as follows: "From the cardiovascular standpoint, the situation is unequivocally critical due to myocardial failure and apparent multiple emboli arising from the left atrium or ventricle. By all rules, life expectancy can be measured in the case in hours only."*

This opinion, in which members of the transplant team concurred, raised the possibility of heart transplantation. Again, a pos-

*J. D. Hardy; C. M. Chavez; F. D. Kurrus; W. A. Neely; S. Eraslan; M. D. Turner; L. W. Fabian; and T. D. Labecki, "Heart Transplantation in Man: Developmental Studies and Report of a Case," *Journal of the American Medical Association* 188 (1964): 1132.

sibly available patient donor who had sustained severe head injury was comatose on a respirator, although there was no way of knowing when his heart would arrest. As we had given extensive and profound thought to the whole problem of donor and recipient, we again had considered the possibility of getting the donor heart from our largest chimpanzee.

The prospective recipient went into terminal shock at approximately 6:00 P.M., with a blood pressure of seventy and virtually without respiration except for the continued use of the mechanical ventilation through a tracheostomy tube. Death was clearly imminent, and it was obvious that if heart transplantation was to be performed, it had to be done at once. The family gave permission for heart transplantation, and they understood that a human heart might not be available—for at that time it was not ethically acceptable to stop a respirator before the heartbeat had ceased.

The patient was rushed to the operating room, and his heart ar-

---

OPERATIVE PERMIT

I hereby give full permission for left leg amputation and heart surgery on Boyd Rush. I understand that any clots present will be removed from the heart to stop them from going to still more arteries of his body. I further understand that his heart is in extremely poor condition. If for any unanticipated reason the heart should fail completely during either operation and it should be impossible to start it, I agree to the insertion of a suitable heart transplant if such should be available at the time. I further understand that hundreds of heart transplants have been performed in laboratories throughout the world but that any heart transplant would represent the initial transplant in man.

Signed (for family) _____
Witnessed _____
Witnessed _____

January 23, 1964

Operative permit for transplantation of the first heart in man.
From Hardy, J. D.; Chavez, C. M., "The First Heart Transplant in Man: Historical Reexamination of the 1964 Case in Light of Current Clinical Experience," Transplantation Proceedings 1 (1969): 717.

rested just as the chest was opened. We began cardiac massage immediately and soon had the patient on the pump. Meanwhile, the tranquilized chimpanzee had been anesthetized.

At this point there was sharp discussion among the members of the transplant team. We were all well aware that any transplantation of a heart in man would be followed by public consternation and major criticism. We also knew that the use of a chimpanzee ("monkey") heart would augment the criticism immeasurably. It was a profoundly sober moment for all, and an agonizing moment for some. Therefore, I polled each of the five primary members of the transplant team individually, and their votes were recorded. Four voted to proceed with transplantation, even though the chimpanzee heart had to be used. The fifth abstained. In view of the early success achieved with the chimpanzee kidney transplants in New Orleans, I felt that this transplantation was morally justified: no human heart was available and the patient was being kept alive solely on the heart-lung machine. At best, he might rally with the transplanted lower primate heart; in any case, we would not have risked the life of a patient who might otherwise have lived days longer.

With this decision behind us, we proceeded without any particu-

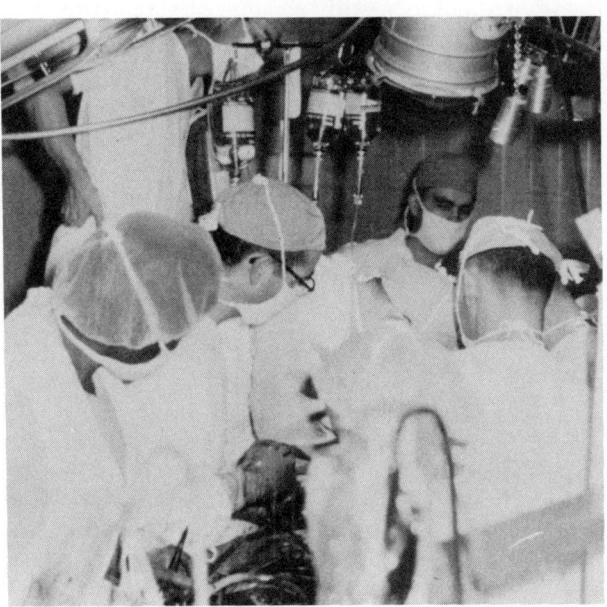

Transplantation of the first heart in man, January 23, 1964

lar problem. The arrested heart of the recipient was removed. It was an awesome sight to see the empty space in the recipient's chest where his own heart had been. The heart of the large chimpanzee, taken by the other team in the adjacent operating room, was transplanted. To my immense relief, the transplant began at once vigorously to exhibit disordered ventricular fibrillation, as soon as release of the clamps permitted its perfusion by the patient's own oxygenated warm blood. A single shock with the electrical defibrillator produced a normal heart rhythm. A pacemaker was sewn onto the surface of the heart, in case it should be needed postoperatively, and the pump support was discontinued. The transplant sustained the blood pressure at between 90 and 100 mm Hg for about an hour and a half, but thereafter the pressure gradually declined. The entire operation had been recorded on film. The donor heart was requested by, and ultimately donated to, the Smithsonian Institution in Washington. Success has a long yardstick, with an infinitely graduated scale.

In retrospect, and on the basis of subsequent research all over the world, the patient could not have been expected to live indefinitely, considering the far advanced state of his metabolic deterioration preoperatively. We later showed, in animals, that the heart of an animal dying of shock is readily capable of supporting a new host, when transplanted to a normal chemical environment. But our human recipient did not afford a normal chemical environment for the donor heart. Moreover, a larger heart for transplantation would also

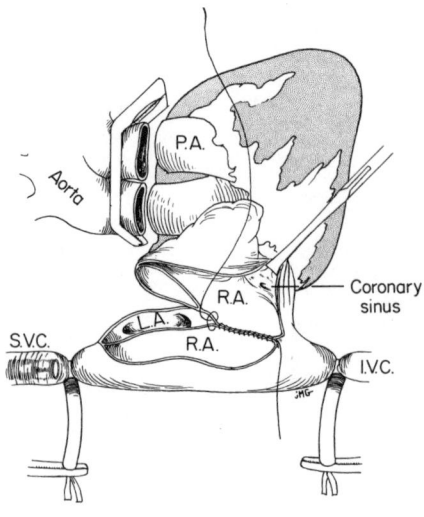

Technique of heart transplantation. From Hardy, J. D.; Chavez, C. M.; Eraslan, S.; et al., "Heart Transplantation in Dogs: Procedures, Physiologic Problems, and Results in 142 Experiments," Surgery 60 (1966): 361.

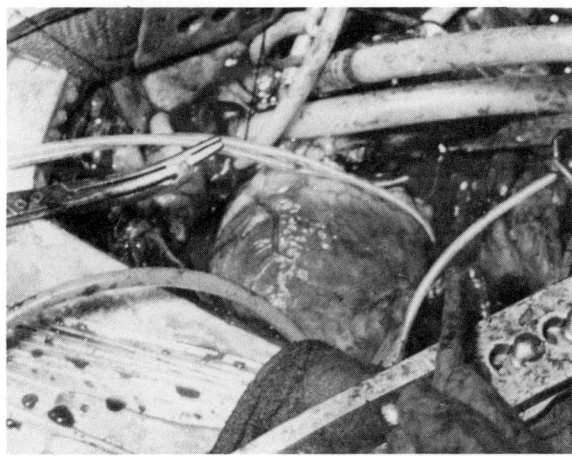

The first heart transplant in man.
From Hardy, J. D.; Chavez, C. M., "Transplantation of the Heart," in Hardy, J. D., ed., Human Organ Support and Replacement (*Springfield, Ill.: Charles C Thomas, 1971*). *Courtesy of Charles C Thomas.*

have been desirable. Nevertheless, we had demonstrated that the procedures of heart transplantation, so long practiced in the animal laboratory, were readily transferrable to man—that the heart could be removed from one primate and inserted into another primate (man) without difficulty. We had also breached the massive intellectual and emotional barrier which had previously prevented heart transplantation in man. Furthermore, we had achieved this substantial advance in knowledge and human philosophical horizons without shortening the life of a patient or incurring the then unacceptable ethical position of removing a still-beating human donor heart. The coronary arterial supply of the patient's own (excised) heart was found to have been 90 percent occluded when carefully studied by the pathologist. This was well before the development of heart vessel angiography and coronary bypass.

The resulting publicity would be impossible to describe here. Public media reporters from around the world seemed to come out of the woodwork. At this stage, Mrs. Maurine Twiss, Director of Public Information and a thoroughly experienced journalist, was of the greatest help and support to our group. We had never been exposed to such massive public interest, and it was her wise counsel that kept the situation within bounds, though at times these bounds were sorely strained.

But the worst was yet to come. The Sixth International Transplantation Conference was meeting in New York at the Waldorf-Astoria two weeks later. We had two papers on the program already, but I was now asked to join a hastily arranged panel on transplantation of the heart. The moderator of the panel was Willem Kolff, inventor of the artificial kidney in Holland during the Nazi occupation in World War II and also the inventor of the artificial heart which was the direct prototype of the one inserted into Barney Clark at the University of Utah Medical Center two decades later.

Dr. Keith Reemtsma spoke first, about his chimpanzee kidney transplants in humans at Tulane University. Kolff called my name to speak next, but before I was allowed to begin, he said to the large audience, "In Mississippi, they keep the chimpanzees in one cage and the Negroes in another cage, don't they, Dr. Hardy?"

This introduced into the equation, and the occasion, the huge problem of the bitter integration struggle currently raging in Mississippi, along with the use of a lower primate heart for the transplantation. I frankly admit that, for one of the few times in my professional career, I was taken aback and did poorly. The audience was palpably hostile, after the moderator's opening remarks and attitude. I gave our experience as it had happened, but there was not a single hand of applause thereafter. The remaining panelists, including Norman Shumway of Stanford and William Holden of Case Western Reserve University, said some positive things about the transplant, but it was a dismal day.

Kolff later asked me if I had not realized he was joking. I answered, "No, and I don't think that the worldwide audience knew you were joking."

The Society of University Surgeons met about the same time in Philadelphia. The council had voted to recommend that the annual meeting be held in Jackson several years later. After attending the council meeting I had returned to Jackson to a commitment, but at the full business meeting on Friday, the members rejected the council recommendation and refused to come to Jackson because there were several black members. This reversal of the council's recommendation was virtually unheard of. It was especially embarrassing to me, since I was still on the council by virtue of having just recently been president of the society. Just how much of the problem was the integration situation in Mississippi, and how much the heart transplant, one could not know.

A few months later Thomas Starzl of the University of Colorado and I were both speaking on a postgraduate program at the University of Minnesota. He was a world leader in kidney transplantation and *the* leader in liver transplantation. "Jim, you didn't do too well there in New York," Tom said. "It was the only time I ever saw you flustered. You know, you and I are absolute pariahs in American surgery."

He went on to say that a nationally ranked surgeon had called him a few nights before, quite late and obviously a bit in his cups, and had blasted him for transplanting the liver in man. Apparently the caller had followed up his call with an apologetic and conciliatory letter a few days later. "But," Tom said, "*in vino veritas.*"

The American Surgical Association met later in the spring. Dr. Ravdin came from a meeting and remarked, "Jim, someone said a while ago that your transplantation of the heart was not merely *immoral*, it was *amoral*." He went on to say that there had now been enough of this sort of thing, that it was time to begin the counterattack.

And yet, although I was considerably depressed and had certainly learned who my friends were (they were far fewer than I'd thought), I still felt that we had achieved an important milestone under acceptable ethical and moral circumstances. During the summer vacation I happened to read a biography of Disraeli. It seemed that he had written a novel, *Vivian Grey*, clearly based on an intimate knowledge of acquaintances in London, and it had caused a major outcry. To get away from all the turmoil, he had accompanied a friend to Italy and Spain. When he reached those countries, he found that his novel was not only widely accepted but thoroughly praised. He stopped apologizing.

When I traveled in Europe, I found that our heart transplant was known everywhere, and instead of all the carping and criticism going on in the United States, many surgical scientists in Europe simply wanted to know why we had not gone right ahead with another one. The answer was that Dean Marston could protect me just so far; beyond that, the opposition might well force the loss of my academic post. And I had noted that when one loses an academic post, for whatever reason, one's chances of getting an equal or better post elsewhere are seriously diminished. It seemed prudent not to transplant another heart, what with the prevailing public opinion in the United States, and it was obvious that Norman Shumway and his group at Stanford felt the same way. This left the door wide open for Christiaan Barnard in Capetown, South Africa—who had done far less laboratory work than a number of groups in the United States—to take a human recipient in fair condition and the still-beating heart from a head injury victim, and to successfully perform his human-to-human heart transplant in 1967. Thereafter, within the year, there were a number of heart transplant centers going forward in the United States, and we then transplanted another heart with ease. Incidentally, it is much easier to transplant a heart from one human being to another than from one dog to another. The structures to be sewn—the atria, the aorta, and the pulmonary artery—are much larger and less fragile in the human than in the dog, and it is easier to monitor and support the human patient in the recovery room postoperatively.

But the aftermath of the first heart transplant was a searing experience for me. It was the first time my clinical integrity had ever been challenged, as Kolff had challenged it in New York. It hardened me forever, and never again was I to be shaken at a podium.

Meanwhile, life did go on, but it was as if there had been a recent bereavement in the family, for the lung and heart transplants were never mentioned by friends. Actually, the circumstances were probably not as unfavorable as they seemed to me personally. By invitation, I gave a substantial paper at the annual meeting of the American Surgical Association, reviewing our extensive experience with lung transplantation. At the same meeting I was elected a member of the American Board of Surgery, the major examining group in American surgery.

In July I wrote Professor Brent, who was Peter Medawar's colleague, as follows:

July 6, 1964

Professor L. Brent
Zoology Department
University College
University of London
London, England

Dear Professor Brent:

In looking back over a somewhat tumultuous year, I find that one matter remains outstanding and I wish to write you about it.

You may recall the panel in New York when Doctor Kolff abruptly turned to me and made a series of extremely derogatory accusations which left me all but speechless. Actually, he later asked me if I had not realized he was joking. I replied that I had not realized he was joking and that I did not believe the members of the audience had realized he was joking. But in any case, I was perhaps understandably taken aback by this novel experience of having my clinical integrity thus assaulted.

In rebuttal, I noted that you and your colleagues took now a position that had been substantially modified since clinical kidney homotransplantation had been initiated some years ago. I mentioned your group without any special reason except that most of us in this country consider yours the outstanding theoretical unit in existence. My point was that the views of all do change with the unfolding of events and experience—that thus liver, lung and heart transplants might well be looked back upon differently with further changes in human imagination and acceptance.

Yet, the reason I write is that, given time to reflect upon what was a most disturbing moment for me, I realize that my mention of your group might have appeared indelicate and even discourteous to a distinguished visitor. If so, I regret it and ask that you view my reference as derived from profound respect rather than from any desire to draw you into a domestic controversy.

Respectfully yours,

He replied:

14th July, 1964

Professor James D. Hardy, M.D.
The University of Mississippi Medical Center
2500 North State Street
Jackson, Mississippi 39216

Dear Professor Hardy,

Thank you very much for your letter of July 6th. I appreciate the fact that you have written to me about this matter, but I assure you that not the slightest offence was taken at the time, and that you need not give it any further thought so far as we are concerned.

Yours sincerely,

L. Brent

Finally 1964 drew to a close. The heart transplant in January, and the murder and burial of three civil rights workers beneath a newly constructed dam near Philadelphia, Mississippi, had generated about as much news as Mississippi could stand for one year. And yet, in the civil rights and integration struggle, the closing months of 1964 probably represented the true turning point and ultimately the end of public segregation in the state. It was clear that the FBI had managed to infiltrate the Ku Klux Klan and had begun to get reliable information regarding the collaboration between law enforcement, the Klan and the white Citizens Councils. One incident stands out in my mind which illustrates brutally the changing state of affairs at that time. Leaving the hospital one night through the emergency room about nine or ten o'clock, I was accosted by a sheriff from a rural county who asked, "Doc, are you in charge here?"

"Well," I said, "I am the head of surgery here."

Pulling me into a nearby treatment room and closing the door, the sheriff said, "Doc, you got to help me save my deputy. The FBI is everywhere, but nobody knows where. Doc, things have got so bad you can't even shoot a nigger no more."

For years our splendid cook, child helper, and housekeeper, Mrs. Sarah Gray, a matriarch in charge of various generations of her family, had said that colored people were often more afraid of the "polices" than they were of the robbers. This emergency room vignette was my first real face-to-face encounter with the possible truth of her statements.

Another example: a Ku Klux Klan team was intercepted as they were placing explosives at the home of a Jewish businessman in Meridian. They were captured and the female driver of the getaway car was killed. She proved to be a well-known young public school teacher in Jackson.

The integration fight and resulting national scorn were taking a debilitating toll of the medical school faculty. Before he left for a chair at the University of Texas in Galveston, Dr. Artz had advised his colleagues that if they did not want to be buried in Mississippi, they had better get out while they still could. Julian Youmans in neurosurgery said, "The segregation fight has cut down the academic front-runners here." It was clear that he planned to make a move, and soon he did.

1965: Bitter harvest but hopes for spring

All things considered, we had managed to stay above water in 1964. Silence had been our public policy, amidst all the publicity and vituperation, but I did lash out once. The *Annals of Internal Medi-*

cine published an arrogant and viciously critical editorial regarding our human lung transplant. I had become accustomed to similar articles in that journal, but this particular editorial went beyond the pale. Although having had no contact with organ transplantation, the two authors had proceeded to pontificate extensively. I wrote a letter to the editor which was direct and to the point. The editor of the *Annals* was an old research friend at the University of Pennsylvania. He acknowledged that the authors' criticisms had been harsh and perhaps misinformed, but that they had been honestly made. I replied, with some asperity, that the *Annals* seemed to be especially hospitable to such manuscripts attacking the new field of organ transplantation.

By 1966, the storm of criticism was beginning to give way to the more sober realization that the heart is nothing more than a pump. Personally, I had decided that I must preserve my own self-image: that my self-respect could not be a reflection of others' opinions; that I could not be offended unless I allowed myself to be offended; that under the circumstances in which we had performed the first heart transplant in man, demonstrating the feasibility of this procedure, it had been morally acceptable and as successful as possible; that given precisely the same set of circumstances, at precisely that point in time, I would have done the same thing again. It was clear, however, that to successfully transplant a heart in man, it must be possible to obtain a still-beating heart from a brain-dead donor and to put it into a recipient who is not in terminal shock at the time he is taken to the operating room. Even so, years later it was to be shown that the healthy heart from a brain-dead patient, if cooled quickly, could be stored in ice for several hours and then transplanted successfully, as with the kidney and liver.

An important source of support to me was a senior surgical statesman who had himself felt the lash when he had done something new. Dr. Lester Dragstedt, chairman of surgery at the University of Chicago for many years, came to visit our laboratory in 1966. He had introduced vagotomy for the relief of peptic ulcer, and for this he had been bitterly criticized until vagotomy became the standard surgical treatment. He watched us do a canine heart transplant, from beginning to end, over a period of several hours. "Jim, I have seen a miracle here this morning. My warmest congratulations. I just wish my career was beginning now and could go forward with the development of this great new field of organ transplantation. Now let me say this to you. Just go around the country and tell your story, over and over again. Everything will be all right."

Dr. Dragstedt was proven correct when I was invited to give our original experience and to preside over the opening session of the Second World Heart Transplantation Congress in Montreal on June 6, 1969. And with the years came vindication. Moreover, at this writing an infant at Loma Linda University is surviving on a baboon

---

Scientific Programme

FRIDAY MORNING, June 6th 1969

SITE: Man and his World, Auditorium Ste-Hélène
9:00—GENERAL SESSION
"THE WORLD'S EXPERIENCE"
Chairman: James D. Hardy, M.D.,
University of Mississippi, Jackson, Miss., U.S.A.

Panelists

1 GROOTE SCHUUR HOSPITAL, Cape Town, South Africa.
Christiaan N. Barnard, M.D.
2 STANFORD UNIVERSITY, Palo Alto, Calif., U.S.A.
N.E. Shumway and E.B. Stinson, M.D.
3 TEXAS HEART INSTITUTE, Houston, Texas, U.S.A.
Denton A. Cooley, Grady L. Hallman, M.D.
4 MEDICAL COLLEGE OF VIRGINIA, Richmond, Virginia, U.S.A.
Richard R. Lower, Eric Kemp and Walter H. Graham, M.D.
5 BROUSSAIS HOSPITAL, Paris, France.
Charles Dubost and J.P. Cachera, M.D.
6 MONTREAL HEART INSTITUTE, Montreal, Canada.
Pierre Grondin and Gilles Lepage, M.D.
7 UNIVERSITY OF SAO PAULO MEDICAL SCHOOL,
Sao Paulo, Brazil.
E.J. Zerbini and Luiz V. Decourt, M.D.
8 METHODIST HOSPITAL, Baylor University, Houston,
Texas, U.S.A.
Michael E. De Bakey, M.D.
9 GUY'S HOSPITAL, London, England.
Donald Ross, M.D.
10 UNIVERSITY HOSPITAL, Ann Harbor, Michigan, U.S.A.
Donald R. Kahn, J.A. Walton and Herbert Sloan, M.D.
11 UNIVERSITY OF TORONTO, Toronto, Canada.
W.G. Bigelow, M.D.

Second World Symposium on Heart Transplantation, June 6–8, 1969, Montreal

heart, which genetically is considered to be further away from the human than is the chimpanzee.

A heart is transplanted in Capetown

I remember exactly when I first heard the news. It was the night of our 1967 annual departmental Christmas party. My wife and I had just walked to the top of the stairs of the River Hills Tennis Club when an assistant, who had worked with me in the animal laboratory so diligently with heart transplants, came up to me and said, "I heard on the radio driving over that somebody had successfully transplanted a heart in Capetown, South Africa. Dr. Hardy, we should have done that *years ago!*"

I confess my disappointment was enormous, though not so much for myself personally, for I knew that Shumway's group at Stanford had done the most extensive and best work in the field. We had long been waiting for them to transplant a heart in man, following which we planned to transplant another. Hanlon's group in St. Louis had also been in the field, as had Blumenstock at Cooperstown, New York, and other groups. Then why had none of us performed another heart transplant following our first three years earlier? The reason was public and professional opinion in the United States, along with the national governmental committees within committees, protecting the public from "experimentation." These had become so burdensome and severe that we simply could not risk another transplant: should the patient fail to live at least a few weeks, as well he might under the American strictures of not being able to remove a still-beating heart and requiring a terminally ill recipient, the results could prove disastrous, both professionally and with regard to grant support from Washington, upon which all of us were heavily dependent. We would have been longer in getting our own open-heart work in patients going in Jackson had we not been able to take the heart pump and other equipment from our experimental laboratory to the hospital to perform the human open-heart surgery. Again, our hospital did not then have funds to pay for such expensive instrumentation; it had to be purchased with research funds.

Nevertheless, the South African transplant was a bitter pill to swallow, since the United States had spent so much money in this field over the years. Christiaan Barnard had spent some time with one of Shumway's previous associates, Richard Lower in Richmond, and then had gone back to Capetown and simply done it, with very little animal work and with no publications indicating such work in his laboratory. He was a well-known heart surgeon, however. The United States had only itself to blame for loss of this major opportunity.

A few days later I called the team in Capetown to learn details of the operation. It was obvious that opinion in the United States had changed overnight and that it was now possible to transplant hearts in this country, even though we had let the first successful heart transplant go to South Africa. Christiaan Barnard was away speaking, but his brother Mario Barnard, also a member of the transplant team, told me they had drawn carefully upon our published experience with the heart transplant and that they appreciated the guidance it had given them. Curiously, some months later, Christiaan Barnard himself wrote me that our heart transplant in 1964 had not in fact been the first heart transplant in man. Although offering no documentation, he actually claimed to believe that the ancient Chinese had successfully transplanted hearts centuries ago. Presumably, those ancient heart transplants had been performed without anatomical knowledge of the circulation of the blood, blood transfusion, suture materials, proper instruments, anesthesia, the heart-lung machine, or modern physiologic support and postoperative management.

The attitude of our national governmental institutions changed overnight. All the transplant teams in the United States, plus outstanding heart surgeons who had not been interested in transplantation, were called by the National Institutes of Health to a meeting at O'Hare Airport on December 28, barely two weeks after the heart transplant in Capetown, to plan for the future. Barnard reviewed the details of his case. Once again I was besieged by reporters and telephone calls asking for a review of our 1964 heart transplant. This time there was none of the adversarial hostility that had characterized such interviews in 1964.

Quite aside from its human application, heart transplantation per se proved very useful as an experimental model in animals. As noted previously, we were able to show that in animals dying of shock from induced infection or blood loss, the heart could be removed from the dying animal and transplanted into a normal recipient successfully. That is, the heart of an animal dying in shock was readily capable of functioning effectively if transplanted into the normal metabolic (chemical) environment of a healthy recipient. This supported our belief that, had the human recipient not been in shock at

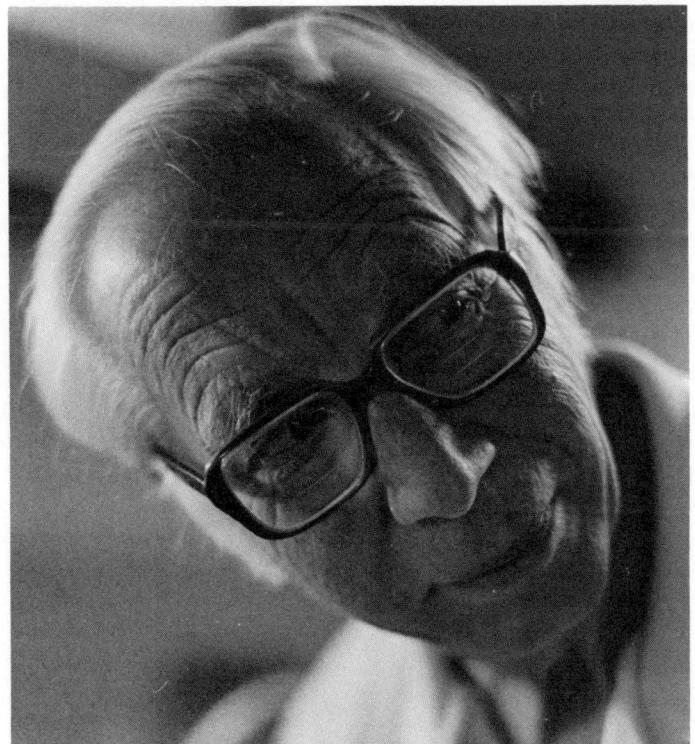
Willem J. Kolff, inventor of artificial kidney and artificial heart

our first heart transplant in man in 1964, the heart of the large chimpanzee might well have been able to support the patient until rejected.

The artificial heart

Dr. Tetsuzo Akutsu, who had developed the first artificial heart prototypes with Dr. Willem Kolff in Cleveland in 1958,* had joined our department in 1966. His ten-man group was financed by the National Institutes of Health. They had progressed from having nearly every calf recipient of one of their various artificial heart models die on the operating table, to achieving several weeks or months of sur-

*T. Akutsu, and W. J. Kolff, "Permanent Substitutes for Valves and Hearts," *Trans. Amer. Soc. Artif. Intern. Organs* 4 (1958): 230.

vival in almost every experiment. Moreover, the artificial heart provided a useful model for differentiating the effects of circulatory drugs upon different elements of the circulation: for example, the specific drug administered could have no effect on the mechanical heart itself, and thus any changes noted in the blood pressure had to be due to effects of the drug on the blood vessels of the circulation. Kolff later continued his artificial heart development at the University of Utah.

Denton A. Cooley was the first to insert a total artificial heart replacement in a human, but recently William C. DeVries has replaced the human heart with the current model and with a fair amount of early success.

The major complications of the *artificial* heart were, and remain, fatigue and subsequent breakage of the materials, blood clotting on the artificial surfaces, with loosened particles embolizing to various arteries of the body, and infection where tubes must pass through the chest wall. The heart *transplant's* major problems rest with the homograft reaction and the drugs necessary to prevent transplant rejection.

CHAPTER 17

The Developing Department of Surgery: Further Progress

The departmental activity had moved forward very satisfactorily for several years, until 1971.

Another anesthesia crisis

Anesthesia coverage at the University Medical Center had improved considerably with the arrival of Leonard Fabian from Duke University as chairman. However, the electrical anesthesia research emanating from our surgery laboratory had stimulated much national interest among anesthesiologists, and speaking tours began taking much of Fabian's time. His department suffered, and problems arose in the absence of adequate anesthesia coverage and consistent administrative leadership. The current dean, Robert Blount, had tried repeatedly to reason with him, resulting in Fabian's threatening to resign on several occasions. Growing discouraged, the dean suggested he resign in writing and then filed his letter without comment. With the next "resignation," however, the dean said that he would not need another letter, that the one on file would suffice. Dr. Fabian was stunned. He had felt secure, what with the national scarcity of academically oriented anesthesiologists.

We were again faced with a severe anesthesia crisis, for the anesthesia staff was very small. There were few residents, and almost all the registered nurse anesthetists had been phased out. It was in this critical situation that I was able to make one of my most gratifying administrative adjustments.

The first priority was to get someone capable of giving safe anesthesia for the open-heart operations. For this we were able to attract a superb cardiac anesthesiologist from the heart surgery service of the University of Tokyo—he wished to work in the United States for a year to improve his English. He arrived promptly and served admirably in that capacity. In addition, our general surgical residents were able to give limited service. We had always rotated them through anesthesia for three months during their training, so that they would understand the problems of the anesthesiologist and because there were rarely enough residents in anesthesiology to cover the needs. Further, I learned that a Turkish surgeon who was learning lung transplantation in our animal laboratory had been an anesthesiologist at a university hospital in Turkey before entering the army and then going into surgery. Leaving the laboratory temporarily, he was able to perform general anesthesia under routine and carefully circumscribed circumstances. Fikri Alican, another Turkish surgeon who had come to us from the University of Istanbul to do transplants, knew of a young anesthesiologist at his home university. She was already well trained but wished to learn more English and observe American anesthesia practices. She came and also served admirably. Dr. Jesse Mullins, a solid member of the anesthesiology staff, gave support to the trainees and the nurse anesthetists. We thus moved forward until James Arens arrived from the Ochsner Clinic in 1972. He soon had with him an outstanding group of academic anesthesiologists, the like of which I had not seen since leaving Philadelphia many years before. It was a privilege to work with his group over the next few years, before they again scattered. Hospital-based anesthesiologists are highly mobile, since they immediately have a monopoly without having to build up a private practice.

Storm clouds gathering

The internal struggles in the Department of Surgery—first with neurosurgery, then with orthopaedics, and twice with anesthesiology—had inevitably taken their toll on my political support. Regardless of the merits of the case leading to a confrontation, each of the principals inevitably loses something in the exchange because both have friends and supporters, and the enemies generated by these conflicts tend to coalesce.

True, I had been much in the public eye, too much in many ways. My opposing neurosurgery's becoming a separate department still rankled in some quarters, though ultimately my position was going to be vindicated. Critics said that Dr. William Enneking had been "run off" in orthopaedics, and that the head of anesthesiology had been treated in the same manner—completely disregarding the fact that the latter had a separate and coequal department of the medical center and that he had resigned. It was a time for proceeding carefully.

Anticipating imminent attack, two of my senior residents, Martin McMullan and Joe Ed Varner, came to warn me privately that it was a precarious time, and that I should try to pull back on all fronts. They said that some of the younger members of the clinical faculty, who felt that a change should now be made in the leadership of the Department of Surgery, were meeting secretly. I had been told of one meeting, in which a perennial opponent in another department had suggested that two members of my own department, who were present at the meeting, should take over a segment of the operating activity which I had developed from scratch. This suggestion apparently was quickly squelched by one of my staff who reportedly said, "Your suggestion simply goes to show that you don't know Dr. Hardy at all. You just don't do that to him. He tries to treat everyone fair, and he expects the same in return."

Then a member of still another department of the medical center requested an appointment. Hardly had he seated himself than he said abruptly, "We are going to get rid of you. You have served your time."

"That's a straightforward statement, to say the least," I replied. "Fortunately, I work for the dean, the chancellor, and the Board of Trustees of the Institutions of Higher Learning. I serve as the chairman of the Department of Surgery at their pleasure. Then there is of course the tenure problem, and it would take you a considerable amount of time to overcome that obstacle."

Thus the spring of 1971 was an unsettled period due to multiple factors, some beyond my control. It was true that I had been away from the university a fair amount, though always with the permission of the administration. Also, early in the 1960s we had all been on the front end of the learning curve with kidney transplants and open-heart surgery—as were the majority of surgeons beginning such work. We had lost the occasional kidney transplant patient, but this was due, in part, to the fact that we did not have timely blood dialysis and had to resort to peritoneal dialysis, which was not safe from infection or truly effective at that time. It was still a time when transplant surgeons chose to increase the anti-rejection drugs to a level that risked fatal infections, rather than to remove the failing transplant early and save the patient by recourse to the dialysis. We had also lost an occasional open-heart surgery case that would not have been lost with further experience. However, we at times had had badly inexperienced anesthesia for the pump cases, we had a small anesthesia recovery room but no intensive care unit, and experienced nurse coverage for these patients had been almost nonexistent. We considered that, under the circumstances in which we'd had to work, the results had been reasonably good. The transplant patients had usually had no other choice, for long-term, chronic renal dialysis was just developing in our medical center.

It was clear that both clinical and political parameters needed to be strengthened. To this end, we redoubled efforts to get competent anesthesia, which we achieved with the recruitment of James Arens. Next, Dr. Akio Suzuki was brought from Cleveland, where he had participated in a massive volume of open-heart surgery for twelve years. We insisted on space in which to form a surgical intensive care unit. The nurses were trained, and this unit was functioning within the year, thanks largely to the untiring efforts of Dr. Hilary Timmis. The hospital laboratory made arterial blood gas values and other supportive chemical analyses promptly available on a twenty-four-hour basis, for the first time. Finally, after mending political fences, the overall atmosphere turned around and was essentially back to normal by the year's end.

Winds of change

The gradual turnaround for the better was external as well. The state of Mississippi had finally integrated with a remarkable degree of acceptance, albeit with much pressure from the federal government. A true social revolution had taken place since the Ole Miss crisis a decade before. This achievement, though imperfect and incomplete to be sure, had substantially improved the capacity of the University of Mississippi Medical Center to recruit new faculty members, academicians who would not have considered coming ten years before.

I could think back on all that had transpired in the seventeen years since the medical school and hospital had opened in 1955. Truly, "mine enemies had grown older." Most of the formidable medical politicians who had so opposed the medical center originally had long since turned into friends, if perhaps not close ones; we were all now more concerned with getting on with our lives.

The Mississippi Surgical Forum

With the student and intern-resident educational programs fully established, we turned attention to our obligation to offer postgraduate education to surgeons in the surrounding area. We had brought in visiting lecturers and professors from other parts of the country, and each year, from time to time, two or three guest lecturers had been invited to join our local school staff in presenting a three-day course on topics of current surgical interest. However, although some of our guest speakers were known throughout the world, attendance had been poor, even of surgeons right in the city of Jackson. We really had no good ideas as to how to improve the attendance. Funds were not available to invite a large number of out-of-state speakers, as the program was free to any surgeon who wished to come.

While participating in the University of Minnesota's postgraduate course, in which almost six hundred people enrolled, I mentioned our poor attendance. Dr. Richard Varco said that their courses had been going for twenty years or more, with many people attending more than once. They rotated the subject matter so that any surgeon attending the course each year would cover most phases of current surgical knowledge and practice, and they charged a tuition fee, both to pay speakers and to exact appreciation.

The information that helped us most in making our course a success, however, came from Dr. Wiley Barker of UCLA, when we were both speakers at a similar course put on by UCLA at Palm Springs. "I bet you send your circulars only to surgeons in your state and surrounding states," he said. "You must send them nationwide. We mail out thousands of brochures. Furthermore, it is important to have quite a number of out-of-state speakers, for local and regional surgeons consider that they already know what the faculty of their nearby medical school knows."

We decided to put a substantial amount of money into a trial effort to achieve a successful course. If the results were unsatisfactory, then we would drop the effort. We invited nationally and internationally known lecturing surgeons and paid them expenses and a decent honorarium, mailed brochures to thousands of surgeons throughout the United States, and charged a fee, as did Minnesota and UCLA.

The results were spectacular. Surgeons from approximately forty states attended the Mississippi Surgical Forum, and the number who applied exceeded the four hundred that we could accommodate in the lecture hall. Year by year after that the subject matter was rotated. The recommendations of those attending were carefully analyzed and employed, and there developed a sustaining group who came year after year. The annual course became a rallying point for graduates of the University of Mississippi Medical Center, from both the medical school and our residency training program.

The orthopaedic uprising

I was at home revising a manuscript one evening (July 1, 1976, to be exact) when Vice-Chancellor Norman C. Nelson called to ask me to come down to his office right away. He would not say over the telephone what the problem was. I could not imagine what administrative problem could be of such gravity that he would neither mention it over the telephone nor let it wait until morning. Curious, I went right down to his office, where I found him, the university lawyer Carl André, the attorney William Winter (later governor), the chief of orthopaedics, Paul Derian, and the chief resident in orthopaedics. The chief resident, representing the orthopaedic residents, accompanied by Winter, had come in to throw down the gauntlet: All eleven residents in orthopaedics at the University of Mississippi Medical Center would resign immediately unless certain conditions were met. The principal condition proved to be that the chief of orthopaedics, the only full-time member of our orthopaedic staff, must be relieved as chairman of the Division of Orthopaedic Surgery immediately. There was even discussion that he be fired, but this was not only completely inappropriate but also unrealistic, as he was a tenured professor. While there are grounds for firing anyone, a tenured professor is rarely released without considerable documentation and even legal advice. Dr. Derian was accused of inadequate teaching and leadership in a wide range of specified activities.

The residents' move abruptly brought to a head a situation in orthopaedics which I had long realized was an unhappy one, although I had not known the depth of the problem. Ever since the previous chairman of orthopaedics had left, the affairs of orthopaedics had been tacitly handled by the new chairman's direct communications with the current dean, rather than communications through departmental channels in the usual way. If this was the way that the university administration wanted to handle orthopaedics, it was the administration's privilege to do so. But I had sought clarification as far back as 1970. I had written to Robert E. Blount, then dean, as follows:

Dear Dean Blount:

I was truly disturbed to call Dr. Derian about a matter and find that he had been in Europe for two weeks and will be there for a week or so longer. Dr. Derian is a member of the Department of Surgery and Dr. Carter [a previous dean] asked me to please pay more attention to what Dr. Derian and his group were doing. I cannot do this with the present administrative arrangements. I would request that we return to standard practice and have all requests for travel, or any other items which must require administrative and Board of Trustee support, sent through this office—if this is satisfactory with you.

Dean Blount had answered with a handwritten endorsement to the effect that he completely agreed that all such administrative items must pass through my office to keep me informed. However, this had not been done. I now assured the current dean and vice-chancellor, Norman C. Nelson, that whatever might be wrong with orthopaedics, I would do my best to help.

The fact that Mr. Winter was there, retained by the residents, was in itself a sinister development, since this was the first time in my memory that a group of residents had engaged legal counsel before presenting a complaint to their own medical school administration. Moreover, since Mr. Winter's legal work involved few cases such as this, some wondered about political overtones, inasmuch as the wife of the chairman of orthopaedics, Patricia Derian (who later went to Washington with President Carter as Assistant Secretary of State for Human Rights), was considered a political rival.

The attorneys for the two parties, Mr. Winter for the orthopaedic residents and Mr. André for the University Medical Center, went into another room and drew up an agreement which was then signed by both lawyers and the vice-chancellor. I did not see the agreement, but the thrust of it was that Dr. Derian would step down as chairman of the division and a new chairman would be brought on board as soon as possible. Dr. Derian readily agreed to this, to my surprise, but I sensed he realized that this course was the better of two unhappy alternatives. Moreover, at the time he was deeply distressed over an unrelated personal problem. The residents were to return the next morning and take care of their patients—whom they had abandoned abruptly in leaving without notice.

As head of the overall Department of Surgery, I became *de facto* acting chairman of the Division of Orthopaedics, though my management of such cases had long since been discontinued. Interestingly, the members of the Mississippi Academy of Orthopaedics met in urgent session and mailed a protest that orthopaedics was being administered by a general surgeon (me)—although they well knew that, had there been an orthopaedist available, he would have been appointed on the spot.

Meanwhile, we general surgeons provided emergency coverage of the in-house orthopaedic patients during the night, expecting the orthopaedic residents to be present the following day. To our surprise, however, the residents did not appear. Later on in the day, if memory serves, they turned to television and the newspapers to make additional demands, ignoring the signed agreement. With this development, it was obvious that bad blood existed to the extent that other arrangements were going to have to be made. With two general surgery residents, I surveyed every orthopaedic patient currently in the hospital and promptly discharged those who could safely go home. Moreover, since the orthopaedic outpatient clinic was huge, we quickly went through these patients and reduced the number to an absolute minimum. The orthopaedists in town were apparently too busy with their practices to assist with emergencies, and the orthopaedists at our Methodist Rehabilitation Center were discreetly unavailable. Newspaper coverage was extensive.

The massive and bitter public assault on the chairman of orthopaedics cut in many directions. First, either Winter was in accord with the continuing absence of the residents, or he had lost control and there was no one with whom the university could readily deal. The rock-hard uniformity and cohesiveness of the eleven orthopaedic residents was impressive and surprising, until it was alleged that they had commonly been allowed, themselves, to select the new residents coming in—a selection usually made by senior staff members. One had to admire the care and time the residents had clearly expended over the months prior to their ultimatum. Most of them had already lined up tentative residency positions elsewhere.

Eventually, the chief of orthopaedics elected to practice in another city. The residents agreed to return only if the entire group was taken back as a unit, with complete amnesty. The university, bruised by all the unpleasant publicity and the secret and legal approach by the residents, offered to consider the residents' applications individually. Actually, we were willing to reinstate all of them, for we knew they had courageously addressed a serious problem. However, we felt that the administrative integrity of the institution would be compromised if their all-or-none ultimatum were accepted. They all left for positions elsewhere.

In a few months James L. Hughes, from Johns Hopkins, had re-established the residency program and had recruited a strong staff of able academic orthopaedists.

The ENT-plastic surgery struggle

A controversy was steadily growing, not only in our institution but throughout the United States, between the specialties of otorhinolaryngology and plastic surgery, over which group would operate for what problems in which patients.

Ear infections, infected tonsils, and sinus problems had been so common and serious for so many years that the ear, nose, and throat specialists had all the work they needed. With the advent of increasingly effective antibiotics, however, operations for sinus problems and infected ears and mastoids became relatively uncommon, as indeed did tonsillectomy. As the specialty of ENT continued to dwindle in scope, it was apparent that if it were to survive and thrive, it must begin to treat other disease conditions. Thus ENT began to encroach upon the long-established domain of plastic surgeons, who naturally defended their turf with vigor.

Early on, we had had part-time attending coverage of both these services in our University Hospital, but there had been little competition because we had no full-time surgeons in either specialty. However, Godfrey Arnold had come from New York to develop a program in ENT, and had recruited an associate, Myron Lockey, who had done much head and neck surgery. This group began to do a lot of surgery that ENT had never done before in our hospital. When Michael Jabaley arrived from Johns Hopkins to be full-time chief of plastic surgery, we expected there would be conflict, and there certainly was.

They would meet separately, to try to agree on a definite list of operations that would be allocated specifically to one service or to the other, and then I would meet with them to firm up the document. However, each arrangement lasted only a few months, and then another agreement had to be worked out, almost always with further encroachment of ENT upon the domains of plastic surgery. It was not a happy time for me. Although my own general surgery service had done much of the head and neck surgery during our early years in Jackson, this work had long since been given over to plastic surgery. They simply did a better job, especially with the reconstructive procedures which were so time-consuming and demanded expertise beyond the command of the usual general surgeon.

The national battle between ENT and plastic surgery over the purview of each specialty reached a crisis in our medical center in 1979.

Disregarding all the many agreements made, dating back to 1966, the ENT residents began surreptitiously to perform even face-lifts, the quintessential operation of plastic surgery. Neither Dr. Arnold nor Dr. Lockey had ever done face-lifts and they were not doing them now. We had several times offered to allow the ENT residents to learn face-lifts and related plastic procedures by rotating on the plastic surgery service or by scrubbing with surgeons out in the city of Jackson. Actually, very few face-lifts were done in the University Hospital anyway, but here a basic administrative principle was involved. The two full-time ENT staff members had repeatedly assured me that they would permit no face-lifts to be done on the ENT service, either at the University Hospital or at the closely associated Veterans Administration Hospital. The whole issue came to a head when, despite a discussion less than three weeks before, the residents in ENT deliberately defied the agreement we had made and, in effect, challenged my authority over the Department of Surgery.

This was beyond acceptance. Without further consultation with the ENT staff, who had failed to maintain discipline among the residents in their division, I wrote each resident in ENT that, should he perform any such operation in the future, the penalty would be instant dismissal. Simultaneously, I wrote the director of the operating suite not to "set up" for any such operation by anyone in the ENT division, either staff or residents. This was a drastic action, but it was taken only after the most extreme provocation. Actually, I was not certain that I had the authority to do this, but I suspected that I probably did have—or that even if I did not, the other side would not know whether I did and hence would not challenge it.

Dr. Arnold was at retirement and really was not entering the conflict, but Dr. Lockey had been expected to take over the chair. My action finally brought the whole problem out in the open, and Dr. Lockey requested of the hospital Executive Committee a formal hearing where he would defend his rights to perform the proscribed plastic operations. In most *community* private hospitals, almost any surgeon who has the training may do almost any operation; I held, however, that a University Hospital must have regulations that preserve an adequate teaching environment in all disciplines. These regulations build fences between different services to preserve discipline, standards, and "turf." For example, most general surgeons could perform an adequate hysterectomy, but in a University Hospital hysterectomies are the province of obstetrics-gynecology so that this department can develop and maintain an effective teaching and training program.

Dr. Lockey maintained that the patient who had precipitated the whole problem was technically his private patient ("Medicaid pending"), though actually operated upon by residents, and that he was free to do with his private practice as he pleased. However, with the advent of third-party payers in the form of Medicare and Medicaid and other sources that covered the majority of patients, virtually every patient could now be classified, to some extent, as a private patient. Thus ENT could theoretically capture virtually all the disputed patients, regardless of the service to which they would otherwise have been assigned—if ENT were vigorous enough in finding these patients first.

The sorely vexed Dr. Lockey made an effective and temperate presentation of his case to the Executive Committee. I was proud of him. He was an excellent surgeon, and I liked him personally, although I did *not* like his aggressive pursuit of the national objectives of the ENT specialty at our expense.

The most difficult decision I had to make was just how much ammunition to use in presenting my case. I did not wish to be excessively heavy with argument and facts; on the other hand, the issue was too important to risk losing the vote for lack of force. Therefore, I developed my presentation with care, referring to events dating back fourteen years to 1966 and before. First, I played a conference tape made five years before. Someone remarked that the tape could just as well have been made yesterday, since the problems remained exactly the same—which they did, not only in Jackson but throughout the United States. Next, I showed lantern slides of numerous printed operating room schedules listing the plastic operations which had been done by the ENT residents. All the various agreements that had been made, almost year by year for sixteen years, were cited.

I summarized the presentation with "The Three Issues": 1. The constitutional issue: Is the University of Mississippi a guest in its own hospital? Can the hospital staff dictate to the university? 2. Does the university have academic authority over its University Hospital? That is, can the university, through academic appointments, control its university hospital? 3. The otolaryngologist's personal conduct: Was it disruptive to the operation of the hospital? Had he failed to honor administrative assurances by aiding and abetting face-lifts by ENT residents? Had he failed to provide moral leadership for his residents? Had he attempted to destroy the ENT service? (He had apparently written critical letters to a number of centers in the United States, before ever talking to us seriously about his plans.) Finally, had he challenged and disregarded departmental authority? Yes, he had.

I alleged that these facts constituted *contumacious conduct*. The dictionary defines contumacious conduct as perverse in resisting, stubbornly disobedient, rebellious, insubordinate, and irreconcilable. Under university policy, one of the circumstances under which a person's contract could be terminated was contumacious conduct. The members of the Executive Committee voted unanimously with my position. Although several successive committees were appointed to look into this matter further, this vote was never changed. Accordingly, Dr. Lockey soon informed us that he would be resigning, as he had made clear he would do from the outset, should he not be supported by the Executive Committee.

But this was only the beginning of the problem.

It was necessary to alert the residents at once (as if they did not know already) that there might well be inadequate staff coverage of their residency training program after July 1, and that they should feel free to begin looking elsewhere for residency positions. Gradually they did leave, one by one.

Then, on November 1, 1979, virtually all of the ENT specialists in the state of Mississippi went public including a message to the Board of Trustees of Institutions of Higher Learning, to the chancellor, and to members of the legislature. They claimed that Dr. Hardy was imposing strictures on the specialty of ear, nose, and throat that would make it impossible for future young physicians to train adequately in this specialty.

A letter to the university signed by virtually every trained ENT surgeon in the state of Mississippi contained a long indictment of Dr. Hardy and his policies against ENT. This letter, bearing so many signatures, proved ultimately to be a major legal mistake that redounded to the advantage of the University of Mississippi Medical Center and its legal defense against the lawsuit in federal court.

Early in 1980, the university was informed by legal counsel for the American Academy of Facial, Plastic, and Reconstructive Surgery (the "Academy") that legal redress would be sought in federal court unless the university policies in question were changed. The Academy's legal counsel in Chicago retained the impressive Jackson firm of Wise, Carter, Child and Carraway to conduct the lawsuit against the university at the local level. The University Medical Center had no choice but to address this legal issue, since the ultimate responsibility and accountability of the university to conduct its affairs was thus threatened. In addition to retained counsel, the university enlisted the services of the Brunini law firm. This was going to be an expensive proposition for both sides.

The most pressing immediate problem was that the ENT patients had to be treated. Fortunately, plastic surgery and general surgery could together readily cover the vast majority of ENT patients. (This was a far different situation from that which had existed in the orthopaedic crisis.) Nonetheless, the national ENT specialists seized this opportunity to break the resistance of the University of Mississippi Medical Center, trying to establish, nationally, a precedent that would give ENT open access to face-lifts and cosmetic procedures, which had thus far been performed largely by plastic surgeons. Therefore, all possible pressure was brought to bear upon us in Jackson.

But the outside forces did not prevail. The more than thirty state ENT specialists who had signed the original letter to the University—threatening professional, political, and legal measures—were presumptive parties to the lawsuit, including a special lawsuit for the ENT residents themselves. Clearly, it was going to be necessary for the university's state-supported legal defense to take exhaustive and very expensive depositions from each of these thirty ENT surgeons who had entered the fight. Ultimately, the issue died under the burden of legal expenses, and the ENT group withdrew the lawsuit.

No one took any satisfaction from this crisis, least of all myself. When I became president-elect of the American College of Surgeons, it was threatened that the approximately three to four thousand ENT members would consider dropping their membership in the organization unless the Board of Regents of the American College of Surgeons at least censured me. The regents had no thought of doing so, nor did anyone believe seriously that most of the ENT members would resign, but this embarrassment diminished the pleasure of being president of the organization. My effort to maintain administrative principle was vindicated, however, and I took the abuse as part of my job, though my wife was much less philosophical.

The ENT service was soon restored and, indeed, markedly improved upon.

Sixty years: a fateful age

Even I had to acknowledge that reaching the age of sixty was a certain milestone. My twin brother Julian said, "James, we've got to admit that we're now beyond middle age." Sadly, he died within the year following a coronary bypass.

A surgeon's patient referrals tend to fall off rapidly after the age of sixty, much more so than those of internists. His referral circle of physicians is reduced by retirements, younger surgeons are perceived as more able to withstand the stress of long operations, and the older surgeon is less enthusiastic about accepting emergencies at night. At sixty it occurred to me that I had been taking night call since 1942, a total of thirty-six years, and while I still did, it was obvious that the residents did not call me at night, unless it was unavoidable, but would call my junior associate instead.

We had also changed "Sunday School Rounds," after almost twenty-three years, to seven o'clock Wednesday morning, since the operating room personnel had been given this hour for in-service education. Thereafter we continued to make Sunday rounds, but less formally.

Not that age sixty provided respite—the pace picked up, if anything. Dr. C. Rollins Hanlon, director of the American College of Surgeons, called me one Sunday afternoon about a "chore." "The Board of Regents has elected you to fill Curt Artz's unexpired term as second vice-president. [Dr. Artz had recently died.] Obviously, the reason I am calling is to learn whether or not you will accept."

Both he and I knew (I had once been on the Nominating Committee of the American College of Surgeons) that the office of second vice-president in the college was generally considered a dead end, with little or no authority or function. To tell the truth, this honor was not overwhelming to one who had just a year or so before finished the office of president of the American Surgical Association.

But it certainly indicated that the Board of Regents, the group that conducts the affairs of the ACS, held me in high esteem, and the untimely death of Dr. Artz was the only circumstance in which the Board of Regents had the authority to appoint such an officer. Thus, they had especially honored me. Without hesitation, of course, I said that I would be most pleased to serve. While it was highly unusual for a second vice-president to achieve higher office, it was unlikely in my case anyway, since I had not served as a regent or even as a governor.

To illustrate the limited importance attached to this office, at the next meeting at the ACS headquarters in Chicago I could find no seat that was reserved for the second vice-president, although all the regents, the president, and the first vice-president had name plates on their desks. Finally, I slid into an empty chair adjacent to Professor Mark Ravitch of Pittsburgh, the first vice-president, whereupon he leaned over and whispered in my ear, "Now, never forget for an instant, Jim, that you are only one heartbeat away from the office of first vice-president."

Curiously, I felt almost a release at this appointment, for it meant my official travel for the college would soon be at an end, after the

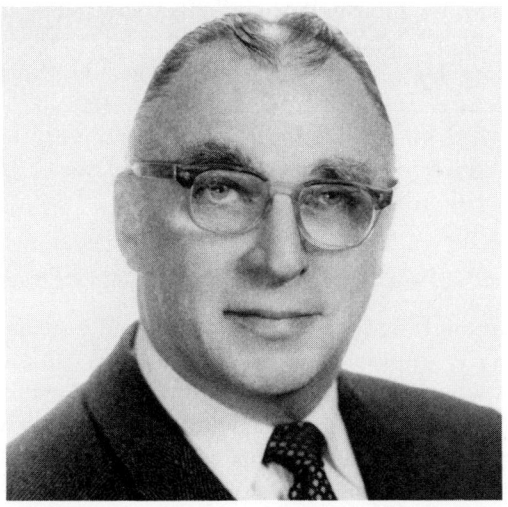

Mark Ravitch, surgeon, historian, linguist, and editor of A Century of Surgery, 1880–1980: The History of the American Surgical Association for 100 Years *(Philadelphia: J. B. Lippincott, 1981).*

unexpired term had been completed. However, this belief proved premature.

New lease on tenure

The United States Congress in 1978 passed a measure eliminating all age limits for government service. Although tenured professors were temporarily excluded, the law provided that after 1982 academic personnel could serve until age seventy. The state of Mississippi adopted the same policy, and the Board of Trustees of Institutions of Higher Learning interpreted this to mean that departmental chairmen in the medical school could serve in their administrative role until the age of seventy.

The news caught me off guard. I had reflected, from time to time, on what I would do to occupy my time in retirement. To be sure, with several of my surgical books current and selling reasonably well, I could be occupied with the inevitable new editions. But I would be separated from assistants who had been associated with the books, not to mention from the crucially important first-class typists who had worked with me through the years. But most of all, I knew I would sorely miss the daily routine of patients, associates, interns, residents, and medical students. Now, all of a sudden, five new years were available, but it took me a while to readjust my mental orientation. I was distinctly surprised at how this more distant enforcement of retirement enhanced my spirits and day-to-day enthusiasm. I had not expected this, but it was very real. Virtually overnight, future planning took on a longer range, larger dimensions, greater depth.

Elected president-elect of the American College of Surgeons

When my appointment to fulfill the unexpired term as second vice-president of the American College of Surgeons expired, I was next elected first vice-president—a highly infrequent promotion. Then, at the 1979 ACS meeting, Dr. C. Rollins Hanlon, executive director of the college, came into a meeting and asked me to step outside. It was only then, after all possible committee meetings and objections had been hurdled, that he could tell me the great news that I would be proposed to the membership as the nominee for president-elect of the college. At the annual business meeting this nomination was made official and was voted on favorably by the members. Having been a member of the Nominating Committee some years earlier, I was fully aware of the extensive discussions and various echelons through which my nomination had passed successfully. Clearly, the Nominating Committee had felt I met the "size-quality-force" test. I felt a great pride and pleasure over this huge honor in American and, indeed, world surgery. The American College of Surgeons has about forty-five thousand members and has chapters in numerous countries around the world.

Happenings, Books, and The ACS Presidency

My work—the usual teaching, clinical surgery, research, national and international travel, lectures, writing, and all the rest—continued at as fast a pace as I could maintain. Therefore, when a group of outstanding vascular surgeons had put together the Southern Society for Vascular Surgery, I already had more obligations to attend meetings than could reasonably be fulfilled in a responsible way. I had respectfully declined both the original invitation to join and the others that followed. Having for years been a member of the national Society for Vascular Surgery and the International Cardiovascular Surgical Society, the addition of still another vascular membership would require more time away from the University Medical Center than could be justified. I had managed to get away with this tenuous position for several years until John H. Foster, pioneer vascular surgeon and a strong member of the Southern Society for Vascular Surgery, called and pointedly reminded me that it was going to be very difficult to certify vascular fellowships at medical centers where the chief of the service was not a member of his regional vascular society—in this case, the Southern Society for Vascular Surgery.

"John," I said, "for the very first time I see what an outstanding organization the Southern Society for Vascular Surgery has suddenly become. Believe me, my membership application form will be in the mail tomorrow, for we are just now making application for certification for our vascular training fellowship!"

John laughed, "Jim, I just knew we could count on you."

I flew to San Juan for the meeting: I was the only inductee with gray hair, and the only active member who was instantly eligible to become a senior member and never pay dues. (Actually I did pay dues, since even senior members were "permitted" this privilege.) Everyone got a chuckle out of the situation, but our fellowship for vascular surgery training was approved without delay.

Books

Over the years, my relations with medical book publishers provided me with an additional, thoroughly enjoyed, professional dimension. Collecting books on medical history provided still another literary diversion, as well as the pleasure of pursuing sought-after volumes in second-hand bookshops in cities around the world. My interest had been especially quickened early by Dr. Abraham Rosenbach, rare book dealer. He had told us exciting experiences in chasing library sales across the ocean, in Dr. Ravdin's home one evening during my residency.

My first book, *Surgery and the Endocrine System* (1952), was mentioned earlier; there was a real need for it, as there was for *Fluid Therapy* (1954). One book, *Critical Surgical Illness* (1971), was written to move our Department of Surgery toward a somewhat more clinical, as opposed to an experimental, orientation. I produced other books for still other objectives, but always the writing represented both diversion and continuing self-education, for one must truly know a subject to write about it and then *sign one's name* to it. A letter to a friend in 1970, states the case:

May 12, 1970

Dr. Paul Nemir, Jr.
Philadelphia, Pennsylvania

Dear Paul:

I have thought a lot about our discussions. Again, during the worst days of unrest and travail here in Jackson years ago, I found the detachment of writing useful review articles or books to be very helpful in maintaining equilibrium. In addition, I learned an enormous amount about a lot of different things. Furthermore, this is one area in which the individual has absolute control of the situation and initiative, and publishers are eternally avid to secure good manuscripts.

Otherwise, as Carlyle put it, the problem is "to do what lies clearly at hand." I am sure that the reorientation which you have achieved during the last two years will gradually begin to be ever more rewarding. It was a most difficult shift to make, and few people could have done it as well as you have done it.

From 1979 through 1983, our office group produced new editions of three substantial books: *Critical Surgical Illness* (W. B. Saunders, 1980, 2d edition); *Scientific Foundations of Surgery* (London, William Heinemann Medical Books Ltd., 1981; I was co-editor of this British-American book with Professor James Kyle of Aberdeen, Scotland); and *Complications in Surgery and Their Management* (W. B. Saunders, 1981, 4th edition). In addition, I finished the initial work on and organization of a new textbook of surgery entitled *Hardy's Textbook of Surgery*, which Lippincott published in 1983. This represented a large amount of work on the part of a number of people. In addition to writing some chapters in each volume, I was also the single editor for three of the books.

Why on earth would anyone take on this much writing in so few years? The reasons were simple: first, the new editions were due; and second, at that time retirement from my academic post was obligatory at the age of sixty-five. I had long planned the continuation of these books, through various editions, as a means of occupying my time, once mandatory retirement had arrived in 1983.

President of the American College of Surgeons

The 1980 annual Clinical Congress of the American College of Surgeons met in Atlanta, only about four hundred miles from Jackson. The able secretaries and technicians who had had so much to do with my achieving the presidency were invited to attend the meetings, exhibits, the convocation, and to hear my presidential address. A number of our family were there, in the handsome suite provided by the college. There were the usual nightly parties and banquets to attend, but the big moment was the convocation, where the approximately sixteen hundred new members from the United States and around the world, in their mortarboards and robes, were initiated into membership in the college. After honorary fellowships had been conferred on several distinguished surgeons from various parts of the world, the final event of the evening was the presidential address.

I had given much thought to what direction my remarks should take. They must not be controversial. Much of my year as president-

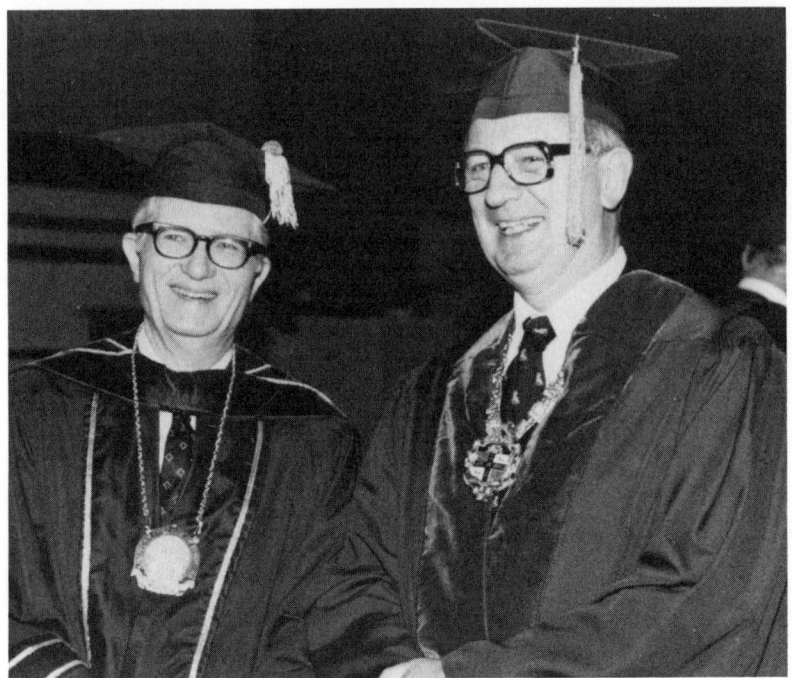

JDH (left), president of the American College of Surgeons, and Sir Alan Parks, president of the Royal College of Surgeons of England

elect had been plagued by the continuing hassles and skirmishes with ENT groups at the local and national levels. ENT had strong representation within the college, on the Board of Governors, and indeed on the Board of Regents, with whom I sat several times each year. The lawsuit in federal court had continued, and this was no time for any message that might cause any segment of the college membership concern. Ultimately, I decided to speak directly to the new initiates before me, with the message being couched in terms that applied equally well to anyone in the audience of two or three thousand people. The address informed the sixteen hundred new initiates of the methods by which the American College of Surgeons functioned in its teaching and regulatory activities, which were extensive and far-reaching. I then went on to current issues before American surgery, and closed the address with my own career experience and basic philosophies regarding surgery, its practice, its morality, and its future. I closed with a brief verse, which was simple but profound, one that had served as a compass for me and which I hoped might serve as a compass for them:

> One ship sails east,
>   And another sails west
> By the selfsame winds that blow;
>   It's not the gale,
> It's the set of our sail
>   That determines the way we go.   (After Ella Wheeler Wilcox)

With that, Weezie and I embarked upon the busiest year of travel of our entire experience. The president of the American College of Surgeons does not have the major administrative authority, as does the president of the American Surgical Association. Because of the massive size of the American College of Surgeons, the administrative authority is vested in the Board of Regents, of which the president is a member. The president represents the college at many meetings and functions in the United States and not infrequently

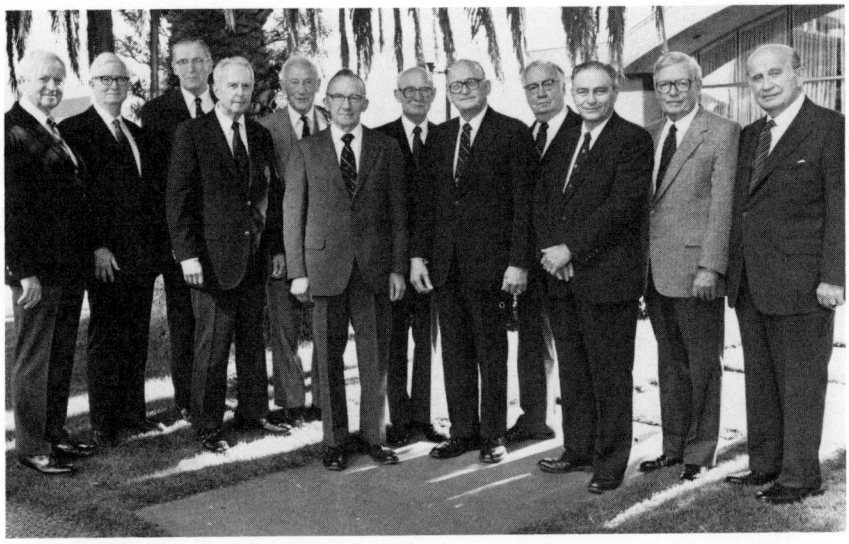

Past presidents of the American College of Surgeons: (left to right) *George R. Dunlop; JDH; Jonathan E. Rhoads; H. William Scott, Jr.; Claude E. Welch; C. Rollins Hanlon (Director, ACS); Charles W. McLaughlin, Jr.; William H. Muller, Jr.; Frank E. Stinchfield; G. Thomas Shires; William P. Longmire, Jr.; Robert M. Zollinger*

abroad during the year. The college defrays the expenses of the president and his wife in their extensive travels to these various meetings and other obligations at which the college must be represented or at which the president is invited to speak. In addition to speaking at numerous state chapters of the college during the year, our travel took us to Europe, Puerto Rico, and South America. The college headquarters in Chicago assists and protects the president from excessive drains upon his time. For example, should the president have a conflict, the college headquarters will offer an alternate speaker or representative.

The decision of whether or not to attempt at least a few words of greeting in the native language is always a tricky one. In Paris, as president of the college, I did close the American part of the joint meeting in carefully rehearsed French, and it went off fairly well. (I simultaneously showed slides in English for the Americans.) But in Mexico City once, my practiced Spanish phonics precipitated an awkward situation. I barely knew what I was saying as I told the large, enthusiastic audience from North, Central, and South America what a wonderful time I had had in Mexico City on my honeymoon (the Americans were wearing translation earphones). The phonics, provided by a Mexican colleague, must have been accurate, for the president of the Mexican chapter of the American College of Surgeons, chatting with some of us Americans, announced to the group that his English was poor and that he would drop back and converse with Dr. Hardy in Spanish!

As president, I presided at the 1981 Clinical Congress of the college in San Francisco, where our Fairmont Hotel, atop Nob Hill, had already been exquisitely decorated for the Christmas season.

Editor of the "World Journal of Surgery"

At the conjoint meeting of the French surgical societies and the American College of Surgeons in Paris in 1981, Drs. Martin Allgöwer of Switzerland, Maurice Mercadier of France, and Vincentzo Speranza of Italy—the executive subcommittee of the Executive Committee of the International Society of Surgery—met in emergency session and urged me to take on a new project. The previous editor of the *World Journal of Surgery*, upset when his recommendation to go from six to twelve issues per year had been denied, had abruptly abandoned the journal. The group asked if I would undertake to reestablish the periodical. This seemed a worthwhile challenge, and I was confident that, with our superior editorial staff in Jackson, we could pull it off. If so, it would be a nice coup. I said yes. The

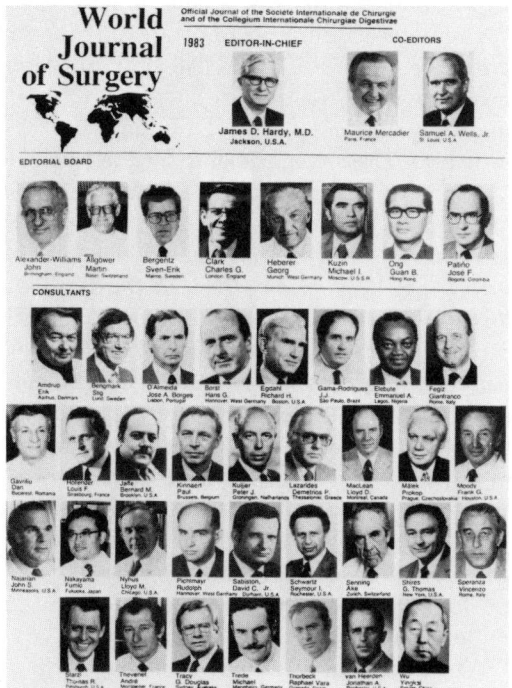

Official publication of the International Society of Surgery (Société Internationale de Chirurgie)

journal was reestablished on a regular publication schedule within six months. However, there were two particular problems: first, the time required to mail manuscripts back and forth to distant parts of the world, and second, the fact that a good many of the manuscripts had to be rewritten in better English.

A day with President and Mrs. Reagan in Washington

While I was in office, the president of the ACS was invited to attend the induction of Dr. Loyal Davis of Chicago at the Irish embassy in Washington. Davis, Nancy Reagan's stepfather, had been a prominent figure in American surgery for fifty years and editor of the journal *Surgery, Gynecology and Obstetrics* for almost that long. He was to be awarded an honorary fellowship by the Royal College of Surgeons in Ireland. He had been invited to Ireland a year before, but his health was poor and he was unable to go. Instead, since his son-in-law was now president and his stepdaughter the first lady, the entire council of the Irish Royal College of Surgeons had flown to Washington to award the honorary fellowship in the Irish embassy.

The Irish embassy was not a large building, but it was attractive and nicely furnished. The salon available for the formal exercise was itself probably no more than thirty feet wide and eighty to ninety feet long. This sharply limited the number of people who could attend. The hall had been filled with chairs, the front two or three rows reserved for the leading members of the Royal Irish College and for President and Mrs. Reagan and their immediate associates. Weezie and I originally sat near the back of the room beside Mr. and Mrs. Roger Mudd, who graciously moved to make room for us. However, a messenger was sent back and I was told that I was to come up front, although there was not room for my wife. I found myself in the third row, between political advisor Lynn Noffzigger and an ambassador who had not yet arrived. In the row ahead of me were Michael Deaver, Edwin Meese, and James Baker. Mrs. Reagan was soon escorted in and seated in front, to our left. Mr. Noffzigger and I chatted together for a few minutes, as Mrs. (Ambassador) Walter Annenberg, seated just behind me, leaned over and asked Mr. Meese, "Who's keeping the store?"

When everything had been arranged, with the Irish members in formal robes and the ancient staff of the college in place, President Reagan himself was escorted in, along with Dr. Davis. The president was seated with his wife and Davis was seated separately a bit forward. The ceremony conferring the honorary membership was then conducted. A champagne reception followed, during which President and Mrs. Reagan stood around, shook hands, and spoke with all the guests. The Reagans invited the Irish contingent to come by the White House late that afternoon.

That evening, there was a formal dinner in Decatur House, a converted mansion near the White House. Perhaps a hundred guests were seated at tables of eight or ten each. Edwin Meese was on my right. He was an easy conversationalist. I commented about the two-hundred-year-old induction ceremony. "Yes," he said, "it was impressive. When we came east to Washington we decided to put some pomp and ceremony back into the presidency, not have the president shown carrying his own suitcase [as with Mr. Carter]. What do you think about it?" I replied that I tended to favor formality.

President Reagan made fine remarks about Dr. Davis, who responded in kind. I am sure the president made points at home, with all the time and attention he had devoted to Dr. Davis that day.

CHAPTER 18

Called Urgently to Peru

With the battles I had fought and the offices I had held, I had no illusions that academic medicine was remote from politics. Even so, I was surprised to receive a telephone call on Friday afternoon, February 23, 1973, from the State Department in Washington: "Can you leave for Lima immediately?"

Peru, he meant, not Ohio.

"For what purpose?"

"There is a serious illness there, and they have requested that you come."

"Well, I am of course concerned about sick people everywhere, but resources are limited. What's wrong with the patient in Lima? It may be some disease I don't treat."

"It's said to be a ruptured abdominal aneurysm. By the way, how did they ever get *your* name?" (This man has a limited future as a diplomat, I thought to myself.)

"They probably remember me from my lecture on the subject in Lima on at least two occasions, possibly three. Yes, I do treat aneurysms."

"Then will you go? At least, will you speak to the ambassador at the Peruvian embassy?"

"Yes, I will be glad to do that."

"Then stand by and the Peruvian embassy will call you right back."

The Peruvian embassy called and I asked who had the aneurysm.

"We are not allowed to say, but the problem extends into the presidential palace."

"Then it must be the president, for his wife would be unlikely to have a ruptured abdominal aortic aneurysm."

It would be possible to leave Jackson in about two hours for Miami, and then go on to Peru. However, I urgently warned the Peruvians in Washington that the patient might well not survive until I could reach Peru, if he in fact did have a ruptured aneurysm. I urged that they marshall all the possible local talent and operate on him at once. I requested that Pompeyo Chavez, chief of surgery in one of the largest hospitals in Lima and a long-time friend, be contacted to stand by at the telephone when my plane reached Miami. I asked that the consul in Miami meet my plane there, and together we would call Dr. Chavez in Lima. Dr. Chavez was not a vascular surgeon who did aortic surgery, but he was a well-trained general surgeon with long experience. Surely he would know what vascular surgeons were available in Lima. Incidentally the president, Juan Velasco Alvarado, was formerly a general in the army.

The consul met the plane in Miami, and we called Pompeyo Chavez at once. He said that President Velasco had just gone into profound shock and that they were rushing him to the operating room. Suffice it to say, the talent available operated on the president, and the aneurysm was replaced with a fabric graft. One or two unfortunate maneuvers, due to limited experience, resulted in problems that might have been avoided by a more experienced vascular surgeon, but the important thing was that, using thirty-six bottles of blood, they had got the patient through the operation in fairly stable condition.

It required eight or nine hours to fly from Miami to Lima. As the plane approached the city, a stewardess announced in both Spanish and English that no one was to move until Professor Hardy of the United States had disembarked. They hustled me off the plane and there, at the foot of the steps, was a small convoy headed by a high-ranking army officer. We went through the city of Lima with sirens wailing, the traffic parting like the Red Sea, straight to the hospital. Pompeyo Chavez met me at the door of the recovery ward and outlined the overall situation. The president had survived the operation, though his right leg was cool. His blood pressure was reasonably stable, he was putting out urine, and he was recovering from the anesthetic. The fact that a good volume of urine was being excreted was a very favorable sign. It meant effective heart action, adequate blood volume, and probably good kidney reserve.

After examining the president myself, I decided that the most pressing consideration was whether or not he would lose his right leg unless further surgery was done immediately. There was no discernible pulse at the right groin, but a fairly good pulse on the left. It was apparent that clot blockage existed within the abdomen in the iliac artery to the right leg. The surgeons had already attempted to remove clot from the right side and had in fact removed some clot. But even so, the condition of the right leg remained somewhat precarious. All things considered, however, with the patient having undergone all that he had, it seemed preferable to observe the right leg closely and not to do any further operating at the moment, even if amputation ultimately became necessary. In consultation with the operating surgeons present, as well as with Professor A. Magee Harvey, head of the Department of Medicine at Johns Hopkins University Hospital who had been summoned as consulting internist, we elected to observe the right leg and to do a fasciotomy on the lower leg later in the day if this became more clearly indicated by leg swelling.

Just then it occurred to me that no one had even asked about my passport, and that I had forgotten my bag in the excitement of getting away with the military escort. I need not have worried. The protocol officer assigned to me, Colonel Velasquez, said that the bag was already in my room at the hotel.

Next, a far more general conference was held in a large room without furniture, consisting of, by my count at that time, thirty-one physicians. This included ten sent, uninvited, from Cuba by Castro.

The Peruvians did not know quite what to do with the Cubans but did not want to offend them. A stenographer and a tape recorder were present, and the remarks and recommendations of each of these physicians were then duly recorded, taking at least an hour, probably longer. I was invited to speak first. I sincerely congratulated the team of surgeons who had brought the president through to this point. Apparently, the president had been seized with severe left flank pain while in the receiving line at a formal evening reception. The cause had at first been obscure, but with increasing evidence of severe blood loss and no blood showing by vomiting or from the rectum, his physicians had decided that he could have a ruptured abdominal aortic aneurysm.

I next briefed the group on the patient's overall condition with respect to circulation, respiration, and kidney function. The critical status of the right leg was emphasized. Each of the other physicians made their remarks. Pompeyo Chavez stood at my side throughout, translating both from English into Spanish and from Spanish into English for my benefit. This huge consultation was in itself most illustrative of the problems that the president's case posed, for every physician wanted to have some role in his treatment. He thus got too much treatment. No single physician was in charge. Being a general in the army, he had been hospitalized at El Hospital Militar.

At last I was free to go to the hotel, take a shower, and get something to eat. It was a brilliant summer day, not hot but infinitely pleasant, with the oleanders and bougainvillea blooming on the terrace adjacent to the dining room. I was overwhelmed with the peacefulness of the place, and was reminded of my residency days when I would fly from snow and ice in Philadelphia to the warm sea breeze in Charleston, South Carolina, with the oleanders blooming along the road leading from the airport into the city.

In the early afternoon, about two o'clock, a staff car took me back to reexamine the president. By this time a fasciotomy was definitely indicated, and the local surgeons asked me to perform this operation. I recommended that we not move him from his monitoring station in the recovery ward, but that we perform the operation right there with him in bed. The purpose of this procedure, performed under local anesthesia, was to divide the strong fascia along two sides of the lower leg. This would allow the swelling, due to long-standing inadequate blood flow, to bulge through the incisions and relieve the pressure on the arteries and nerves within the closed compartments. The foot would receive more blood flow. The patient remained stable throughout this straightforward procedure. Thereafter, the color of the foot was definitely improved, and the president was able to move his toes and could feel touch and a pin prick. While not robust, the blood flow through the leg now appeared to be enough that the leg would survive for the time being. Another operation could always be performed later to improve the blood flow still further. At this time, and again that evening, I met and talked with the president's wife, Consuelo. She was an attractive, dark brunette of about forty or fifty, with quick intelligence, poise, grace, and charm, though she was obviously worried. She was taller than most of the other Peruvian women about her. We agreed to meet again at 9:00 P.M. to review the entire situation, which we did. Meanwhile, I called the hospital back around 5 P.M. and again about midnight.

The first twenty-four to forty-eight hours are crucially important in the survival of a patient who has gone through what the president had endured over the past twenty-four hours. At the evening meeting at the hospital, I urged that the number of physicians writing orders for medication and treatment be strictly limited. As often happens when prominent people are ill, the management of his case was going to be less than optimal if this discipline were not enforced.

I received a call from our United States ambassador to Peru, inviting me over to the embassy for a meal or just a drink, if possible. He also volunteered to come chat with me at the hotel. I thanked him but emphasized that I needed to spend most of my time with the president.

Needless to say, the public media were everywhere, flashbulbs popping and television crews shooting. The newspapers showed me being met by the officer and his retinue at the airplane.

By Sunday afternoon it was clear that the president's recovery was progressing satisfactorily, and I had a speaking engagement in Washington on Monday. The Peruvian government used a bit of persuasion with the airlines and soon had cleared me all the way through.

Meanwhile, Lieutenant Colonel Felix Vilela Carrillo had appeared and was my escort for the day. He was a career army officer, clean cut and engaging and apparently assigned to the battalion of some seventy-five tanks around Lima. He had been with the president for many years and was clearly close to both him and Señora Consuelo Velasco. To entertain me, he offered to show me the president's palace and offices, and they proved interesting. For example, the president's own private office had five doors leading to individual rooms around its perimeter. I asked why there were so many doors, and Colonel Carrillo said that it was to accommodate incompatible groups: "For example, last year he had the Red Chinese waiting in a room through that door, and the Americans waiting in a room through the other door. Neither group knew before or after that they had both been here at the same time." This was at a time when China and the United States were still at arms length.

This gave me an idea. At the University Medical Center we were just then drawing up the plans for the new clinical science building, in which would be housed the various clinical departments such as medicine, psychiatry, obstetrics and gynecology, and surgery. On my return to Jackson, I changed the architectural plans of my own office so as to have four doors—one entering from the hall, and each of the other three leading to different secretaries with different responsibilities. It proved convenient and efficient.

Colonel Carrillo drove me to the Army Officer's Club, Central Lima. It was a splendid facility. We dined in a very large hall and were virtually alone until the Cuban delegation came in and waved from across the room. Colonel Carrillo was interested in the United

States' reaction to General Velasco's military regime, which had taken over U.S. companies, and so forth. He went on to say that they wanted Peru for Peruvians, and that they had no resentment toward the United States otherwise. He had ordered wine, but when it came, he tasted it and refused it with some vehemence. The startled sergeant sped away and returned with another bottle, which the colonel considered satisfactory. Following dinner we drove to the airport, where we conversed in the VIP Room until the plane was announced. Just as we approached the steps of the plane we were all bade stop. Out of a side door of the airport strode a tall military officer in white uniform and much braid, who saluted and brought best wishes from the president himself. And then he and Colonel Carrillo and the airport authorities receded as the plane departed. What an eventful thirty-six hours in Peru!

I got back to Washington in time to give my report to the trauma meeting at the National Institutes of Health at precisely 3 P.M. Monday, as had been scheduled.

Some weeks later I received a call from the Peruvian ambassador in Washington inviting me to come to the embassy on a specific date to receive the Order of the Sun, apparently the highest award which could be given by Peru under the circumstances. Unaware of the dimensions that the ambassador envisioned for the occasion, I replied that it was not really convenient for me to come to Washington at that time, but that doubtless some other requirement would bring me to Washington later in the year. He did not inform me that Dr. A. Magee Harvey, the physician from Johns Hopkins who had also been in attendance upon President Velasco, was to be decorated at the same time. As far as I knew, all I had to do was to go by the embassy sometime and pick up the medal. Thus the "ugly American" is sometimes ugly out of sheer ignorance of what is expected.

The date of May 30 was agreed upon, and by this time considerably more information was available. It was apparent that a formal reception was to be held. Engraved invitations were sent, inviting members of my family and friends in the Washington area whose names I had supplied.

When we Hardys entered the front door of the embassy, we were taken aback by the large number of people, dressed to the hilt, who were there for the award. In addition, there were newspaper reporters and television crews. The ambassador, resplendent in his official dress and elegant manner, made a superb speech to me in front of the grinding television cameras and the large assembled audience. It was most impressive. Then, stopping abruptly, he turned expectantly to me. In that instant, I realized I was expected to make something in the nature of an equally eloquent reply. Caught completely flat-footed for one of the few times in my life under such circumstances, I managed to say a few appropriate words, but they were by far second to the splendid address of the tall ambassador, the Honorable Fernando Berckemeyer. He placed the beautiful, large medal, the Order of the Sun, with its red ribbon around my neck, and gave me a lapel emblem which he said would open any door in Peru. I was required to sign the formal book register for persons who had received the Order of the Sun from Peru. The ambassador and my family stood in line and received all the guests prior to cocktails and a buffet dinner.

CHAPTER 19

National and International Participation and Awards

Physicians in academic medicine have the opportunity, and often the obligation, to participate in national and international education. In the process, they may become involved in a wide range of activities, which can absorb a great deal of time and energy unless kept firmly in perspective.

My appointment as chairman of a department in a medical school, along with prominence in research and writing, resulted in a steadily increasing flow of invitations to participate in meetings and organizations of national and international significance. I became thoroughly familiar with the phenomenon of the visiting professor, the named lecture, and surgical organization committee work. I was eventually to speak in more than forty states and twenty-five foreign countries, many times in some of these places.

The visiting professorship can be the most time-consuming of these obligations, if for no other reason than that so many invitations may arrive. Moreover, when a colleague calls from his university and names a date a year away, it is hard to say no—especially if the friend has just spoken for you or has written a chapter in your recent book. In recent years the traditional three-day stint of lectures, clinics, conferences, operations, and evening banquets has been shortened. Eventually, I myself almost never agreed to more than two days at a time.

Whether or not a particular invitation was accepted depended, of course, on time available, prestige to be gained (mine or the university's), time away from Jackson and practice, airplane schedules and access, and obligation to the prospective host. It is flattering to be invited, but selections have to be made. I learned not to accept on receipt of the initial telephone call, for it was awkward to ask baldly if travel expenses were paid, even if I were certain that the date did not conflict with something else. Surprisingly, many medical societies, especially state medical associations, did not even offer to pay travel until they were asked. Curiously, academic surgeons may be considered teachers who automatically must go and teach, whether paid for time and expense or not. This gradually changed, however. I certainly was not going to have the University of Mississippi pay for such travel, and eventually delayed accepting invitations until personal travel expense was assured. On occasion my wife's travel was provided as well. In fact, inclusion of travel expense for the wife almost ensures acceptance, for surgeon and wife often see more of each other at such meetings than at home.

Travel

The foreign visits were for me the most memorable. Although there were many, it will be sufficient to recall just a few here.

In 1958, the American College of Surgeons held a regional meeting in Stockholm in conjunction with the Swedish Surgical Society. It was at this occasion that the International Surgical Club was organized in Edinburgh. Sir John Bruce, president of the Royal College of Surgeons of Edinburgh, was host. Twenty-five surgeons from the United States and Canada, and twenty-five from Western Europe and Scandinavia, were to be invited. I was much honored to be included in such distinguished company, for I had been a surgery department chairman only two years when invited. Jonathan Rhoads took exception to the name "club" and suggested we substitute "group," as the name International Surgical Group might be more acceptable to the U.S. tax authorities.

At first, the meetings were to be held every two years, but John Gibbon, inventor of the pump-oxygenator, insisted that a yearly meeting was essential to achieve and maintain continuity. I privately planned to attend only every second year. The group was to meet twice in Europe and then once in North America, on a rotating basis. The British were initially firmly opposed to inviting German members, but eventually its roster represented many of the most outstanding surgeons of the time. They came to know each other well, as papers were given and information was exchanged.

At the American College of Surgeons meeting in Stockholm, Dr. Ravdin had advised me, "Jim, you are now well known throughout the United States, and you should concentrate more on placing articles in the foreign literature and in getting yourself known abroad."

This was not my plan, however. In the first place, the situation in Jackson was more tenuous than anyone outside the state was aware, and the cloud of the integration fight was now much larger than the proverbial man's hand. Without a firm home base, little can be accomplished. And anyway, Pasteur's policy had always seemed a sound one to me. When asked if he were disappointed at having been passed over that year for membership in the French Academy of Science, Pasteur was reported to have replied, "No. Perhaps the time may come when they will have to explain why I am not a member." That is, if I were truly eligible, I probably would be acknowledged anyway.

After transplanting the first heart and the first lung in man, I was invited many places, and one commitment I made was to participate in the International Congress on Respiratory Diseases in Turin, Italy, in 1965. Several preliminary events, however, complicated my departure from the United States. As it happened, we transplanted two cadaver kidneys a day or so before I was scheduled to depart, and I hated to leave the recipients, even though they were well covered. I also had to attend the regular meeting of the American Cancer Society Committee on Clinical Research in New York before leaving for Italy.

Armed with a phrase book of the Italian language, I visited the usual sights of Rome before proceeding north to Turin (Torino). I found there much interest in our work. At the formal banquet on the last evening, the master of ceremonies suddenly stood up at the raised head table and announced in English, "Ladies and Gentlemen, the American astronaut, John Glenn, has just landed safely in the Pacific Ocean." From the thundering applause, it was apparent that every person in that great banquet hall, from whatever country, took personal pride in this achievement of man. I went on to Paris, where I gave a talk on heart and lung transplants through an interpreter before returning home.

Our best-remembered family trip was when in 1965 I went as visiting professor to the teaching hospitals in Honolulu. Our four girls were old enough to read the map and to pick out our itinerary by car through the west, the Grand Canyon, and on to Los Angeles, where we stored the car near the Los Angeles airport. The garage was near Watts, which burned while we were gone, but fortunately our car was spared. Although my days in Honolulu were completely filled with lectures, operations, and conferences at the three hospitals—Queens, St. Francis, and Kuakini—Weezie and the girls saw everything available. We had rented an apartment just a block from Waikiki beach. Two of the girls were so captivated by the area that, for several years, they planned to grow up and go back and teach in Hawaii. Japanese names became almost as familiar to us as Smith. The most singular remembrance was a weekend trip to the island of Kauai, where much of the movie *South Pacific* had been shot.

Only a night or so after we had got settled in Honolulu, I received a call from Queens Hospital around midnight with the news that a young sailor had run his motorcycle under a truck and had severed his leg above the knee. Would I please come right over, inasmuch as I was a transplant surgeon? Rushing over, I found that the leg was attached by only the sciatic nerve. Nothing else of substance remained intact. I called for the orthopaedists to stabilize the bone fracture, and after a great deal of irrigating to remove the cinders and dirt from the wound, over a period of six hours we did reestablish continuity of the arteries and veins and the other nerves that could be found. To our considerable gratification, the leg became pink. While obviously not normal in blood flow, it certainly appeared likely to survive. However, three weeks later, significant infection became evident and the leg was amputated to avoid the risk of generalized systemic infection.

One of the most select groups of clinical surgeons in the United States is the venerable Society of Clinical Surgery, an elite surgical travel club. It was founded to give surgeons the opportunity to visit each other's operating rooms, and to learn how operative procedures and management were carried out in other clinics. The programs were put on by the individual members' hospitals, most of which were university medical centers. The society met with us in Jackson in 1965. To put on a good program before this highly critical and discriminating group was a stern challenge for the members of our department, but it went off well. On Friday morning various staff members performed different operations in the operating suite, beginning at 7:00 A.M. My own team used two operating rooms, and I performed two open-heart cases, a mitral valve and the closure of an atrial septal defect, as well as resecting a large abdominal aortic aneurysm—all before our talks began at 10 A.M.

Weezie and I made the grand tour in 1966. The National Heart Foundation of Australia (Western Division) had extended an invitation, and we visited Tokyo and Hong Kong before arriving in Perth. The Royal Australasian College of Surgeons and the Research Society were to meet there in a few days, and my active participation in these meetings was a part of the overall arrangements. Several of those attending had worked in our laboratories. We were housed near the University of Western Australia Medical School and its teaching hospital. All expenses were paid by the hosts. I spoke many times during those three weeks, with emphasis on organ transplantation and cardiovascular operations. Clinical organ transplantation was not yet under way in Western Australia, and there was great interest in this subject. While the Australians were of course peculiarly Australian, they were closer to the average American than people in almost any other country I ever visited. Incidentally, two of Mississippi's problems pursued us there. First, the *Perth Daily News* ran a large front-page photograph of James Meredith lying on the ground, shot on the highway from Memphis, captioned "Negro Civil Rights Man Shot Down." On another day, the same newspaper featured the Jackson Country Club, where the sheriff and his deputies were carrying out cases of whiskey from the annual major social event, the party after the King and Queen's Carnival Ball. Mississippi was still a dry state at that time, but Governor Paul Johnson had decided that the time had come to terminate the hypocrisy by clamping down on illegal liquor, and thus forcing those who were having it both ways (voting dry for political reasons but partaking as desired) to abolish prohibition in Mississippi, the last holdout in the fifty states. Shortly thereafter, the legislature voted in local option, so that counties could vote individually on whether or not they wanted to have beer and whiskey sold legally.

We left winter in Perth for tropical Bombay by way of Ceylon. I spoke at the medical center of Professor P. K. Sen, the same man who had worked with me in the laboratory in Philadelphia some years before under the auspices of the Rockefeller Foundation. My topic at the Seth Edward Hospital and Medical School was organ transplantation, with the emphasis on the heart and the lung. After bringing Sen to the United States, the Rockefeller Foundation had established a cardiac surgery unit in Bombay. He had an excellent group.

Back at home, summer was occupied with routine medical school and hospital duties, but I was again on the travel circuit at the beginning of September. Dr. Carlos Chavez, a colleague originally from Lima, and I fulfilled lecturing obligations with the First Argentine Congress of Angiology (1 Congreso Argentino de Angiologia) organized by the Argentine Society of Angiology. Dr. Chavez acted as my interpreter, but on one occasion (and perhaps on others?) he exceeded his role, I thought. In the course of giving a lecture, which Dr. Chavez was interpreting into Spanish at intervals when I paused, I realized I had omitted a very important point a few sentences back. I asked Dr. Chavez to tell the audience. "Don't worry," he replied. "I told them when we passed. Keep moving!"

Buenos Aires impressed me as a highly sophisticated city, containing not only peoples of Spanish origin but large contingents of Italians and Germans—witness the collaboration of the Argentine government with German and Italian submarines and warships during World War II. Argentina seemed oriented more toward the continent of Europe than the United States in cultural and postgraduate medical interests. In contrast to much of Mexico City and Lima, Peru, for example, Buenos Aires itself seemed to be a progressive city with attractive architecture and modern facilities in general.

From Argentina we went to Peru. Because our plane was delayed, a delegation of about fifty people waited until two o'clock in the morning before they finally gave up and went home. The lecture, which was to have been given the next morning at a meeting in Lima, is the only scheduled lecture of any significance that I ever missed. We did reach Lima the next day, however, and I gave talks on the transplantation of organs and the management of abdominal aortic aneurysms. As related in the previous chapter, the latter lecture was to have special consequences a few years later.

One of my most pleasant assignments in the fall of 1968 was to participate in the celebration of the two-hundredth anniversary of the University of Lund in Sweden. En route my wife and I flew to West Berlin by way of Hamburg. The purpose was to speak and to visit the hospital and laboratories of E. E. S. Bucherl, whose group had done outstanding research in lung transplantation. Next we proceeded by way of Copenhagen, Denmark, to Malmö, Sweden, crossing the water by hydrofoil. There we were met by a group of medical students in nautical dress, and were driven to nearby Lund where we were housed at the Hotel Lundia. The weather was brisk in late September, but there was no ice or snow yet. The theme of the scientific program, before the formal commemoration ceremonies, was once again the transplantation of organs. At the formal banquet there was nearly a riot by several hundred students who protested the use of funds to celebrate the anniversary. They thought the money should have been sent to feed the starving natives in Biafra. For a brief time the lights were cut off from the outside. This ominous disturbance was corrected eventually, upon the arrival of adequate police reinforcements. Professor Philip Sandblom—formerly chairman of surgery but now president of the University of Lund—and his wife Grace were our principal hosts.

The Marnoch Lecture, which I gave in 1969 at the University of Aberdeen in Scotland, was to be related to cancer. George Smith, who had visited us in Jackson some years earlier, was chairman of the Department of Surgery there. I had chosen the title "The Systemic Effects of Non-Endocrine Tumors (Why Cancer Patients Die)." Much more was now known about the general effects of cancer than when I had first told Dr. Ravdin in 1946 that I wanted to investigate cachexia. Most cancers had now been shown to produce chemical substances that interfered with normal body metabolism.

A particular problem was that, having traveled so rapidly from plane to plane and airport to airport, my baggage had been lost. As always, the speaking slides and manuscript were safely with me in my briefcase, but the days passed and my bag did not arrive at the home of the Smiths, who were my hosts. Professor Smith asked one morning, "I say, Professor Hardy, what are you sleeping in?"

"About what you'd expect."

He gave me a pair of pajamas.

Incidentally, in Europe, to be addressed as "Professor" commonly implies more prestige than "Doctor," whereas in the United States the opposite may be true.

I went next to London for the first joint meeting of the Surgical Research Society of Great Britain and our own Society of University Surgeons from the United States. This was a rewarding meeting for me personally since, at my presidential address before the Society of University Surgeons in Cleveland back in 1962, one of my major points had been that we should look into the possibility of meeting with similar international groups, such as one then soon to be formed in Great Britain.

My mission to Greece came about in the following way. Dr. Alton Ochsner called me from New Orleans in the summer of 1969: "Jim, you are going to be invited to participate in a commission, which will go to Greece in the early part of next year to evaluate and make recommendations for the reorganization of Greek medical training. The reason I am calling is to alert you to this invitation and to urge you not to turn it down."

In distinguished company, Weezie and I departed New York's Kennedy Airport on Saturday, February 14, 1970. We visited the

University of Athens, which had about four thousand medical students, and the medical school at Salonika, which had two thousand students. We met with prime minister George Papadopoulos and later with the minister of education. A number of us on the committee also gave lectures. Among other things, we recommended that the number of medical students be drastically reduced; the minister of education replied that open admissions was the European custom. We wondered about taking so many Arabs, about whose previous education little was known; the minister replied that in the Mediterranean area a country needed all the friends it could get. We noted the remarkable extent of nepotism in the medical schools; the minister replied that in Greece it was a matter of personal honor to get one's relatives in after one had got in himself. The minister, an attractive, intelligent, and knowledgeable man, clearly was doing his best under the circumstances.

Russia came on the travel agenda in 1971 because of the joint meeting in Moscow of the International Society of Surgery and the International Cardiovascular Society. After several days in Helsinki and Leningrad, we arrived in Moscow on August 21, and were put up in the Rossiya Hotel, a huge building said to contain six thousand rooms. We had had a splendid young female guide in Leningrad, who had been an English major, spoke excellent English, and taught in a college as her regular work. She was thoroughly conversant in English literature and would have been a credit to any country. The churches in Leningrad, with their round, onionlike Byzantine domes, were spectacularly beautiful, though few if any of them appeared to be in active use. (We did enter a functioning church in Moscow.) The Hermitage Museum and the circus were also extraordinary. For example, a large bear would come out and perform some trick or feat and then would applaud when the audience applauded, as is the Russian custom. The bear would then hold up one of his front paws to indicate when the applause had been sufficient.

Moscow was far more serious than Leningrad. There was little opportunity to dine in Moscow other than in precisely the same hotel restaurant, at exactly the time specified on the schedule, without exception. Our tour guide was either Russian or had Russian relatives in Moscow. He told us, as did the new female guide who was with us on almost all our trips, that we could go about pretty much as we pleased so long as we avoided places we were told not to visit and were circumspect with taking photographs. He also said that almost as much money had probably been spent on bugging each of the six thousand rooms in the hotel as had been spent on the hotel itself.

The surgery meeting began the next day, and we signed up for visits to various hospitals in Moscow, generally referred to as institutes, in addition to attending the main sessions of the meeting. Not aware that one had to rush quickly to get a card to go to the institute of one's choice, I found that only the cancer hospital remained open to me. Fortunately, my colleague William Glenn of Yale, then president of the American Heart Association, took me under his wing and I was carried along in the official car that spirited him to the Heart Institute. Their volume of open-heart surgery was not large, but they had postoperative examples of most of the usual types of such surgery. The question of the use of blood drained from cadavers, so often spoken about in connection with Russia, was brought up. One of the female physicians told me that it was rare indeed that cadaver blood was actually given to a patient. On another occasion, I remarked to a guide that we had always been told that perhaps two-thirds of all Russian physicians were women; where were they? The guide smiled slightly and replied, "Out in the provinces." Certainly the institutes we saw were run by men.

The director of the Cancer Institute spoke quite passable English, and when I asked him where he had learned it, he said proudly, "I taught myself from books. Is it good?" I assured him that his English was readily understandable and that I was surprised that he had

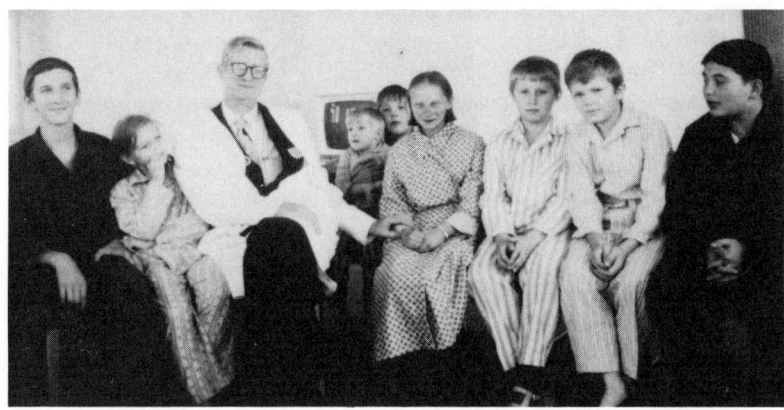

JDH with heart operation children at Vishnevsky Institute, Moscow

been able to learn from just books. Had he traveled abroad? He said that he had left Russia for a day or two to attend some international meeting, but that he had never spoken English outside his country.

The one institute that I had been especially interested in attending was the Vishnevsky research center, but the cards to this institute had gone quickly. However, the next day when I gave my formal address, "Transplantation of the Heart and Lung: Current Status," a small delegation was waiting for me at the foot of the stage. Two young men in their mid-thirties, both of whom spoke English, were there to extend an invitation to come to the Vishnevsky Institute the next day. With them were two lung transplanters known to me through the literature but who did not speak English. An official car called for me at the hotel, and I spent a rewarding morning touring the laboratories of this world-famous research institute. They showed me a computer with which they were experimenting making diagnoses from the patient's symptoms, the immediate example being a patient in faraway Vladivostok who had been correctly diagnosed as having appendicitis.

At noon we went to join Professor Vishnevsky and perhaps a dozen other surgeons largely from Russia, East Germany, and the Balkans. They were speaking German, little of which I understood. At the close of the luncheon one of the English-speaking surgeons rose and indicated that I was to stand, as did Professor Vishnevsky. The young surgeon interpreted for Vishnevsky. He made some congratulatory remarks and ended with the following lines: "Dr. Hardy, a lot of water has passed under the bridge since you performed the first heart transplant in man and the first lung transplant in man. But remember this, *no words can ever be taken from a poem, or notes from a song.*" It was then clear to me that I was the honoree of this luncheon. Professor Vishnevsky presented me with two medals to commemorate the two transplants.

One particular scientist whom I most wanted to meet in Moscow was Demikhov. He had transplanted organs in dogs as early as 1947, but these studies were not known in the United States until much later when his reports had been translated into English. To my inquiry, the information person at his institute said that he was down at the meeting giving a paper. To this I replied that he was not even listed on the program for that day. Quite unperturbed, she then blandly changed her story and said he had left on vacation. At this point an Englishman at my elbow said to me, "What she means, old chap, is that you are not going to see Demikhov in any case. Apparently Demikhov is in disfavor here." And he must have been right, for we were never able to locate Demikhov during the week.

Some of the meetings were held in the Kremlin itself, and to everyone's admiration, almost a thousand surgeons and spouses were served a buffet dinner one evening. The heavily laden tables, with about twelve place settings each but with no chairs, provided a splendid meal which was quickly consumed.

One evening P. K. Sen of Bombay had arranged with the Indian embassy to give a reception and buffet dinner for friends of his from throughout the world. We had his invitation with the address printed on it, and without too much difficulty, we obtained a taxi in the early evening. After rattling through the streets for quite a distance, it was obvious to Weezie and me that the driver could not find the place. Somewhere, someone had told me that Russian children were now required to learn English. As the thought came to me, I saw sitting on some stone steps a boy of about twelve years, with a mature woman who I supposed was his mother. Tapping the driver on the shoulder, I motioned him to stop. Walking over to the boy, I asked, "Son, do you speak English?"

"Yes, some English."

"Then would you please ask your mother where the Indian embassy is?" I said as I showed him the invitation.

He spoke in Russian to his mother and she smiled, stood up, and walked about a block ahead of us to a park. Pointing across the park to a brightly lighted building several hundred yards away, she indicated that that was the Indian embassy, which her son confirmed in English. Truly, English has become the Latin of our time.

A Viennese surgeon guided us through the subway system and back to the Rossiya Hotel late that night.

At midweek I came down with some infection which caused me to have high fever for about forty-eight hours. Although missing one or two functions, Weezie and I still got to most of the evening sessions, and I managed to be present at the scientific meetings that I had really wanted to attend.

Russian surgeons who spoke English seemed to have no reluctance to discuss political matters or anything else. I asked why they had thrown out Khrushchev. I had always rather understood him after I heard the story that, when asked why Stalin had tolerated his son's antics and alcoholism for so long, Khrushchev had replied simply, "You don't turn your back on your children."

The Russians replied that Khrushchev was an ineffective administrator, the country had been doing poorly economically, and a more stable and experienced hand was needed at the helm. They pointed out that Khrushchev was living without restraint in his own dacha near Moscow, free to come and go as he pleased.

When I returned home, I scheduled a report on Russia for surgical grand rounds and the notice had been placed on the bulletin boards. Just before my talk, a man appeared in my office who showed his badge and identified himself as being with the CIA. He asked if he might listen in.

"Certainly you may listen, as may anyone else. But tell me, how could I have learned anything in Russia that you folks in the CIA wouldn't already know far better?"

"You'd be surprised. You probably were shown medical procedures and operations and hospitals and details that we would have great difficulty in getting in to see ourselves. How would you compare the Russian surgery you saw with similar American surgery at this time?"

He came and sat throughout the hour, taking notes. He then disappeared just before the audience rose and was not seen again.

Another interesting interlude occurred during the fall of 1973. We arrived in Rio de Janeiro and were met at the plane by Dr. Daltro Ibiapina Oliveira, our host and constant escort during the visit. He whisked us through customs. Dr. Daltro spoke English, but for some reason he found it easier to understand my wife's English than to understand mine. Thus he asked her to ask me if I would be willing to operate on television for the large medical congress of which my own addresses were to be a part. I agreed to do so, assuming that the operations proposed were ones that I commonly did. Then, to my surprise, it developed that the printed program already distributed to the members attending the congress stated specifically that I would operate on television for the congress. If my memory is correct, the precise operations were named. These included first a cholecystectomy and then a vagotomy and resection of the stomach. In addition, a thoracic aneurysm was scheduled for the last day of the visit. I declined to operate for the aneurysm, though it was a short one situated precisely in the center of the aorta as it descended through the chest; I was unwilling to leave the patient without my postoperative presence.

Not knowing the Portuguese language, I was concerned that the presentation of the operations on television before the large audience of the congress might not turn out very well. Nonetheless, undaunted and having operated in many university hospitals on such visits in the past, I laid out on the table all the instruments that I would need for the operation, and then simply pointed. Dr. Daltro was present throughout the operations, standing beside me looking over my shoulder. He had taught me the Portuguese words for hemostat, forceps, scalpel, and scissors. In five or ten minutes the suture nurse and I understood each other well enough, and the operations were completed in short order.

My principal lectures had to do with postoperative respiratory insufficiency and unruptured and ruptured aneurysms, and in addition there were all the usual conferences and ward rounds in various hospitals. Everywhere, the audience wanted to wait after the lecture to see the two films depicting the first heart transplant in man and the first lung transplant.

I had been elected a councillor for the international Transplantation Society. The council met in London in August of 1977 to make final plans for the meeting in Rome the following year. The president of the Transplantation Society was Leslie Brent, Nobel prize winner Medawar's colleague. The meeting was held at his laboratories at the St. Mary's Medical School and Hospital.

The sessions lasted two days. The chairman of the local committee on arrangements was Raffaello Cortesini. At one point he announced that the pope himself had agreed to address the opening session in Rome. I asked him, "Doctor Cortesini, how does the pope feel about organ transplantation? You know, some religions are still opposed to human transplants. What if the pope comes out flatfooted against organ transplantation in man? Won't that cast a shadow over subsequent events?"

"Dr. Hardy," Cortesini said, "the pope is for anything that works."

At another point Cortesini pointed out that the funds that had originally been allocated to him were now inadequate because of the inflation that Italy and all other countries had experienced. One of the council members from Belgium remarked, "Why don't you just get the money from the Bank of the Vatican? It is the richest bank in Italy."

To this, Cortesini replied simply, "It is blessed."

National committees

Almost every head of a department of surgery will be called upon sooner or later to serve on various national committees. National time tithing, it has been called by someone. These committees range from those within surgical societies per se to committees of a decidedly different nature. The surgical society committees will be mentioned elsewhere. Suffice it to tell here about service with the American Board of Surgery, the National Board of Medical Examiners, the National Institutes of Health, and the Clinical Research Committee of the American Cancer Society. Participants are generally unpaid, but travel expenses are reimbursed.

The American Board of Surgery was established in 1937, and it has the responsibility of examining surgical residents after they finish their residency and awarding certificates of competence. Procedures change, but during my six years on the board, I traveled six or eight times each year to some city or university to conduct oral examinations, leaving on Sunday afternoon and returning Tuesday night. The candidates for these oral examinations had already had the required four to five years of surgical residency and had passed the tough written examination. From time to time the oral examinations were criticized as being too subjective on the part of the examiners, and it was suggested that they ought to be discontinued. The other side of this, however, is that the experienced examiner can assess not only the candidate's store of information but also his thought processes and reaction to the unexpected. Finally, someone observed dryly, the examiner can also note whether or not the surgical candidate has two hands.

The National Board of Medical Examiners tests medical students both during medical school and after they finish. Moreover, questions derived from the national boards are used to test foreign physicians seeking to enter the United States. I served on the Surgery Examining Committee. I learned how extraordinarily difficult it was to develop a question for which all five members of the committee could agree that there was only one really correct answer—someone could usually point out some other answer as an at least plausible alternative.

Many medical academicians serve on the study sections, the training grant committees, and the councils of the National Institutes of Health. Here the government does pay a nominal stipend per day, but payment for travel expense is the main consideration. I served on the Surgery Study Section for four years, later the Anesthesiology Training Grant Committee for over three years, and still later a committee on artificial medical devices for almost as long. The responsibility of the study section was to evaluate pertinent grant applications that had been submitted to the NIH and to rec-

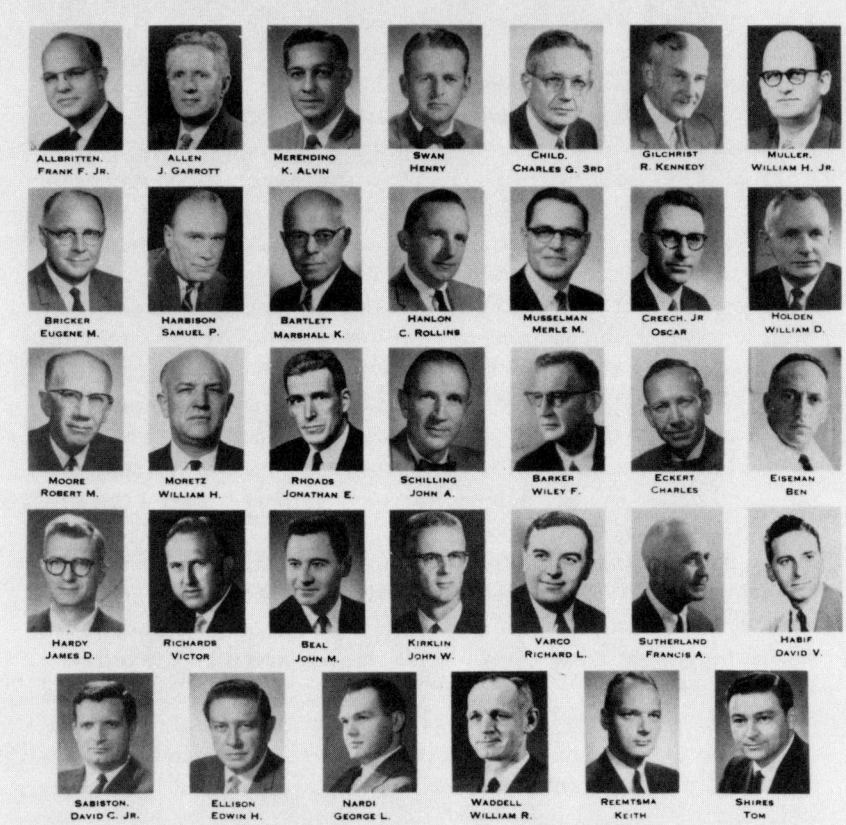

The members of the American Board of Surgery are responsible for certifying that surgical residents have achieved the appropriate residency training and knowledge of surgical practice.

ommend which should be supported and for how much. Still higher echelons also evaluated the requests and made the final decisions. The Clinical Research Committee of the American Cancer Society had a similar function.

The Anesthesiology Training Grant Committee had been established to try to increase the number of anesthesiologists. Congress had apparently declared anesthesiology, pathology, and radiology "disaster areas" because so few medical students elected to enter these specialties. The anesthesiology committee, on which I was the only surgeon with about fifteen academic anesthesiologists, was charged with receiving and evaluating requests from academic training centers for funds with which to improve their training facilities and to pay anesthesiology residents' salaries. Frankly, I was surprised at how limited the anesthesia personnel were at many of our best-known universities. We awarded very substantial grants, and there was a temporary increase in resident and staff recruitment. On the whole, however, the results did not match the cost. In later years, however, perhaps because of some great cycle or even perhaps because of the funds we did recommend for training, the specialty of anesthesiology became much sought after by medical students, as in fact did pathology and radiology.

Presidencies

One commonly accedes to the presidency of an organization by serving faithfully in lower offices, by having "paid one's dues." The office of secretary is a signal position, for this officer is commonly nominated with an eye to promoting him or her to possible higher office in due course. This was the route by which I had ascended to most of my leadership positions. I was elected president of the Society of University Surgeons after first serving as secretary for three years, an office that allowed me to know the rising young academic surgeons of the United States and Canada better than I ever would again. This was a young man's organization, for one became a senior member at forty-five, but the presidency was an office of distinction just the same. The title of my presidential address was "The University Surgeon and His Society: Reflections and Perspectives."

With the Society for Surgery of the Alimentary Tract, my election probably came about through my having served as program chairman during the first years after it was founded. It was initially named the Society for Colon Surgery, but I found it hard to attract enough good papers to develop a challenging program devoted solely to the colon. I proposed that we become the SSAT, which allowed the program committee to include papers dealing with any aspect of the alimentary tract, including even the liver, pancreas, and spleen. This strategic change allowed the society to grow into an important national surgical organization.

My rise up the ladder in the International Society of Surgery began with my election as secretary of the United States chapter for four years, during which we finally cleaned up the Augean stable of the outdated membership rolls. Also I was given increasingly important assignments on the biennial programs.

The presidency of the Southern Surgical Association came as a happy surprise. I had never served in any lower capacity in this venerable and widely respected society, except to participate in the program almost every year. My presidential address was entitled "She is Risen." It was a panorama of the current South and its great progress. The closing lines were: "When I was a boy, my grandmother used to tell us about how the Federal troops had burned everything when they came through. And men would often say, 'Hold on to your Confederate money, boys, the South will rise again.' Ladies and Gentlemen, she is risen." The address got mixed reviews. My point that qualified minority surgeons should be elected to membership found favor with some but not with others. In fact, it was suggested that approval for publication of my address with the other association papers in the *Annals of Surgery* be withheld unless mention of the composition of the membership was deleted. However, I pointed out that a nationwide audience had heard the address; that it was not feasible to omit mention of the membership paragraph entirely. An acceptable modification was proposed and accepted. Actually, a black member was proposed for membership the following year but he failed to be elected. He subsequently became a member of the American Surgical Association, president of the American Cancer Society, and secretary of the American College of Surgeons. (The first black was elected 12 years later, in 1985.)

The diversity of opinion was not too surprising, though some opinions were a source of deep dismay to me. Everyone was entitled to his position, but so was I.

As with the Southern Surgical Association, my election as president of the American Surgical Association (which someone has called the priesthood of American surgery) was truly a surprise, both because I had served in no lower office and because the presidency of the ASA is the greatest professional honor that can come to an American surgeon. This, the 1975 meeting, was held at the Le Chateau Frontenac Hotel in Quebec City, Quebec. I was almost overwhelmed, but I did manage to pull myself together to make the usual acceptance remarks. Since 1976 was national bicentennial year, I chose for the presidential address "American Surgery—1976." The ASA itself was just approaching its hundredth anniversary, and I thought that perhaps the speaker in 2076 might want to look back in the records and review my address, as I had reviewed the addresses of many previous presidents.

Ascending to the presidency of the American College of Surgeons was described previously. To achieve the presidency of this college, including as it does almost forty-five thousand members from all the surgical specialties, one truly must have participated in many roles in the ACS over a period of many years. I had served on numerous committees, had given many papers, participated in panels, and presented movies and exhibits, had served on editorial assignments, and had also served as second vice-president and then first vice-president.

Honors and awards

After mentioning the presidencies, it may appear offensive to cite honors and awards. I do so only to note derivations. When one gives an honorary ("named") lecture, one is often given a medal and a certificate attesting that one is now an honorary member of that society. The "name" is usually that of some distinguished former member of the society or a university professor. In the course of time one may receive a substantial number of these awards as visiting professor, each and every one appreciated. The first named lecture I gave was the First Horace G. Smithy Lecture at the Medical University of South Carolina in Charleston. Dr. Smithy was a surgeon who had mitral stenosis, and he had worked desperately to devise an operation for this. He had died just before such surgery was initiated in the late 1940s.

> Ihr bringt mit euch die Bilder froher Tage;
> Und manche liebe Schatten steigen auf.*

*You bring with you the pictures of earlier days, and many cherished memories come to mind. From the prologue to Goethe's *Faust*.

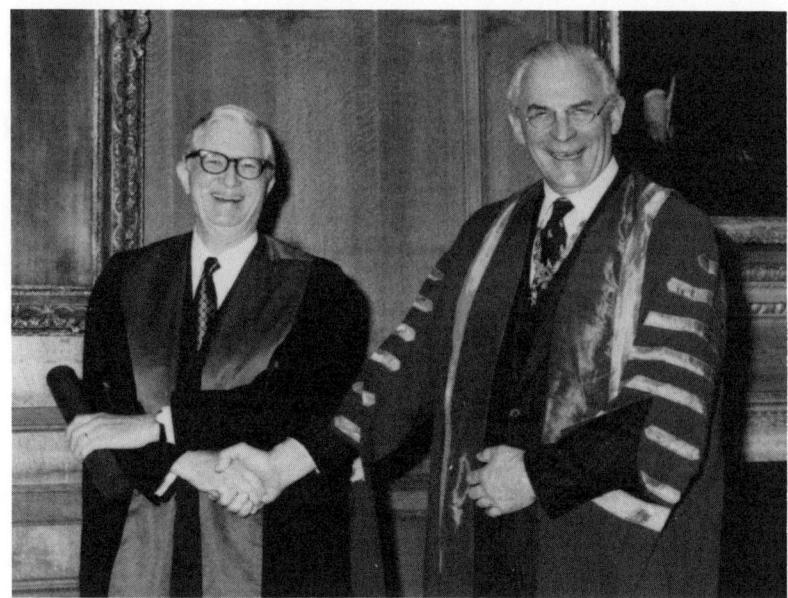

JDH (left), on award of honorary fellowship in the Royal College of Surgeons of England, on occasion of the annual Hunterian Lecture, with Geoffrey Slaney, president, Royal College of Surgeons.

One of the most gratifying named lectures I gave was the first Julian Johnson Lecture in Thoracic Surgery in Philadelphia. "J. J." had trained me in thoracic surgery, and before the large Penn audience, I presented transplantation of the lung and heart.

As for awards and citations, there were many, including not only those in Mississippi but also honorary memberships in the French Association of Surgery (Association Française de Chirurgie), the French Academy of Medicine (Académie Nationale de Médecine), and the Royal College of Surgeons of England in London. Of much importance to me was the First Federal Award in Mississippi. This honor was given each year to three outstanding Mississippians at a large banquet to which leaders from all over the state were invited. I was indeed gratified to have been selected. My appreciation of the true magnitude of this honor was increased no end, however, when in December our youngest daughter, Katherine, said soberly, "Daddy, it's been a great year for the Hardy family. You made First Federal and I made cheerleader."

CHAPTER 20

The 1970s: The Practice of Surgery Is Changing

The financial parameters of surgical practice reflect social and economic changes in the country at large. The original surgeons in England and France were designated "barber surgeons." They were barbers who also did limited surgery, and the elite of the medical profession looked down on them. In the 1800s surgery became a more specialized and accepted calling, though few surgeons had had training to elevate them above the general practitioner who did surgery on the side. This state of affairs persisted well into the 1900s, but the advent of the American Board of Surgery in 1937 meant the end of the informal apprenticeship. The board required a minimum of four (later five) years of approved formal surgical training after graduation from medical school before the resident was permitted to take the written and then the oral examination to gain board certification.

The board-certified surgeon required support in anesthesiology, pathology, and radiology, plus modern technical instrumentation. These requirements, in addition to the young physicians' reasonable expectation of an adequate financial return to justify the long years of training, increased the cost of giving better surgical care. After World War II, medical students, especially military veterans, often married in college or in medical school, had children, and ran up a substantial debt, which made income imperative. (In my own class in medical school, in contrast, perhaps fewer than fifteen students out of 140 were married.) The young surgeons were still willing to work long hours, but they were far more determined to get paid for it promptly than once was the case.

The advent of third-party payments—first Blue Cross–Blue Shield and later many others, but above all federal Medicare–Medicaid—opened Pandora's box. Medicare proved far more expensive than most people had expected, though physicians were not really surprised. Prior to third-party payment, surgeons and other physicians had treated indigent patients without charge—it was expected and accepted. When suddenly the government began paying hospitals and physicians for the care of this large segment of the population, the indigent plus the elderly, it was a true bonanza.

Furthermore, the government made what many believed was an ill-considered policy of paying hospitals "charges plus 10 percent" instead of a flat rate. Not only was there no incentive to economize, but there was every incentive for the hospital to charge as much as possible. The fees paid surgeons were more nearly fixed, but even so there were wide variations among individual surgeons and among geographical regions of the country. The procedure was wide open to costly abuse by all involved—hospitals, physicians, and patients.

The patients, often contributing little or nothing out-of-pocket as the third party paid through the mail, felt free to see the doctor and get admitted to the hospital almost as a convenience. Everyone benefited except the taxpayer as the cost of medical care soared. Interns and residents now were paid a fairly reasonable salary, and the salaries of nurses, traditionally low for their education and training, increased considerably, as did those of hourly wage earners. Expensive coronary artery bypass became one of the commonest if not the commonest operation in many major hospitals.

The American College of Surgeons became concerned with the steadily increasing costs of medical care. Over the years this organization had substantially eliminated ghost surgery (where a trained surgeon is brought in by the practitioner and operates without the patient's knowledge), fee splitting (essentially a kickback to the referring physician), itinerant surgery by a surgeon living at a distance (resulting in inadequate preoperative and postoperative care, and discouraging young surgeons from locating there), and surgery by untrained physicians. It had sought to reduce the startling cost of malpractice insurance (sometimes forty thousand dollars or more per year) by measures to reduce the number of medical malpractice lawsuits. And in the 1970s it turned its attention to containing costs, including exorbitant surgical fees. It would be accurate to say, however, that little headway was made with the last.

Enter DRG (diagnostic related groups).

In the late 1970s, the state of New Jersey initiated prepayment. Instead of paying after-the-fact "charges plus 10 percent," the hospitals were to be paid a flat fee, as for a gallbladder operation, for example. If the patient could be discharged sooner than the specified number of days, the hospital made money; if the patient stayed longer than the days allowed, the hospital lost money. About two-thirds of the cost of medical care is represented by hospital costs (and about two-thirds of hospital costs are for salaries and wages). This pilot study was then embraced by the federal government for Medicare, and other third-party carriers were expected to move in this direction. While open to abuse, the DRG policy included computerized safeguards against fraud; against hospitalizing a patient for convenience, or altering the date of onset of symptoms to make a patient eligible for insurance payment, disability procedures, or workman's compensation; against excessive testing, unnecessary operations, or misrepresenting the patient's diagnosis to record a more serious disease for which payment would be higher.

The hospitals and ultimately the physicians are the principal targets of the DRG policy, but patients themselves will probably feel the tightening controls. For example, there may be a greater out-of-pocket charge to the patient. It has been shown many times that the patient who must pay at least something each time he visits the physician or hospital is much less likely to abuse the system than is one who pays nothing.

The DRG policy poses problems that will be explored as experience accumulates. For one thing, the policy will bankrupt many marginal hospitals, often convenient to local citizens, which may have kept patients in as long as possible in order to keep the occupancy rates high enough to pay the hospital's costs. The DRG is certain to raise problems between the hospital administration and physicians who use the hospital: Will the surgeon who orders too many tests, takes too long in the operating room, keeps patients in the hospital too long, and has too many complications (and threatened lawsuits)—will this surgeon be denied privileges by an increasingly powerful hospital administrator who must preserve the solvency of his institution? And what will DRG payment do for teaching hospitals, which as tertiary or highly specialized institutions care for an inordinately large percentage of critically ill patients while bearing the additional burden of educational costs? Will fewer tests or early hospital discharge of patients with undetected complications that appear later at home—will these result in still more malpractice lawsuits against surgeons? What will be the effect on manufacturers of sophisticated hospital equipment, or on pharmaceutical sales and expensive development of new drugs?

Clearly, there will be a "doctor's dilemma." After having been free to use every drug and technological facility to fight for the life of a critically ill patient, the physician may now be called upon to make judgments: Who should live and for how long? Can the CAT scan be omitted? Will this omission possibly lead to a lawsuit?

Few problems have had more impact on the surgeon's use of sophisticated testing equipment than have lawsuits. Patients have come to expect that every aspect of the operation must be perfect. If it is not, there may be litigation, urged on by the huge number of lawyers who graduate annually in the United States. While careful attention to details and full discussions with the patient and his family can be helpful, all these considerations still may not prevent a lawsuit. For example, the single suit filed against me over the years was brought by a patient and family who had left the hospital saying gratefully, "Doctor, we'll never forget you." They didn't.

I had come in as the good Samaritan in an emergency, performed a long and difficult operation at night, attended the patient intensively thereafter, and ultimately turned the patient back to his original surgeon. The complication had been a minor one which cleared up, and the suit was eventually dropped; but it had not only taken time, it had reminded me once again not to let my malpractice insurance lapse.

The steady increase in the number of American physicians has already resulted in greater competition. Aggressive advertising, once derided, has been tacitly accepted in some areas. Young surgeons are much more willing to accept salaried positions with practice groups or hospitals. Professional practice audits, peer review, second opinion requirements, the high cost of liability insurance and of the opening of an office have all contributed to changing attitudes. The entrepreneurial fee-for-service approach, especially for a solitary practitioner, is being replaced by a preference for collective safety and security through still further specialization. The patient will better know comparative costs, hospital and physician credentials and quality, and the multiple treatment choices available.

Above all, there is already a vast trend toward managing every illness possible without admitting the patient to the hospital. Witness the mushrooming of outpatient surgicenters and walk-in immediate care clinics.

Surgical practice is changing. It will be challenging. It will be different. But it will always be rewarding, in many ways.

CHAPTER 21

The Surgeon Becomes the Patient: My Own Operations

My year of the presidency of the American College of Surgeons began in October 1980. It was continually eventful, and so much time was involved that at least one of my predecessors had taken sabbatical leave the entire year, so that he would be free to come and go without constraint. Clearly, it was going to be a busy year covering all the responsibilities.

Added to these professional considerations was a possible personal problem. Some months before I began my tenure as president, while standing in my office gazing out the window one Saturday morning as I prepared to thumb through some unread surgical journals, I had an abrupt blurring of vision in my left eye, with a feeling of faintness. I quickly sat down in a chair and the attack passed off in a few moments. Having routinely performed surgery on the four neck arteries which supplied the brain, I knew at once that I might have had a cerebral transient ischemic attack (TIA)—momentary blockage of a small artery to a segment of the brain. This brief deficit could have been caused by a small particle of old thrombus in a carotid artery breaking off and passing into the brain. Since the symptoms did not afford a conclusive diagnosis, however, and as they had occurred only once, I simply acknowledged this as a possible warning. Then, again, on a cold night in January 1981, I went down to the office to do some work, started to hang up my topcoat with my left arm as usual, and suddenly found it weak. There seemed to be no loss of sensation in the hand. No pain. This event, too, passed off within a few moments and there were no other symptoms then or thereafter. Nevertheless, the previous eye problem, plus the current arm weakness, could well presage a serious situation. I resolved to check it out. However, as I was just now beginning my year as president of the college, it was not convenient, or advisable from a political standpoint if no other, to go into a hospital in the United States to have definitive studies performed, including arteriograms.

The Executive Committee of the International Society of Surgery required my travel to Basel, Switzerland, twice a year, and the next visit was less than a month away. I asked Dr. Robert D. Currier, chairman of our Department of Neurology, to try to arrange arteriograms in London. It developed that he knew Sir Roger Bannister (the original four-minute miler but now a neurologist) at the National Hospital for Nervous Diseases. Dr. Currier wrote Dr. Bannister and alerted him to the fact that I would be in touch with him:

January 22, 1981

Sir Roger Bannister
The National Hospital for
 Nervous Diseases
Queen Square
London Wc1N3B
England

Dear Doctor Bannister:

Would it be possible for you to arrange an arteriogram for a friend, Jim Hardy, who will be in London February 5th and 6th? He is a 62 year old man who had loss of vision transiently in the left eye (or a left visual field defect) two years ago and then an episode of weakness of the left arm two days ago. He is otherwise quite healthy.

He wishes to have the arteriogram done there rather than here for reasons he will explain. It is not to take advantage of the National Health Service; he will be a private patient.

I realize this is an unusual request and apologize for the short notice, but hope it can be fitted into your schedule. He and I will be quite grateful.

He plans to go on to Germany after leaving London.

He plans to call your office before leaving the States (around February 2nd or 3rd) to see if such an arrangement is possible.

With best regards,

Robert D. Currier, M.D.
Chairman, Department of Neurology

After giving the letter time to arrive in London and be considered, I called Dr. Bannister. He assured me he would be glad to take care of me as the private patient I wished to be. He went on to say, however, that he could not allow me to have the arteriograms one day and then fly on to Germany the next day. At the very least, I would have to plan to be in the hospital before the arteriograms and for two and preferably three days afterward, to be observed for any late complications.

He was right, of course, but I could not afford this kind of time under the circumstances and I was willing to take the risk incurred by leaving the hospital early. He wanted to know why I did not have the studies done in the United States. I told him that with my current political status as president of the 45,000-member college, there was hardly any hospital I would be willing to enter where I might not be known to the surgeons. My symptoms had been minimal, and I considered it safe to postpone investigation, if it had to be done in the United States. Certainly, it was not convenient for me to spend a week in London at that time, with the various speaking commitments that loomed immediately ahead. He cautioned me not to put off the studies too long, lest a stroke occur. Fortunately, there were no other symptoms until possibly an event that happened at the end of the year, well after my responsibilities as president of the college had ended. Throughout the year, I took aspirin on a regular basis to reduce the risk that further clumps of blood platelets would form in the carotid arteries and embolize to the brain.

My turn as a patient

At about 6:45 A.M. on December 4, 1981, I was driving to the hospital, as I had countless times over the years. The next thing I knew I was asking one of our surgery interns, who was looking down at me on the examining table, what was going on. He answered, "You've been in an automobile accident, Doctor Hardy." Apparently I had been driving through an intersection with the light in my favor when a car coming from the opposite direction had cut quickly in front of me. Both cars were traveling at perhaps thirty miles an hour, and my small Mercedes had sustained massive front-end damage. I was told that I got out of my car, as people stopped and came over, and announced that I was all right and did not need to go to the hospital. At that hour of the morning, nurses were changing shifts in the various hospitals, and one of our University Hospital nurses recognized me. An ambulance was called and a young physician waited with me until I was delivered to our own emergency room. Of all this I remembered nothing. The neurological specialists call this a traumatic regressive amnesia. They told me then that I might never remember anything of the accident. I still don't.

I had a number of fractures. A great burst of activity centered around various examinations and X-rays. Head X-rays and a CAT scan disclosed no skull or brain damage, though my head had hit the windshield (at that time I was not yet routinely wearing a seatbelt). I had multiple fractures in the right hand, some in the left hand, and the right patella was broken. A marked slowing of the heart rate developed (my chest had struck the steering wheel), and for a day or so serious consideration was given to the insertion of a pacemaker for heart block, at least temporarily. The cardiac monitor was strapped on, but with a gradual increase in the heart rate, the need for a pacemaker receded.

The care I received from our nurses was superb. I had known they were good, but seeing them through the eyes of the patient, I was even more impressed and was grateful.

There remained in the back of my mind the possibility that I might have had another transient ischemic attack which permitted the accident. All observers in the fairly heavy traffic at that hour said that the driver of the other car had cut directly in front of me against traffic. However, had I been completely alert, would I not have been able to take some evasive action to avoid the head-on collision? Therefore, we proceeded to perform the cerebral arteriograms which I had sought in London almost a year before.

The vascular radiologist passed the catheter through a leg artery and up to the arch of the aorta. Then the radiopaque dye was injected quickly and multiple films shot rapidly to record the contour of the flow through the carotid and cerebral arteries. The dye caused a sharp burning in my head for a few moments, but this discomfort diminished quickly after the material had passed through the brain.

These studies showed that, while the narrowing was not severe, there was ulceration in the right carotid with approximately 50 percent blockage of that vessel. Moreover, it was my left arm that had been symptomatic, as would be expected with a right carotid lesion. The blockage itself was not sufficient to cause a serious problem, but the irregularities could represent the type of particles that might have broken off and gone into the brain.

The first priority was to take care of the fractures. Our orthopaedic group had already managed these lesions, though it was necessary to wear casts on the hands and right leg for some weeks thereafter. Eventually, there remained the question of whether or not to have an operation on the right carotid artery. Some of my colleagues favored only permanent aspirin therapy to diminish blood platelet aggregation. No one but I, myself, was enthusiastic about having surgery on the right carotid artery. I well knew that the actual findings at operation were often much more extensive than the X-rays had indicated. Moreover, since I did not care to live my life taking chances with simply taking aspirin, I resolved to take the risk and have the operation as soon as the various fractures would permit.

Although I had been "unconscious" (though awake) for a period of time, the worst part of the accident was not the severe headaches, which steadily diminished in intensity, but the onset of truly extreme nausea and vomiting. This was probably due to temporarily increased intracranial pressure (in the "tight bony box") or some such brain disturbance, but it responded promptly to an antivertigo medication.

Where to have The Operation? My preference was to have it in our own hospital, performed by Robert R. Smith, chairman of the Department of Neurosurgery, and Seshadri Raju, my daily vascular colleague. However, I was not satisfied with the anesthesia available and resolved to go elsewhere—though this would surely be viewed, both locally and nationally, as reminiscent of the cafe manager who hung up a sign "out to lunch" when he went across the street to eat.

In the end, I chose Jesse E. Thompson, vascular surgeon at Baylor University Hospital in Dallas. Since we had two daughters in Dallas (at Parkland Hospital), Drs. Katherine Hardy Little and Bettie Winn Hardy (Story), I elected to go there. Weezie would have moral support and a place to stay. Also, I knew that Dr. Thompson almost routinely used a shunt to maintain blood flow through a detour while he was working on the clamped carotid artery in the neck. While such a shunt is not always necessary (some surgeons say never), in my own experience using local anesthesia I had, from time to time, had a patient who lost consciousness when the carotid artery was clamped for surgery, only to recover promptly when a shunt had been quickly inserted and that side of the brain again perfused more effectively. I wanted a surgeon who was prepared for the facile use of a shunt if, after he had surveyed the situation at operation, a shunt appeared indicated. The operation was scheduled for February 18, 1982.

I was admitted to Baylor Hospital with impressive efficiency. A cardiologist gave me one of the most thorough physical examinations that I had ever had. A neurologist also came in. One of the X-ray films made in Jackson had been mislabeled, but this was corrected by comparing it with the fillings in my teeth. The cardiologist listed the various medical problems that I had had, none of them incapacitating or serious: the weak left ankle caused by a severe sprain in England during World War II; the bronchial narrowing caused by the pneumonia in England during the army service, which had left me with a wheeze in the right chest from time to time; a history of mild cardiac arrhythmia occasionally—especially after drinking too much coffee, losing sleep, and perhaps a glass of wine; and a minor prostate operation at the age of fifty. My family history was important in that my father, and my brothers John and Julian, had all died of atherosclerotic disease of the coronary arteries. But, by contrast, I had never smoked cigarettes, was not overweight, did not have high blood pressure or diabetes, and my serum cholesterol level was normal. Thus, the atherosclerotic changes could be due largely to advancing age.

I became introspective toward the operation. While the procedure did not require extensive dissection, it was a delicate operation which, in inept hands, could result in a stroke or death. Carotid artery surgery had been shown to result in some degree of neurological change, not often major, in a significant percentage of patients. I concluded that the most important consideration was that I had confidence in my surgeon. I also liked the businesslike anesthesiologist, for in many operations (hernia repair, for example) the anesthesia constitutes a greater risk to life than the actual surgery. Therefore, I had no fear of the operation, though I knew the risks, of course. Weezie and the girls knew too, but they smiled when they accepted my wedding ring as I left on the litter for the operating room.

The anesthesia was very smooth, and after I had received an injection in the arm I knew nothing until some hours after I had been apparently awake in the recovery room. The term "apparently awake" is used deliberately, because a number of persons had come in and spoken with me, asking how I felt and directing me to move my extremities to check for any weakness. I had answered them, but not one bit of this did I remember later. This explained to me why, when so often I had told a patient in the recovery room that all was well and that in fact he or she did not have cancer, the patient later complained that I had not visited the recovery room after the operation. The amnesia of general anesthesia may last much longer than appearances would indicate.

I was well oriented by mid- or late-afternoon, but sleep would not come again until the next day. The nurses checked me frequently during the night, and their routine included a careful neurological examination deliberately executed once an hour. I read a novel, as well as the morning newspapers as soon as they arrived. In fact, Dr. Thompson was astonished when he called in early to learn my condition. The nurse told him I was sitting up reading the newspaper.

And that was about all there was to it. As is often the case, the pathology met at operation had been much more extensive than it had appeared in the preoperative arteriograms. The quality of the nursing care, both in the recovery room and later in the intensive care unit as well as on the open floor, was outstanding. As it was a private hospital, there were no medical students. The nurses were accorded extensive responsibility, and I found myself depending more heavily upon them than might have been necessary in a university hospital where numerous trainees are almost always at hand. A truly private hospital has its function, and a university teaching hospital has its function. The two are inevitably at variance because of the different missions assigned to each.

My neck was sore, but the sutures were removed on the third postoperative day. We went to Katherine's home for the night, and then Weezie and I drove home to Jackson the next morning, the fourth postoperative day. At no time was there any complication. Best of all, it was now behind me, and I could proceed with my life as usual without concern. "Without concern" is not completely true. The atherosclerosis itself had not been cured and could someday involve other arteries.

Second carotid operation

I had been completely asymptomatic for three years, until the evening of March 16, 1985. Then, upon standing up to leave a social gathering, I felt dizzy, noted some numbness in the right hand, and promptly passed out. Recovering in less than a minute, I knew precisely what had happened: another TIA, but this time due to atherosclerotic changes in the *left* carotid artery. Needless to say, the episode claimed my immediate interest and attention. Dr. Robert Currier examined me promptly, ordered a brain CAT scan the next day (it was normal), and an arteriogram the day after that. The films showed an excellent result from the previous operation on the *right* carotid artery, but ulceration in the narrowed *left* carotid. I decided immediately for prompt operation. My colleague on the vascular service, Dr. Seshadri Raju, performed the carotid endarterectomy, assisted by Dr. William Neely and the vascular fellow, Theodore Perry. There were no complications, and I was home on the third day. Needless to say, I am very grateful to have been a beneficiary of the great advances in vascular surgery. I barely escaped a serious and potentially permanent stroke.

Heart "operation"

On July 18, 1985, I abruptly experienced typical angina pectoris while tugging on the leash of my bird dog. Coronary arteriograms disclosed severe stenosis of the left anterior descending coronary artery. Faced with the imminent September biennial meeting of the International Society of Surgery in Paris, where I was to be installed as president, I chose balloon angioplasty instead of coronary bypass. This procedure was performed successfully by my cardiologist Patrick H. Lehan and his associate Robert M. Ball, with complete relief of symptoms.

CHAPTER 22

Family

With his children, a man becomes placed, in society and in posterity.

By the time our four girls were seven, six, four, and two, their little personalities were already taking form. For example, one night when I was reading a manuscript in the guest room ("the study room"), I decided that Katherine, now about two years old, should begin to obey. I told her to pick up her socks as she went out of the room, where she had been sitting at my feet playing with a doll. She sat down and stubbornly refused. She would look up furtively at me and, once she caught my eye, would look quickly down again. She remained adamant. Finally, I scooped her up and plumped her into her bed and told her that I was not going to kiss her good night. At this, four-year-old Bettie came in and asked anxiously, "Daddy, aren't you going to kiss Kaky good night?"

"No, I'm not!"

"But, Daddy, it was such a little thing." Bettie, always exquisitely perceptive in interpersonal relationships.

As for Julia and Louise, Weezie and I had disciplined them for some infraction of stated rules, made for their own safety with respect to automobiles in the street. They had been thoroughly outraged, and we could hear them planning to run away. They had put on their new dresses, packed their little doll suitcases, tiptoed down the stairs, and were sitting on the front steps debating their next move.

"Now, Julia," Louise was heard to say, "we must leave while Mamma and Daddy are not watching us."

Julia: "But, Louise, what will we eat?" Julia, always the literal and practical one.

Louise: "Don't be silly. We'll marry somebody and make him support us." Louise, always the imaginative one, the dreamer.

Each morning the maid, Mrs. Sarah Gray, a resourceful Negro woman who was with us for many years, would take the four girls

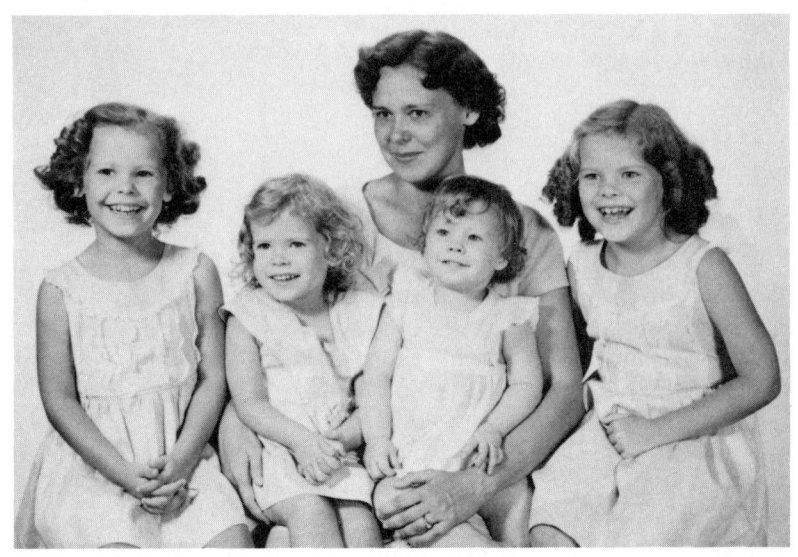

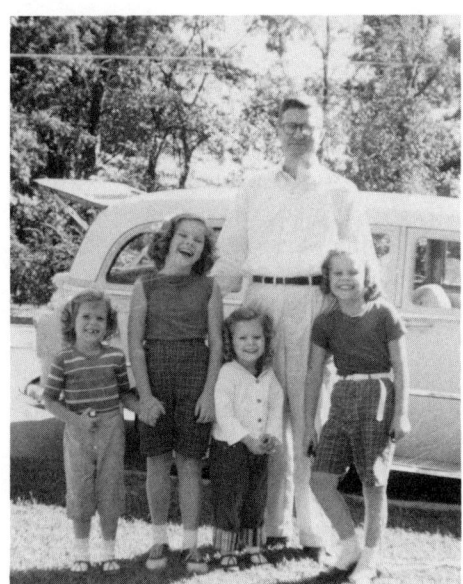

Top, left to right: *Julia, Bettie, Weezie, Katherine, and Louise*

Left: *Going to "spend the allowance"*

around the block, rolling Katherine in her stroller. They encountered a woman and the girls greeted her warmly, as they did almost everyone. The woman said, "Oh, my, four little girls. Are there any boys?"

"Yes," the children answered, "we have one boy."

"How nice," the woman said. "You also have one boy."

"Yes, it's Daddy."

"Well, I thought there must be one somewhere!"

We had taken a lot of ribbing that all our children were girls, and I had probably joined in—but not for long. One day Katherine, sitting on the floor playing at the age of about three or four, looked up at me sad-faced and asked, "Daddy, do you wished I was a boy?"

On Saturday afternoons I took the children to Franklin's ten-cent store to "spend the allowance"—experience in money values, making decisions, respect for property, and honesty.

Every spring the children and I planted a small garden in the side yard. Each girl had her own row, marked by impaling the brightly colored empty seed packet on a stick. Years before, I had read a poignant account by a girl from a farm in the Midwest who now lived in a high-rise apartment in New York City. Each spring, as fond memories of her childhood farm crowded in upon her, she would buy seeds and do her planting in a box of dirt on the windowsill. Now, living far away, our daughters plant a tiny garden each spring.

We built our two-story Georgian brick home in 1961, although the integration battle was in full force and state government threatened to close the public schools rather than to integrate them. But we had already moved from Philadelphia to Memphis, and then to Jackson, and the children were thriving. Although I received a number of inquiries from other universities about this time, we did not want to move again unless the offer was one that could not be declined.

Meanwhile, our work was being acknowledged increasingly in Mississippi and elsewhere. A commendation resolution was voted by the Mississippi state legislature. A steady flow of national and foreign visitors came through our laboratory, and many of them dined with Weezie, the children, and me in our home. The children were usually well behaved when they met surgeons and other scientists, with one exception: If the visitor smoked, they would place small notes in the ashtrays stating "Smoking Causes Cancer." But even this lapse in etiquette we managed to control eventually. It was during this era that my wife was instrumental in developing The International Friends, a group that served to give the wives of our foreign research fellows a chance to get out of the house and meet regularly for visiting and interesting programs.

Breaking the set

September 19, 1968, represented a major departure in the life of our little family. This was the day we drove Louise to Atlanta and to Agnes Scott College in nearby Decatur. It was poignant in many ways, for Louise represented the third successive generation "Louise Scott" who had attended this all-girls college founded by her maternal great-grandfather. A businessman, he had believed that daughters should have a college education as sons did.

Just as we had finished loading the station wagon, the other three girls began to chant to Louise a little tune which was popular at that time and went "And now you are going away." At first we all joined in, but then, like the proverbial ton of bricks, it suddenly hit us all that she *was* going away, and we all choked up and became silent.

We drove her over and got her settled. Her grandmother lived immediately across Candler Street in the large, Victorian, rambling, two-storied ancestral home. However, for reasons which were not entirely fathomable to me, I remained mildly depressed for some weeks thereafter. No other departure, either to college or through marriage, ever pulled so strongly at my heartstrings. In retrospect, I believe it was because this was the first breaking of the set of our little family, which had been close in Jackson because we were new there, were often besieged politically, and had relatively few close friends.

In 1970 I was king of the Carnival Ball in Jackson. By custom, the king and queen were elected secretly by the Junior League. The king was usually a mature man and the queen either still in or just out of college. The invitation was extended, very covertly, late one evening by Mrs. Frances Pat Walton, president, Mrs. Kieta Westbrook, chairman of the ball, and Mrs. Ruth Jenkins, cochairman. I was naturally pleased and honored, yet I had some misgivings; for when Dr. Alton Ochsner had served as king of the Mardi Gras in New Orleans some years before, I had reflected that it was a bit to one side of science and surgery. However, my aides, Mrs. Virginia Parsons and Mrs. Sally Yelverton, were most attentive, and Mrs. Lydy Henley came secretly to our home at night to instruct me in the dramatics of wielding the royal scepter. The Hardy family all enjoyed the excitement and plain good fun of the secrecy, the royal

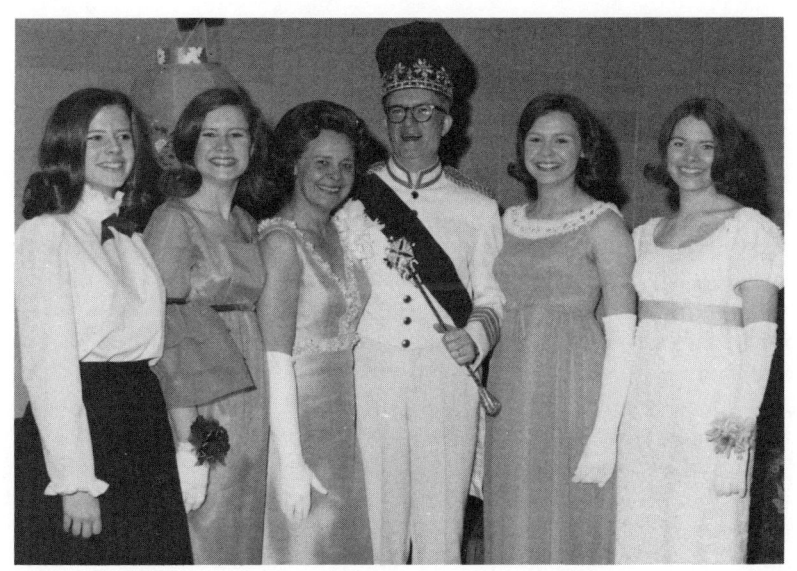

Left to right: *Bettie, Katherine, Weezie, JDH, Julia, Louise*

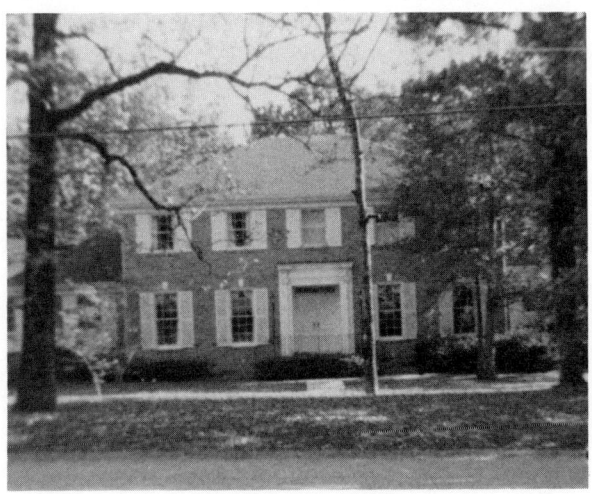

Home

robes and crown, and the final gala evening at the civic coliseum. My queen was the lovely Miss Isabel Lutkin.

Meanwhile, I was grateful to Weezie and the girls for what they had put up with. Many family outings, many a promise to the children, had been blocked by some administrative problem or by the arrival of some emergency patient. In the early days of open-heart surgery, when we would sometimes lose a patient we had hoped we might not lose, the family would accept my silence around the house for a day or so. When a surgeon's children hear that daddy has lost a patient, they know nobody is looking for someone who is missing. The internist usually blames himself for errors of *omission*, but the surgeon usually blames himself for errors of *commission*. As some cynic put it: The internist says, "Oh, Father, forgive us for the things which we have not done, which we should have done." The surgeon asks, "Oh, Father, forgive us for those things which we have done, which we should not have done."

By 1972 our family was progressing well. During the week of May 20, Bettie received all A's from SMU and was to be president of her sorority, Julia got all A's at Vanderbilt and was president of her sorority, Louise graduated from Agnes Scott College Phi Beta Kappa and president of the Mortar Board, and Katherine, still at Jackson Preparatory High School, was head of the Prep Pacers (drill team) and head also of the Prepettes (singers). Katherine was the only one not to graduate from public high school. When she was ready to begin junior high school, the busing mandate required her to attend three different schools in two years, with several hours wasted in the transportation each day. This was just too much, and we put her in a private school. Our first inkling of Louise's making PBK was when she said casually at graduation, "Daddy, if you'll lend me twenty-six dollars I can pick up a Phi Beta Kappa certificate."

Julia graduated from Vanderbilt Phi Beta Kappa and went on to Harvard Medical School. Louise had met Karl-Otto Röska, a German electronics engineer taking postgraduate study at Georgia Tech, and the friendship appeared to have taken a serious turn. She had gone in the summer to the Goethe Institute in Prien, Germany, to study and speak only German. I was not too surprised when they announced their engagement. I had misgivings about my daughter's going to a foreign country and a different culture, but her fiancé spoke English fluently and her German was improving rapidly. She was finishing her master's degree in philosophy at North Carolina in Chapel Hill and later took her Ph.D. at the University of Frankfurt in Germany. In the spring, we drove all the way to Dallas for Bettie's initiation into Phi Beta Kappa at Southern Methodist University and back the same day.

First family wedding

Our first wedding was complicated by Weezie's operation. With Louise's marriage scheduled for June 15, Weezie abruptly developed an inflammatory mass in the right side of her abdomen. She had long known a straight pin, swallowed in childhood, resided in her appendix. Now it had passed through the wall of the appendix and caused an abscess. However, we were uncertain that the lump did not represent cancer. Her surgeon, my colleague William O. Barnett, wisely removed the right half of her colon. Someone asked if I did not want to do the operation myself. The answer was no, for if another capable surgeon is available, a surgeon is well advised not to operate on close relatives. I would not have hesitated to operate had we been somewhere in an underdeveloped country.

Most of the plans and preparations for the wedding had already been made, and it was a splendid occasion. But a father does not change fifteen minutes after he has given his first daughter away. After the wedding pictures had been taken and we had reached the front steps of the church, I took Louise's hand and said, "Come on, Louise, we'll be late for the reception," as I opened the door to my car. But the new husband came over and said gently, "Dr. Hardy, I have my own car."

Our second wedding was Bettie's. She married an S.M.U. classmate, Mark T. Story, who was then in law school at the University of Texas. She herself took her master's and ultimately her Ph.D. degree in clinical psychology at Southwestern Medical School in Dallas. As she and I were just starting down the matrimonial aisle, she said, "Oh, Daddy, they forgot to light the candles!" I looked quickly around for one of my surgical residents, for had one been present those candles would have been lit forthwith.

Katherine, in pre-med at Vanderbilt, had worked with me in the surgical laboratory one summer. When I wrote her that our manuscript had been accepted for publication, she asked that I please write and tell her what it was we had discovered. Julia had done similar work and her paper, too, had appeared in the *Annals of Surgery*.

Katherine came to medical school in Jackson, was elected Alpha Omega Alpha, and entered internal medicine and gastroenterology at Southwestern Medical School and Parkland Hospital in Dallas.

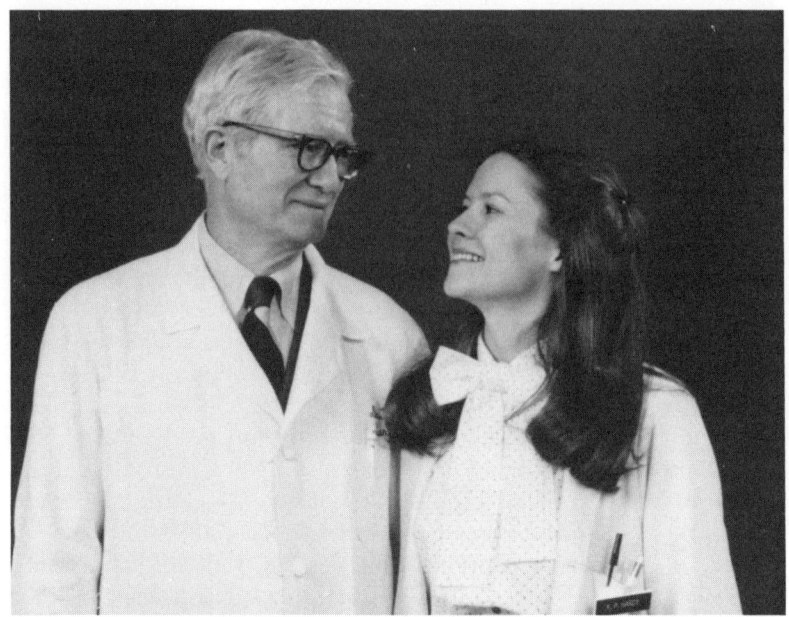

Katherine receiving award in surgery from JDH

She married Louie Little, a Mississippian who had graduated from Mississippi State University, taken his master's degree, and was with the International Paper Company. Julia specialized in psychiatry at Michigan and chose to practice in Ann Arbor.

Death of a twin

After leaving medical school, Julian had returned to do his internship and residency training at the Hillman Hospital in Birmingham, where the new four-year medical school was soon to be established. He married Marion Francis Doughty of Tuscaloosa, whom he had met when he and I were freshmen in college at the University of Alabama. Thereafter they lived in Birmingham, where he had been recognized in numerous ways, including presidency of the Jefferson County Medical Society which included Birmingham. We saw each other perhaps not more than twice a year, but we always felt an immediate intimacy of thought and confident reliance upon each other's trust.

One night, apparently by sheer coincidence, both his son Pat and daughter Anne called me in Jackson to say that they were deeply worried about their father. They said that he did not act like himself and that they thought he was sick, though he maintained that he was not and had seen no necessity to get a checkup. I had known that he had some type of bronchitis or something, but I had had no idea that he was not generally well. Taking the plane to Birmingham the next morning, and a taxi from the airport to his home in the Mountainbrook area, I found him alone at home, lying in bed and staring soberly at the ceiling. This simply was not Julian! Always very active, he clearly was not well. He mentioned a recent chest X-ray. I asked him to get up and get dressed, and suggested we go over to his hospital to see the X-rays that his internist colleague had taken of his chest, though they were more or less perfunctory. I saw a lesion in his right lower lung field, and Julian remarked that he had been very tired lately. He told me, now, that he had had angina pectoris on several occasions. Coronary bypass was scheduled.

He agreed to see a cardiologist at the University of Alabama Hospital. Cardiac catheterization disclosed severe blockage of the left main coronary artery, which could prove immediately fatal should total occlusion occur.

The operation was performed, and he went through it beautifully, being awake and alert by early afternoon. Therefore, in the early evening, I drove back to Jackson to fulfill my own operating schedule the next morning. His improvement continued steadily. However, about a week following his operation, his wife called to say that she was worried about him, though his doctors did not seem to be as concerned as she was.

I went back at once and found a decidedly alarming state of affairs. Unknown to me, he had developed hemorrhagic spots over much of his body, which were now receding. He was extremely weak, he lay listlessly in bed, his pulse rate was 120, his temperature 102° and 103° F, and his nostrils flared when he breathed, usually a sign of some type of cardiorespiratory problem.

It was a Sunday, but I was able to speak with his surgeon at home over the telephone. Soon, the resident on the cardiac surgery service came up to talk with me. He assured me that Julian was really progressing satisfactorily, but that he was not cooperating—they were considering bringing in a psychiatrist to talk with Julian to improve his motivation. This was enough for me.

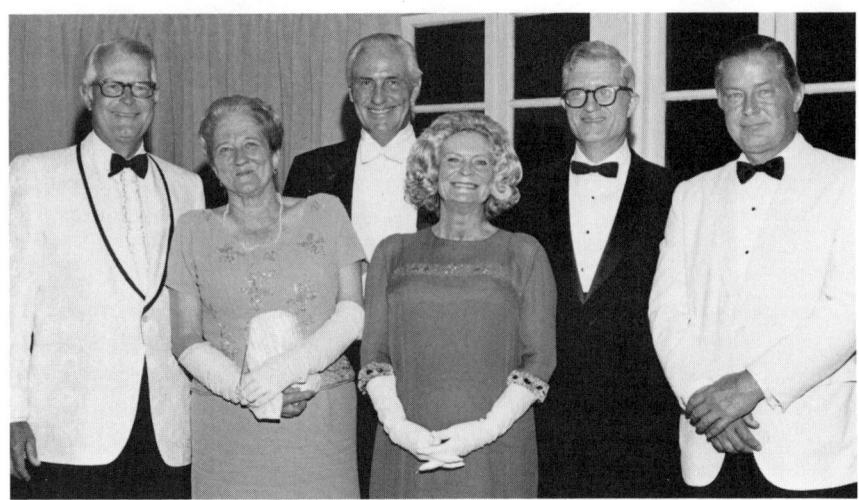

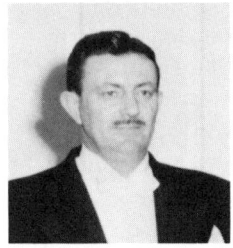

The original Hardy children, 1979 (left to right):
Taylor, Agnes, Fred, Emily, James, Julian

John Morris Hardy

"Doctor," I said, "this man and I have been together now for sixty-one years. He has always been an athlete, he was always the first to take any dare, he would never refuse to cooperate with his physicians, and I think something is very seriously wrong. Just look at him. Note the fever, rapid heart action, dilating nostrils when he breathes, and his profound weakness. This is by no means the normal recovery of a coronary bypass patient. I am alarmed about his condition. In any case, he certainly does not need a psychiatrist."

I called all the family members together. I told them the case could go either way, in my opinion, despite the confidence of his surgeons. However, no major change in his condition appeared imminent.

Leaving Julian that Sunday afternoon was one of the hardest things I had ever had to do. He was so weak he could scarcely get to

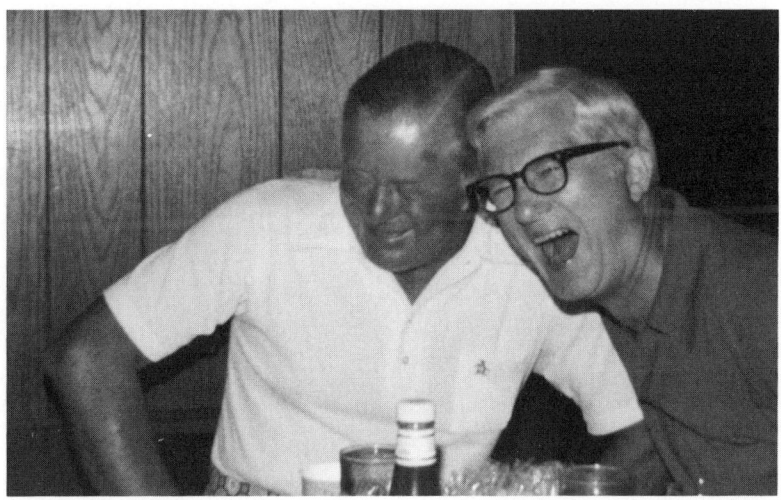

Last photograph of the twins. Julian (left) and James, Destin, Florida, 1979

the bathroom, and then, just before I was going, he asked the nurse, "Where is James?"

I was immediately summoned from the family group down in the waiting room, and I went back and sat with Julian for a while. When I had to go, I could really think of nothing to say to him. Both he and I, being doctors, knew that he was not doing well. What does one say to a twin brother, also a doctor, who knows the score just as well as you do?

I took his hand, always larger, stronger, and somewhat beefier than mine, from his athletics and mild obesity, and we squeezed hands gently. It was the last time I was to see him alive.

Tests showed he was in adrenal failure from the generalized hemorrhages, somehow caused by the anticoagulant he was taking, and he improved promptly on cortisone therapy. A week later everything seemed to be in good condition, and he was getting around in a wheelchair and preparing to go home. I had gone to our place on a lake about seventy-five miles from Jackson. That Sunday morning about seven o'clock, a deputy sheriff came and knocked on the door, there being no telephone. He said, "Doctor, I hate to have to tell you, but your brother just died in Birmingham." Julian had had (another?) massive embolus to his lungs, probably from the deep veins of his legs. It was August 12, 1979.

CHAPTER 23

A Look Backward and a Summing Up

Each man is divided among
the men he might have been
—PAUL NIZEN

As I look back from the vantage point of sixty-seven years, certain major events stand out with a clarity which was not apparent at the time they occurred. *World War II was clearly the watershed of my life.* For the nation, it mobilized a vast, collective, national and global activity, directed with a unified will toward a single goal, victory. For many citizens it represented the single most complete, lifetime break with educational, professional or other civilian routine. It took us out of ourselves, for a time, into infinite dimensions that we were powerless to control. It changed my medical specialty from internal medicine to surgery. It determined the place where I would meet my wife. Always thereafter, events would be "before the war," or "after the war."

Otherwise, the years divide naturally among growing up in Alabama, thirteen years of medical school—internship, residencies at the University of Pennsylvania in Philadelphia—more than three years at the University of Tennessee Medical College in Memphis, and then thirty years with the University of Mississippi Medical Center in Jackson.

Professional activity has been divided, and hopefully balanced, among surgical practice, teaching, research, and administration.

Surgical practice

What changes have taken place over the past forty years. To be sure, standard operations on the stomach, intestine, gallbladder, breast, and thyroid are still performed by the general surgeon—though often now for different indications and with different frequencies. But whereas the general surgeon once treated most of the fractures and soft tissue tumors of the extremities, these are now managed by the orthopaedists, head and neck cancer by the plastic surgeons or the otolaryngologists, colon polyps by the endoscopist, and so on. Drug therapy has reduced the number of operations required for the complications of peptic ulcer. Meanwhile, the general surgeon has evolved to become the vascular surgeon, the general thoracic surgeon, the cardiac surgeon, the organ transplanter, the metabolic surgeon (performing operations to control morbid obesity and hyperlipidemia), and still others.

As for my personal practice, I am grateful that, despite the fact that my career involved as much travel as it did, only twice was I to feel that a postoperative patient I had left behind would have been better off had I been present to care for a complication personally.

General thoracic surgery burgeoned during the 1940s, with tuberculosis surgery made safer with the advent of streptomycin, and subsequently still more effective drugs. And bronchiectasis provided many a lobectomy or segmentectomy for the daily operating schedule. Now, with these diseases essentially controlled with antibiotic therapy, lung cancer and occasional complications of emphysema represent the principal pulmonary operations. Indeed, the number of pulmonary operations has declined so drastically in some medical centers that residents in training have difficulty in meeting their thoracic board requirements. For one thing, many lung cancers that were formerly treated by thoracotomy are now diagnosed without operation and treated otherwise.

But cardiovascular surgery, virtually nonexistent in the 1940s, moved forward in the 1950s to claim a major place in the broad field of general surgery, before cardiac surgery became a clear-cut subspecialty of its own, with peripheral arterial surgery somewhat less so.

Thus, many of the operations commonly performed today had not even been "discovered" when I was in residency training. It is essential that the young surgeon learn to manage change and to grow along with it. Already, many of the cardiac and peripheral artery operations of today are being threatened by the increasingly effective transcutaneous balloon dilatation of many arteries, including the coronaries. Kidney stones are being removed percutaneously, or pulverized with sonic waves, as are some gallstones.

The general surgeon will perhaps now move further into human organ replacement with transplants or artificial devices—while continuing to manage trauma, infections, neoplasia, congenital and acquired defects, and alimentary tract obstructions.

Meanwhile, jurisdictional disputes among the various surgical subspecialties—as to who will do what to whom—will continue to rearrange responsibilities. Statistical studies in Scandinavia indicate that the amount of general surgery, and thus the number of general surgeons required, may be declining. But unlike the phthisiologist, whose tribe now is all but extinct, the long-term survival of the general surgeon can be predicted with considerable confidence. And, incidentally, far more women will be active in the field than ever before.

But with all these changes, the exquisitely sensitive and sometimes fragile element of trust between the surgeon and the patient, who risks his life on the operating table, will never change. The words of an elderly and essentially illiterate black patient, with a very dangerous, large, and painful thoracic aneurysm eroding the spine, put it to me in its purest form. I had briefly told him we would operate the next day, but he called me back. Looking at me steadily but silently with his one eye for a few moments, he then said, "Doc, we ain't talked much, but I'se countin' on you."

Education

Education from birth, in the broadest sense, creates the major cultural and intellectual differences among the peoples of the world. To put this another way, if two newborn infants, whose mothers had been well cared for in the same environment during pregnancy—if these two infants from different races were then reared as twins, assuming essentially equal brain power, they would both be capable citizens, regardless of race. For native intelligence is widely distributed. It has been well said that the greatest waste is a human mind—and few of us ever use even the major segment of the mind's capacity. The problem is, children do *not* receive equal education—not in the home, not among playmates, and not in school. Everything learned may prove useful, or at least interesting, and the sciences of Einstein, Pasteur, Beethoven, and Renoir must all converge somewhere near infinity. Education opens doors to vision, while without it, daily life can afford only limited exaltations. Mere existence should not be enough.

To be sure, our interest here is primarily with medical students.

But what the given medical student has been taught during the twenty-two or so years before he or she is admitted to medical school will substantially determine the student's effectiveness and aspirations in later life.

Once having admitted the student to medical school, the faculty has the solemn obligation to teach him or her as effectively as possible, perhaps to light the spark of idealism, of a higher goal than that previously envisioned. To this end, I have always covered a clinical service, the year around, to remain in daily contact, not only with patients, but particularly with the medical students, interns, and residents. To gain and maintain the respect of trainees, the surgeon must operate—this is his job, and here he is clearly performing his designated function, which no one else on the faculty can do. (And, to paraphrase J. Englebert Dunphy, "No one appreciates a good surgeon more than a sick scientist!")* Far too many of our academic colleagues depart early from the hurly-burly and pressure of the operating theater, virtually always to their loss, in my view.

Research

The investigation of better ways to understand, diagnose, and treat disease conditions must be a significant function of a vital medical center. This is a primary reason for research in a medical school department. But only slightly less important is the educational effect on those doing the research, for once the critical way of thinking of the investigator has been developed in the trainee, he or she will thereafter require that factual information be critically examined before settling on a diagnosis and treatment—whether he or she ever makes a discovery or not. That is, the investigative turn of mind is invaluable in the management of the patient—though, of course, many excellent surgeons simply achieve a trained, even intuitive, turn of mind without any research experience.

Since 1946, when I proposed to Dr. Ravdin that the mysterious cachexia of cancer be investigated, virtually every cancer has been shown to release metabolic products into the bloodstream, which collectively gradually impair body metabolism to the extent that death occurs. As for the endocrine system, the accepted endocrine organs discussed in my slender *Surgery and the Endocrine System* (1952) were the pituitary, the thyroid and parathyroids, the adrenals, the islets of Langerhans (producing insulin), and the ovaries and

---

*J. E. Dunphy, "Presidential Address," *Ann. Surg.* 156 (1962): 327.

testes. It is now known that the gut and its tributaries are perhaps the major endocrine organ of the body, with approximately one hundred of its hormonal substances either identified, or isolated and characterized; a few have even been synthesized. A number of common hormonal substances have been found in the brain, and many additional endocrine substances have been discovered in traditional endocrine organs, such as the islets of Langerhans. The influence of the brain and genetics on human endocrinology and physiology is incalculable.

What of surgical research in the future? It is of course impossible to separate surgical research from that of basic science or the other clinical disciplines. Discovery of all truth must be approached through information and insights gained from many different sources in order to provide the "final" concept. However, having acknowledged this universality of science, one may suggest a few particular spheres of endeavor in which truly significant progress is being made and will continue to be made. These include, for example, organ transplantation for diabetes; artificial replacements for joints, even eyesight and the heart; and remarkable advances in radiological diagnostic and invasive therapeutic procedures. And while it is not surgical research as such, epidemiological studies to determine why certain cancers occur more frequently in different races, or even in members of the same race in different localities, will ultimately reduce disease. Diet restriction and cessation of smoking would vastly reduce cardiovascular disease, lung cancer, and pulmonary emphysema. Immunology is in its infancy.

Thus there is exciting research to be done in the prevention or management of most of the surgical diseases to which man is heir. It is only to be hoped that the research support and medical manpower available will be adequate to the task.

Administration

To paraphrase Lord Byron, administration is for some a thing apart; 'tis others' whole existence. The administration of the department of surgery has afforded me sufficient activity in this area, and I have not accepted the invitation to consider a full-time position as dean. By this, I do not imply for an instant that the post of dean is not extremely important to a medical school; it is simply that, for me, clinical surgery, teaching, and research had laid a prior claim.

Leadership

Administration implies governance, leadership. What is leadership? What are the qualities required? Is it inborn, or can it be acquired? When and in what way should it be exercised?

How many dimensions the word implies, how difficult at times to exert it. A beginning surgical resident is chosen not simply with a view to how well he or she will perform the next year, but rather with an eye to how good a leader the trainee will be as a potential chief resident five years from now. The same could be said for any employee hired with a view to future important advancement.

First, the individual must have already acquired basic human and moral values, for morality is the ultimate reality. Next, a reasonable degree of internal self-confidence, of stability, must be in evidence. Then, competence in medical school reflects not only intelligence but also a willingness to work, for regardless of how bright a person is, the sheer volume of information to be assimilated in medical school requires time and application. These are basic qualities which, when combined with a sufficient volume of adequately supervised surgery, should result in an effective chief resident in surgery five years later. A presentable appearance and a ready facility with the English language are also helpful.

Then what of the administration of a surgery department in a medical school? Basically, it consists of continuing to demonstrate competence as a surgeon, teacher, and hopefully investigator—and then seeking to perceive the concerns of the other members of the faculty and to assist them in achieving their objectives. This support for faculty will most often revolve around matters of office and laboratory space, salary, promotions, supporting personnel, election to professional societies, and related matters. In general, it has seemed to me preferable to give the individual faculty member all possible freedom to expand and grow, as long as it does not encroach on the needs of others. If one can be well liked, so much the better, but it is *essential* to be respected. One must spend time with the person, to know him or her. Like most mammals, people do better with approval.

To be sure, there must be organization and a few clear and consistently pursued departmental policies and goals. Occasionally, the chairman will encounter borderline, if not outright, disloyalty, which if flagrant and chronic, cannot in the long run be ignored. However, this may be quite unintentional, and a candid chat with the colleague will often suffice. Occasionally, however, basic and irreconcilable differences will emerge, and then the problem becomes much more complex. At this point, it is wise to touch base with the dean. One sound policy is to leave every subordinate free to take irreconcilable differences to the dean, if he or she so desires, just so long as the chairman has the opportunity to present his or her views as well. If the colleague accepts this policy, very few irreconcilable differences will arise. But by the same token, the dean who allows the departmental chairman to be privately bypassed, this dean in effect becomes the departmental chairman, and thereafter *he* or *she* must take appropriate responsibility for what develops. To be bypassed costs the chairman authority and prestige, but at the same time it costs the dean the confidence, respect, and support of that chairman.

But, by and large, it is better to be lenient, keep smiling, and wait until all the facts are in and the situation is clear. When, rarely, an unavoidable, hard issue cannot be adjudicated, it must be met head-on without flinching. Optimally, one hopes to lead by example, by representing what most people of good will realize is compatible, not only with their individual goals, but with the welfare of all. Once an issue has been settled, the opposition should be welcomed back into the fold; an opponent today may become an ally tomorrow.

It is hard to transfer vision, but not infrequently vision can be induced. There is some facet, some receptor site, in virtually every trainee, which can be activated to impart the desire to do a better or more responsible job.

A Career Has Run Its Course

By the time this volume is published, my tenure as chairman of the Department of Surgery at the University of Mississippi Medical Center for over thirty years will have virtually run its course. What report can I give on both my institutional stewardship and my personal stewardship?

As for the university responsibilities, my many colleagues and I have revolutionized medical practice in Mississippi. When we arrived in Jackson in 1955, we saw the largest tumors and the sickest patients imaginable. Not a few adults had never seen a doctor (or dentist) in their lives. There were only a handful of surgical specialists in the state, and some counties had no physician at all. Now, every town of even modest size has physicians, at least one hospital,

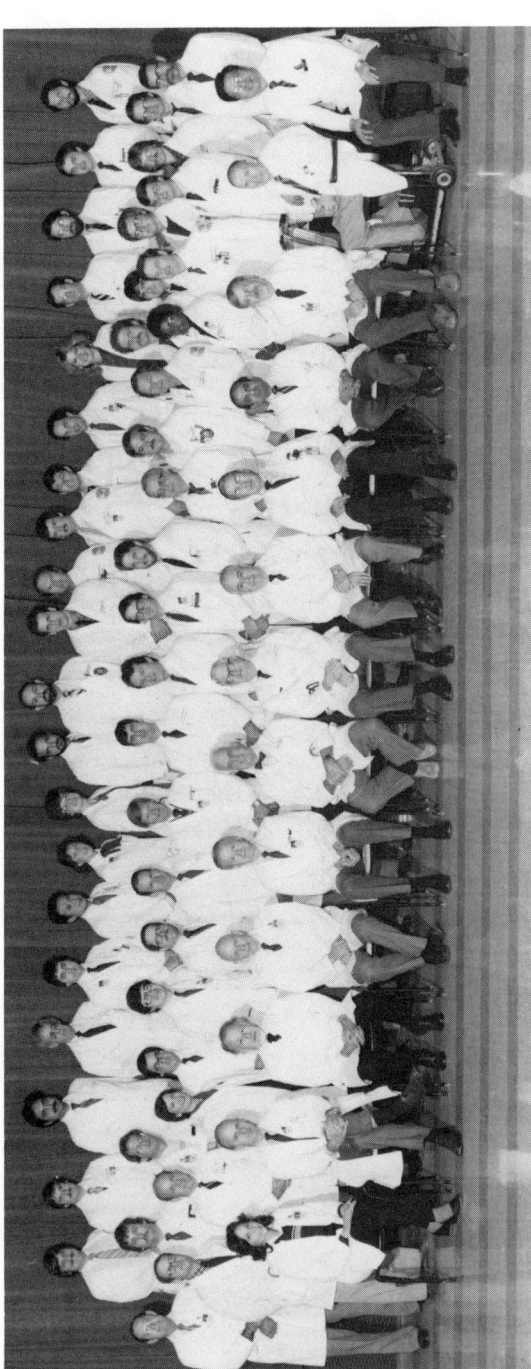

The department of surgery, 1984. Front row, left to right: Karen Morer, Lamar Weems, Samuel Johnson, Richard Miller, Martin Dalton, William Neely, JDH, William Hart, Winsor Morrison, Seshadri Raju, Ojus Malphurs, Judson Farmer, Ching-Jygh Chen. Second row: Don Turner, Scott Houston, James Maher, Fred Rushton, Keith Smith, Connie McCaa, Ralph Didlake, Steve Isbell, Barry Newsom, Douglas Godfrey, David Crawford, Alex Haick, Jeff Budden, Bill Owen, Howell Tucker, Mukadder Cayirli, Stephen Bayne, Barry Sauer, Hunt Bobo, Maxine Eakins, Jim Pennington, Luther Fisher, Bill Mayo, Swayze Rigby, Jeff Cook, Joel Knight, James Peck. Third row: John Tomasin, Joe Moore, Vinod Anand, Ron Krueger, Jim Cotter, Twatchi Yamcharern, Kathy Jackson, Vickie Gerken, Mark Barraza, Lyle Zardiackas, Kirk Banquer, Ron Graham, Marc Aiken, Todd Sherwood, Greg Fiser, DeAnn Smith, John Petro, Ped Hooper, Gray Buck, Jay Miles.

and commonly several specialists. The University Medical Center has graduated 2,550 medical doctors, and the various divisions of the Department of Surgery have trained more than 300 surgical specialists. Since all our medical students must have established residency in Mississippi, a remarkable percentage of them remained to practice in this state. Competent medical care is now available within a few miles, over good roads, from essentially any point in the state. This fact represents the greatest single achievement of myself and all my many colleagues in the University Medical Center over the years: We put together a solid medical school and university hospital, which led the way to vastly improved health care in the State of Mississippi. That was our primary assignment and responsibility. The effort has been staunchly supported by the citizens of Mississippi through their legislature.

As regards my personal stewardship, this judgment must be left to others. But I will say one thing: To myself I have been true. Perhaps some judgments and decisions have been faulty, doubtless they have, but they did honestly reflect the situation as I saw it at the time. That has meant a lot to me.

So the years have scudded by, and now retirement is almost at hand. Are there regrets? There are few regrets relative to professional work. A recent national poll taken by the Gallup Organization revealed that seven out of every ten doctors would choose the same career if they had to make the choice again. Surgeons were the least inclined to do so again, citing long hours, constant pressure, and the sacrifices demanded. But not I. If I have been a prisoner of my career, certainly I have been a willing one. I would do the same thing again. We were brought up on the hard work ethic, and having multiple interesting projects has served only to render life more richly rewarding. What a privilege to arise each morning, with a day of challenging surgery and other activities in prospect. And not rarely, a life is saved. Basically, one simply needs a place to work.

I might have hoped to develop more cohesively a school of surgical disciples, in the academic sense, but this takes time and the development of tradition. Certainly we have developed many first-class clinical surgeons for private practice. Private practitioners represent by far the largest segment of our specialty nationally, and they perform the overwhelming majority of surgical operations in this country. Our trainees know who they are and what they represent. They build their reputations and their careers, day by day.

If there are regrets, and such exist, they have to do with family, things I did not do when I should have. Chekhov, himself a physician, has been quoted as having remarked that physicians have few illusions, which tends to desiccate life. I have not found it so.

On the positive side, retirement will bring a release from certain duties and obligations. For example, there will be no need to make judgments on personnel. No need to progressively harden housestaff against the day when each will face massive hemorrhage alone, the only surgeon present. No need to enforce the discipline of a surgical service, which is essential if consistently good results are to be achieved. And no more recruiting.

And, lastly, there will be a freedom from daily discipline which I have not experienced since childhood.

INDEX

Note: Italicized numbers indicate illustrations.

Abbott, W. Osler, Dr., 73
Adler, Francis, 64
Administration, need to be learned, 366
Affirmative action programs, integration, 238, 239
Agnes Scott College, 79, 354, 356
Ainsworth, Temple, 201
Aird, Ian, 82
Akutsu, Tetsuzo, 287
Alabama College for Women (Montevallo), 8, 22, 27
Alabama State (Bryce) Mental Hospital, 52
Alexander-Williams, John, *311*
Alican, Fikri, 290
Allbritton, Frank F., Jr., *334*
Allen, J. Garrott, *334*
Alley, Frank, 196, 172–73
Allgöwer, Martin, 310–11
Alpha Omega Alpha, 51, 53, 55–56, 65, 68, 196–97, 270, 357
Amdrup, Erik, *311*
American Board of Surgery, 120, 132, 139, 156, 198, 290, 333, 339; members of, *334*
American Cancer Society, Clinical Research Committee of, 333
American College of Surgeons, past presidents of, 309
American Heart Association, 328
American Physiological Society, 147, 184
American Surgical Association, 156
Anand, Vinod, 369
André, Carl, 337, 294–95
Andy, Orlando, 198–99, 203, 222
Anesthesia, electrical, 218
Anesthesiology, recruitment problems, 229

Annenberg, Walter (Mrs.), Ambassador, 312
Arens, James, 290, 292
Arnold, Godfrey, 297–98
Artz, Curtis P., 202, *203–4*, 216, 228, 282, 302

Bach, 143
Bachman, Carl, 191
Bachmeyer, Arthur C., 161, 164
Bahnson, Henry, *161*, 164
Bahnson, Reid, 61
Bailey, Charles P., 159
Baker, James, 312
Ball, Robert M., 350
Ballistocardiograph, for measuring cardiac output, 73
Bama Skippers, dance orchestra, trombone playing in, 16
Banks, Major Gerald, 83–84, 86–87, 90, 94, 97–98, 107, 110
Banks, William Mitchell, 262
Bannister, Sir Roger, 344
Barker, Harold, 83, 86–87, 91, 94, 96, 107
Barker, Wiley F., 293, *334*
Barksdale, Lillian, 13
Barnard, Christiaan, 279, 285–86
Barnard, Mario, 286
Barnett, Ross, 236, 237–38
Barnett, William O., 236, 357
Baronio, G., 240
Bartlett, Marshall K., *334*
Bassett, Henry C., 36
Batson, Blair, 189
Battle of the Bulge, 87; repulsed, 94
Bauer, Walter, 56
Beal, John M., *334*
Beethoven, 62, 94, 108, 364

Bell, Warren, 185
Bengmark, Stig, *311*
Bergentz, Sven-Erik, 311
Bernard, Claude, 159
Billroth, Theodor, 118
Birmingham News, 22, 26
Bittenbender, G. B., 200–201, 203, 228–29
Blake, Thomas H., 201
Blake, Thomas M., xi
Blalock, Alfred, 56, 122, 159, 161, 174
Blount, Robert E., 230, 289, 295
"Blue baby," Blalock-Taussig operation for, 159
Blue Cross-Blue Shield, 339
Blumenstock, David A., 260, 285
Board certification, a major credential, 121
Borges D'Almeida, José A., *311*
Borst, Hans G., *311*
Boswell, Henry, 202
Bounds, Murphy, 87, 90, 98, 105
Breckenridge, C. G., 21
Brent, Leslie, 280–81, 332
Bricker, Eugene M., *334*
Bronk, Detlev, 41
Bruce, Sir John, 321
Brunini law firm, 301
Bryant, Paul "Bear," 20
Bryant, W. Alton, 195, 230
Bucherl, E. E. S., 325
Bunge, Jean, xi
Burnet, Sir Macfarlane, 242
Butler, "Colonel" Carleton, 20

Cachexia, in cancer patients, 132
Cadavers, in gross anatomy, decorum with, 34
Caine, Curtis, 192
Caldwell, Robert, 210
Calne, Roy, 252, 255
Campbell, Gilbert S., 235
Campbell Clinic, 170
Camp Ellis, 83–84
Camp Kilmer, 86
Camp Lee, 82, 84, 85
Camp Patrick Henry, 115
Cardiac catheterization, Nobel Prize for, 159
Cardiac output, decreased in dehydrated patients, 73–74

Cardiac surgery, some American pioneers in, *161*
Cardiovascular surgery comes of age, 159
Carlson, A. J., 81
Carlyle, Thomas, 33
Carmichael, Oliver Cromwell, 10
Carmichael, Patrick Henry, 10
Carr, Duane, 170–71, 177
Carrel, Alexis (Nobel Prize, 1912), 22–23, 163, 242
Carrillo, Felix Vilela, 317–18
Carter, James Earl, 295, 312
Carter, Robert E., 230, 295
Carter, Thelma, 196
Castro, Fidel, 315
Cepellini, R., 249
Chavez, Carlos M., 271, 273–74, 276–77, 324–25
Chavez, Pompeyo, 314–15
Chekov, 371
Chemotherapy, for solid tumors, 216
Chen, Ching-Jygh, 369
Cheney, Roger, 60–61
Child, Charles G., III, *334*
Chimpanzee, genetically close to man, 271
Churchill, Winston, 90, 104, 107, 110
Clarion Ledger, 208
Clark, Charles G., *311*
Clark, Eliot, 33
"Closed Society, The," politics, in Mississippi, 234, 235
Cockrell, Varden, 213
Coggeshall, Lowell T., 178, 179
Cole, Francis, 171
Coleman, James Plemon, 225–26
Columbia Universisty, 8; Alpha Omega Alpha lecture at, 270
Complications in Surgery and Their Management, W. B. Saunders (1981), 307
Comroe, Bernard, 37, 107
Conn, Harold, 213, 228
Cooley, Denton A., 161, 163, 288
Cooper, Theodore, 260
Corley, Karl, 85, 96, 98–99, 101, 105, 110
Cortesini, Raffaello, 332
Cournand, André F., 159
Craaford, Clarence, 159

Crawford, David, 369
Creech, Oscar, Jr., 200, 334
Crile General Hospital, 116
Critical Surgical Illness, W. B. Saunders (1971), 306
Cumbie, Gary, 23, 24, 26
Cummings, Lieutenant, 87, 91, 94, 96–99
Curie, Eve, 22
Curie, Madame, 22
Currier, Robert D., 344, 349
Cushing, Harvey, 54, 72, 271
Cuthbertson, David P., 123

Da Costa, 128
Da Costa Oration, Philadelphia County Medical Society, 128
Dale, Sir Henry, 124
Dalton, Martin, 265, 267
Daltro Ibiapina, Oliveira, 331–32
Damon Runyon Clinical Research Fellowship, 141, 147
Darwin, Charles, 240
Dausset, Jean (Nobel Prize, 1980), 250
Da Vinci, Leonardo, 72
Davis, Loyal, 311–12
Deaver, Michael, 312
DeBakey, Michael E., 152, 154, 161, 163, 200
Decoration, 81st Field Hospital, second battle star, 110
Demikhov, V. P., 260, 329, 330
Demobilization, after WW II, physicians seeking residency training, 121
De Renyi, George, 35
Derian, Patricia, 295
Derian, Paul, 294–95
DeVries, William C., 288
Dewall, Richard A., 160
Diary, wartime, handwritten entry, *109*
Dickson, John H., 196
Disraeli, 279
Divisions of Department of Surgery, University of Mississippi Medical Center, 198
Domagk, Gerhard, German chemist, first sulfonamide (Nobel Prize, 1939), 63
Donald, James, 25, 31
Donnelly, Captain Eileen, chief nurse, 81st Field Hospital, 85, 98

Dorfler, J., 242
Doughty, Marion, 25, 358
Douglas, Lloyd C., 22
Doupe, Joseph, 36
DP's (displaced persons), in Germany, diseases met in, 98
Drabkin, David L., 44, 145–46, 157
Dragstedt, Lester, 122; encouragement to the author, 283, 284
DRG (disease related groups), positives and negatives, 340, 341
Dripps, Robert, 41, 60
Drug addiction, in surgery residents, 232, 233
Dubost, Charles, first successful replacement of abdominal aortic aneurysm with homograft (1951), 164
Dudley, Rispah ("Ripsaw"), 11–12
Duggins, Percy, 80
Dunavant, David, 175–76
Dunlop, George R., 309
Dunphy, J. Englebert, 365

Eakins, Maxine, 369
Eckert, Charles, 334
Education, global, and quality of life, 364
Egdahl, Richard H., *311*
Einstein, A., 364
Eiseman, Ben, 190, 334
Eisenhower, General Dwight D., 104, 116, 124, 132, 172
Elebute, Emmanuel A., *311*
Eliason, Eldridge, chairman of Department of Surgery, University of Pennsylvania, 50, 55, 125–26, 130, 139
Elliott, Glen, 17
Elliott, Lieutenant, 93, 96, 98
Ellison, Edwin H., *334*
Emmerich, Oliver, 234–35
Enneking, William F., 201, 203, 229–30, 290
Eraslan, Sadan, 259, 273, 276
Essential list (of physicians), allowed each hospital during WW II, 67
Evans, Everett, 127
Evers, Medgar, 265
Executive Committee of Hospital Staff, University of Mississippi Medical Center, 298–99
Experience, importance of, in medical practice, 71, 72

Fabian, Leonard W., 273, 289
Faculty Promotions Committee, establishment of, 224, 225
Faculty Search Committee, establishment of, 225
Farm wages, during the Depression, 14
Fee splitting, 340
Fegiz, Gianfranco, *311*
Ferguson, Kreer, 126
Field Hospital, table of organization, 83
Field Hospital, 81st, personnel, at P.O.E. (1944), 88
Fisher, Luther, 369
Fisher, Robert, 35, 61
Fitts, William, 152
Fleming, Sir Alexander, discovery of penicillin, 40
Fletcher, Archibald, 61, 75, 79, 94, 135–36, 139, 156
Fluid Therapy, Lea and Febiger (1954), 306
Foreign language requirements for admission to medical school, 27
Forssmann, Werner, 159
Fortner, Joseph G., 257
Foster, Dr., 25–26
Foster, John H., 305
Foster, Lieutenant, 80
Franklin, Benjamin, 33, 53
Freshwater, Donald, 55, 68

Gallagher, Lillian ("Dean"), 54–56, 76, 78
Gama-Rodrigues, J. J., *311*
Gamelin, Marshal, and fall of France (1940), 42
Gardiner, Evelyn G., xi
Gavriliu, Dan, *311*
General George O. Squier, 112, 113, 115
Gerken, Vickie, 369
Gershon-Cohen, Jacob, early advocate of mammography, 136
Ghost surgery, 340
Gibbon, John H., 128, *160*, 163
Gilchrist, R. Kennedy, *334*
Gilmore, Cliff, 10
Gislason, John, 59, 61
Glenn, Elizabeth, 124
Glenn, John, 322

Glenn, William, 328
Glick, Bruce, 245
Gobel, Charles, 145
Godfrey, Douglas, 369
Godfrey, Lincoln, 35, 59, 68, 73, 77–78
Goebbels, 106
Goldschmidt, Samuel, 124
Grady, John, 11
Graham, Irene, 27
Graham, James, 145
Grand Rounds, major weekly teaching session, 72
Graves, Dean, 40
Gray, Sarah, 282, 351
Gresky, Alan, 17
Gronvall, John A., 230
Gross, Robert E., 159, 161, 163, 242
Guerin, Samuel, 44–45
Guthrie, Charles C., 242
Guyton, Arthur C., 184–85, 188–89, 193, 223
Guyton, Billy, 193

Haick, Alexander, Jr., 369
Hamburger, Jean, 252
Handel, 143
Hanlon, C. Rollins, 260, 285, 302, 304, 309, 334
Hardin, Creighton A., 260
Hardy, Agnes, 8, 145, 360
Hardy, Bettie, 197, 347, 351–52, 355–57
Hardy, Emily (Dolly), 8, 360
Hardy, Fred Henry, Sr. (father), 6, 5–17, 21, 27, 31; death of (1941), 51–52, 348
Hardy, Fred, Jr., 8, 12, 360
Hardy, James Daniel: birth of, 5; twin brother of, 5–6; parents of, 5–9; siblings of, 8; education, elementary, 11–13; choosing a profession, 17; education, high school, 13–18; teaching assistant, biology and zoology, University of Alabama, 23; medical school acceptance at Pennsylvania, 25; Department of German (Alabama), invitation to join declined, 25; graduation from the University of Alabama, 26; medical school study discipline, 33; ROTC, medical school,

fateful decision, 41; Carlisle Barracks (1940–44), 41, 42, 76–78, 86, 105; medical school, junior year, with Julian, 46; Alpha Omega Alpha election, 51; summer extern, Alabama State Mental Hospital, 52; medical school, senior year, 53–57; sarcoidosis, effort to distinguish from tuberculosis, 54; internship application interviews, techniques, 54–55; first publication, effect of sulfanilamide powder on wound healing, 55; oral examinations, experience in taking, 57; medical school graduation, 57, 58; commissioned 1st Lieutenant, 57; internship, Hospital of the University of Pennsylvania, 58; medical resident at Penn, duties and prerogatives, 70; Harrison Department of Surgical Research, 73; hypoproteinemia, impaired amino acid absorption in, 74; gelatin, as plasma expander, research in, 75; acute blood loss, personal signs and symptoms, 77; army induction, Carlisle Barracks (22 April 44), 77; marriage contract, 79; first permanent army assignment, officer's pool, Stark General Hospital, Charleston, S.C., 79; hospital train medical officer, 79; Cushing General Hospital, efficient organization at, 80; McGuire General Hospital, Richmond, assignment to, 80; learning to fly, 80–81; Africa Korps, troops of, transport to Idaho, 82; private pilot written examination, 83; Camp Ellis, Illinois, 81st Field Hospital, assignment to, 83, 84; "Heartless Herman," 85, 116; embarkation, 81st Field Hospital (24 Dec 44), 87; *HMS Vollendam*, 87, 89–91, 122; 81st Field Hospital lands in Scotland, 91; patient in 109th General Hospital (pneumonia), 92; sprained ankle, severe, 93; Channel crossing, on *Sobieski*, Le Havre, France, 95; Chief of Medicine, 81st Field Hospital, Germany, 98; D.P.s (displaced persons) in Germany, diseases met in, 98; Roosevelt is dead ("Ist todt")!, 99; Heilbronn, German Army General Hospital evacuated, 99; Hitler is dead, 102; nicotine poisoning, case of, 103; Germans surrender (7 May 45), 104; V-E Day (8 May 45), 104; Heidelberg, 81st Field Hospital, alerted for movement to CBI (China-Burma-India) theater, 105; twins, a reunion in Germany, 105; St. Victorette Staging Area, southern France, 106; Marseille, residue of war, 106; *Marché noir* (black market), 106; Russia, a new colossus, 107; a French connection, 107; censoring letters, 108; 81st Field Hospital, second battle star, 110; Banks, Lt. Col. and 81st C.O., wounded in head, 110; Moring, Major John B., new C.O. of 81st Field Hospital, 111; "atomic bomb" dropped on Japan, 111; Russia declares war on Japan, 112; embarkation for China-Burma-India theater, at Marseille, 112; Japanese surrender! (14 Aug 45), 113; 81st Field Hospital deactivated (14 Dec 45), 116; Crile General Hospital, Cleveland, 116; Pentagon, the, Washington, 116; ENT, chief of, the Pentagon, 116, 117; decision for surgery instead of internal medicine, 117; residency in surgery finally achieved, 118; surgical resident, Penn, 132; cachexia, in cancer patients, research project, 132; mortality conference, search for truth, 137; chief resident in surgery, 139; cardiothoracic training application successful, 141; marriage, Decatur, Georgia (July 1, 1949), 143; surgery staff, University of Pennsylvania, 144; heavy water measurements successful, for determination of total body water, 145; body composition, measurement of, 146; Damon Runyon Fund, meeting of fellows in New York, 147; "worst case," in Philadelphia, 150; Louise, first child, born (1950), 151; another career decision, academic surgery vs. pure private practice, 151; decision to leave Philadelphia, 152; University of Tennessee, Memphis, decision for,

Hardy, James Daniel (*continued*) 154; American Board of Surgery examinations passed, 156; author of opening paper, American Surgical Association (1952), 156; *Surgery and the Endocrine System*, accepted by W. B. Saunders for publication, 157; Master of Medical Science in physiological chemistry, University of Pennsylvania (1951), 158; the Medical College of the University of Tennessee, Surgery staff member and Director of Surgical Research (1951), 167; Damon Runyon Fund, signal importance of a small grant, 168; national research support, in Memphis, 168; Hardy, Julia Ann, born (1951), 169; West Tennessee Tuberculosis Hospital, thoracic surgery in, 171; mitral commissurotomy, first case in Memphis, 171; surgical consultant to Oak Ridge Institute of Nuclear Studies, 173; "The Cause of Death in Thermal Burns," research grant title, 174; Society of University Surgeons, elected to membership, 176; offered chairmanship of surgery at new University of Mississippi Medical Center in Jackson, accepted (23 Mar 53), 179; Jackson (1955), 181; departmental chairmen in the clinical sciences, search for, 185; town-gown conflicts, 190–93; meetings with Chancellor J. D. Williams, in Memphis, 194; in Oxford, 194–95; contract signed, University of Mississippi Medical Center, 195; Alpha Omega Alpha address, University of Tennessee, Memphis, 197; Surgical faculty, new department of surgery, recruitment of faculty, 198, 200–207; first full-time faculty, Department of Surgery, University of Mississippi Medical Center, 203; administrative organization, Department of Surgery, University of Mississippi Medical Center, 206; nonprofessional personnel, major contribution of, to department of surgery, 207; first patient operated in University of Mississippi hospital, 209; surgical residency training program, University of Mississippi Medical Center, 211–12; hospital affiliations, University of Mississippi Medical Center, 213–14; medical student teaching, University of Mississippi Medical Center, 214; patients, sources of, new University Hospital, 214; research, new Department of Surgery, University of Mississippi Medical Center, 215; research, financial support, University of Mississippi Medical Center, 215–16; chemotherapy, for solid tumors, a first meeting at National Institutes of Health (1956), 216; resident research, manifold values of, 217; electrical anesthesia, 218; laboratory fraud, experiences with, 218–19; departmental finances, 219; departmental financial controls, internal, critical importance of, 220; town-gown showdown, Jackson (1956), 220–23; medical school policies, 223–25; a governor's operation, 225–26; accomplishments and mistakes, early, Department of Surgery, 226–28; drug addiction, in surgery residents, 232–33; first open-heart surgery in Mississippi, 233–34; "The Closed Society," politics, in Mississippi, 234–35; integration of "Ole Miss," impact on Medical Center and the department, 236–37; The William Mitchell Banks Memorial Lecture, 262–63; first lung transplant in man, 264–68; first heart transplant in man, 272; Sixth International Transplantation Conference, bitter criticism, 278; Second World Symposium on Heart Transplantation, 1959, Montreal, 284; a heart is transplanted in Capetown, 285; another anesthesia crisis, 289; Mississippi Surgical Forum, 293; orthopaedic uprising (1976), 294–97; the ENT-plastic surgery struggle, 297–302; Federal lawsuit, ENT surgeons against University of Mississippi Medical Center, 301; sixty years, a fateful age in a surgeon's life, 302; American College of Surgeons, 302;

books by author, selected examples, 306; foreign speaking, decision for using native language, 310; editor, *World Journal of Surgery*, 310; a day with President and Mrs. Reagan in Washington, 311; called urgently to Peru, President Velasco Alvarado, ruptured abdominal aortic aneurysm, 313; fasciotomy, performed on President Velasco, Lima, Peru, 316; Order of the Sun award, Peruvian embassy, Washington, 318–19; organization of International Surgical Group, 321; International Congress on Respiratory Diseases (Turin, Italy, 1965), 322; visiting professor, teaching hospitals in Honolulu (1965), 322; leg reimplantation in man, 323; National Heart Foundation of Australia (1966), 323; Royal Australasian College of Surgeons and the Research Society, Perth (1966), 323; First Argentine Congress of Angiology, Buenos Aires (1966), 324; University of Lund in Sweden (1968), 325; West Berlin (1968), 325; Marnoch Lecture, University of Aberdeen in Scotland (1969), 326; Surgical Research Society of Great Britain and Society of University Surgeons (United States), London (1969), 326; mission to Greece (1970), 326–27; University of Athens, 327; International Society of Surgery, Russia (1971), 327; Heart Institute, Moscow (1971), 328; Cancer Institute, Moscow (1971), 328; Vishnevsky Institute, Moscow (1971), 328, 329; The Kremlin (1971), 330; Indian embassy reception, Moscow (1971), 330; Rio de Janeiro (1973), 331; Transplantation Society, London (1977), 332; American Board of Surgery, service with, 333; National Board of Medical Examiners, service with, 333; National Institutes of Health, surgery study section, 333; National Institutes of Health, Anesthesiology Training Grant Committee, 333, 335; American Cancer Society, Clinical Research Committee, service with, 335; President, Society of University Surgeons (1961), 336; President, Society for Surgery of the Alimentary Tract (1969), 336; President, Southern Surgical Association (1972), 336; President, American Surgical Association (1975), 336; President, American College of Surgeons (1980), 337; International Society of Surgery (Société Internationale de Chirurgie), elected president of (1983), 5; honors and awards, 337–38; first Horace G. Smithy Lecture, 337; first Julian Johnson Lecture in Thoracic Surgery, 338; honorary memberships in French Association of Surgery (Association Française de Chirurgie), French Academy of Medicine (Académie Nationale de Médecine), and Royal College of Surgeons of England (London), 338; the surgeon becomes the patient, 343; transient ischemic attack, 343; Executive Committee of the International Society of Surgery, Basel, Switzerland, 1981, 344; letter to Sir Roger Bannister, 334; concerning automobile accident involving, 345; traumatic regressive amnesia of, 346; fractures sustained by, 346; slowing of heart rate of, 346; pacemaker considered for, 346; Baylor Hospital, Dallas, right carotid endarterectomy, 348; second carotid operation (left), UMC, Jackson, 349; heart "operation," balloon angioplasty, 350; family, 351–61; king of the Carnival Ball, 354; family education and marriages, 356–58; death of a twin, 358–61; a look backward and a summing up, 362–71

Hardy, James Daniel (grandfather), 7
Hardy, James Daniel (physiologist), name identical to that of author, 50
Hardy, John, 8, 12, 211, 348, 360
Hardy, Julia Ann, 169, 351–52, 355–58
Hardy, Julia Ann P. (mother), 5, 6, 7–17, 19, 21, 31, 47, 51, 57, 90, 92, 107, 115
Hardy, Julian Patterson, 5–6, 8, 11, 13, 17–19, 21–22, 25–26, 37, 40, 48, 51,

380 Index

Hardy, Julian Patterson (*continued*) 54–55, 56, 57, 63, 82, 91, 105, 302, 348, 358, 359, 360, *361*
Hardy, Katherine, 197, 338, 347, 349, 351, 352, 353, 355–58
Hardy, Louise Sams ("Weezie"), 79, 81, 138, *142*–43, 144, 147–48, 151–52, 156, 167, 169–70, 177, 179, 194–95, 208, 223, 309, 322, 326, 330, 347–49 351–52, 355, 355, 356–57
Hardy, Louise Scott, 98, 151, 156, 167, 169–70, 351–52, 354, 355, 356–57
Hardy, Taylor, 8, 11, 12, 18, *360*; law school, 37
Hardy's Textbook of Surgery, J. B. Lippincott Co. (1983), 307
Hare, William, 184
Harken, Dwight E., 159
Harris, Seale, 57
Harris, William, 55, 104
Harrison, Samuel P., *334*
Hart, William, *369*
Harvey, A. Magee, 315, 318
Harvey, Major, 92
Habif, David V., *334*
Hayward, Malcolm, 35
Head, John D. ("Jug"), 85
Heaton, Leonard, 127
Heberer, Georg, *311*
Hederman, 210
Heine, 102
Helm, Robert, 36
Helsinki Declaration, of guidelines for human investigation, 249
Hendrix, James H., 176, 201
Henley, Lydy, 354
Hensel, Lieutenant, 105
Hesdorffer, Eugene, 201
Hill-Burton Act, massive hospital building in U.S.A., 121
Hitler, 102
H.M.S. Beagle, 240
Hodo, Henry, 31
Hogue, Mary, 35
Holden, William D., 278, *334*
Hollender, Louis F., *311*
Holmes, Oliver Wendell, 152
Holmes, Verner, 225
Hoover, President, 14

Hospital clinical laboratories, Warren Bell, chairman of, 185
Houston, Frances, 27
Howard, John, 133
Hufnagel, Charles, 251
Hughes, James L., 297
Human organ transplantation. *See* Transplantation
Hume, David, *241*, 251–52
Hunter, John, 121, 123

Integration of "Ole Miss," 236–38
International Friends, 353
International Society of Surgery (Société Internationale de Chirurgie), 5, 310, 311, 336, 350
International Surgical Group, 321
Itinerant surgery, 340

Jabaley, Michael, 297
Jaffe, Bernard M., *311*
Jefferson, Thomas, 107
Jenkins, Ruth, 354
Jobe, Dr., 198
John Gaston Hospital, 170, 174
Johnson, Julian, 126, 130, 132; birth and achievements, 139–40, 141, 150–52, 338
Johnson, Paul, 324
Johnson, Samuel B., 202, *369*
Johnston, J. Harvey, Jr., 192–93
Jones, Edley, 201
Jones, Irene, 27
Justice, racial standards of, 9
Juvenelle, André A., 260

Kassner, James L., 36
Kaufman, Captain, 79
Kaufmann, Berwind P., Professor of Genetics, University of Alabama, 25
Keith, Virginia W., xi, 196, 207–8
Keliher, Alice, 22
Kelly, Officer, 239
Kennedy, John F., 237
Kern, Richard, editor and outstanding teacher, 49
Khrushchev, 330–31
Kidney, transplantation of. *See* Transplantation

King, Gordon, 26
King, Martin Luther, 235
King George, 104
Kinnaert, Paul, *311*
Kirby, Charles, 139–41, 150, 152
Kirchbaum, Bill, 79
Kirklin, John W., 61, *161*, 163
Kitchens, Jim, 39
Kittle, C. Frederick, 260
Kolff, Willem, 251, 278, 280, 287–88
Koop, C. Everett, 64, 75
Krueger, Ronald P., 369
Kuijjer, Peter J., *311*
Kurrus, Fred D., 273
Kuzin, Michael I., *311*
Kyle, James, 307

Labecki, Thaddeus D., 273
Lafferty, Jack, 34
Lahey, Frank, 129–30
Lambertson, Christensen, 74
Landsteiner, Ernst, 251
Lawrence, C. O., 12–13
Lazarides, Demetrios P., *311*
Leadership, dimensions of, requirements for, 367
Le Bonheur Children's Hospital, 175
Lehan, Patrick H., 350
Lewis, Russell, 84, 110
Liefert, Carl, 94, 96, 110
Lillehei, C. Walton, 160, *161*
Lindberg, Charles A., 23
Liszt, 108
Little, Louie, 358
Liver, transplantation of. *See* Transplantation
Lockey, Myron, 297–99, 300
Lockwood, John, 73, 75
Loeb, Robert, 76
Longmire, William P., Jr., 309
Long-Range Planning Committee, 231
"Look rounds," teaching value of, 71
Lotterhos, William E., 221
Love, Jack, W. P., 80
Lower, Richard R., 261, 285
Lowery, A. B., flight instructor, 80–81
Lucas, Marjorie, 129, 149
Lukens, Francis, 74

Lung, transplantation of. *See* Transplantation
Lutkin, Isabel, 356
Lyons, Leonard, 148

MacArthur, General Douglas, 107
McBurney, Charles, 175
McCaa, Connie, 369
McGuire General Hospital, 78, 80, 83
McLaughlin, Charles W., Jr., 309
MacLean, Lloyd D., *311*
McMullan, Martin, 291
Magruder, Thomas, 31
Mahaffeys, 16
Málek, Prokop, *311*
Malphurs, Ojus, 369
Malpractice insurance, 340, 342
Mammography, advent of, 135
Markley, George, 60
Marland, Thomas, 223
Marnoch Lecture, 326
Marston, Robert Q., 230, 232, 238, 248, 264, 269, 279
Martin, Mary, 148
Martin, Walter, 81, 87, 91, 97–98
Mattox, Hazel M., 207–8
Maxwell, George, 97
Mayfield, Peabody B., Tuscaloosa, 52
Mayock, Robert, 36
Medawar, Sir Peter (Nobel Prize, 1960) 242–44; letter from, *244*, 280
Medical fraternities, social centers for unmarried students, 32
Medical school, then and now (1938–42 compared with 1985), 42–44
Medicare-Medicaid, 339
Medicine, Department of, at Mississippi, Robert Snavely, chairman, 188
Meese, Edwin, 312
Mendel, Gregor, 240
Mercadier, Maurice, 310–11
Meredith, James, 236, 238, 324
Merendino, K. Alvin, 334
Merrill, John, 252
Metabolic balance studies, new body composition hypotheses, 123
Methodist Rehabilitation Center, 295
Metras, Henri, 260
Military melancholy, anatomy of, 81

Miller, Richard, 369
Miller, T. Grier, 54, 66–67, 71, 81, 117–18
Mississippi Academy of Orthopaedics, 296
Mississippi Surgical Forum, 293
Mitral valve commissurotomy, 15; first case in Memphis, 171
Monet, 243
Montgomery, "Dr. Jack," 23
Montgomery, Field Marshal, 104
Moody, Frank G., *311*
Moore, Francis, 122, 146, 255
Moore, Robert M., *334*
Moretz, William H., *334*
Moring, John B., 111
Morrison, Winsor, 369
Mortality conferences, at Penn, 137; at Mississippi, 212–13
Moss, Henry, 129
Mounger, William H., 236
Moyer, Carl M., 152, 154
Moynihan, Lord, 120
Mudd, Roger, 312
Muller, William H., Jr., *309*, *334*
Mullins, Jesse, 290
Murphy, Franklin, 51, 76
Murray, Joseph, *241*, 252
Music, in church, 10; in the home, 10; football band, 22; glee club, 22; military band, 22; piano, 61–62; with trombone in dance band and in the University of Alabama concert orchestra, 22
Musselman, Merle M., *334*
Mussolini, Benito, 102

Najarian, John, *241*, 252, 257, *311*
Nakayama, Fumio, *311*
Named lectures, 320, 326
Nardi, George L., *334*
National Board of Medical Examiners, 333
National time tithing, 333
Neely, William A., 196–97, 273, 350
Neer, Charles, 55
Neill, Charles L., 200
Nelson, Colonel, 87
Nelson, Norman C., 230, 294–95
Nemir, Paul, Jr., 306

Neptune, Wilford B., 260
Newala, Alabama, 5, 7
Newton, Michael, 186, 213
Nizen, Paul, 362
Noffzigger, Lynn, 312
Norris, Chaplain, 83, 91
Nyhus, Lloyd M., *311*

Oak Ridge Institute of Nuclear Studies, 173
Obstetrics and Gynecology, Department of, at Mississippi, Michael Newton, chairman, 186
Ochsner, Alton, 326, 354
Olivier, C., 257
Ong, Guan B., *311*
Open-heart surgery, a triumph of, *162*
Operations of General Surgery, Orr, guide to safeguards at operation, 138
Order of the Sun, Peru, 318–19
Ormandy, Eugene, 38
Osler, Sir William, 54, 72, 107, 209
Oulton Park Staging Area, 91, 93, 94
Outpatient surgicenters, 342

Palmer, George, Professor of Chemistry, Atomic Structure, letter to, 24
Pankratz, David S., xi, 178–79; birth, education and achievements, 183–84, 185–97, 198, 202, 204, 211, 220, 222–24, 226–27; resignation of, 229–31
Papadopoulos, George, prime minister, Greece, 327
Parker, Lieutenant, 99
Parks, Sir Alan, *308*
Parsons, Virginia, 354
Parsons, Willard H., 204
Pasteur, Louis, 22, 36, 253, 322, 364
Patiño, José F., *311*
Patton, General George, 93–94, 132
Payne, Franklin, 50
Pearl Harbor attack and World War II (1941), 51
Pediatrics, Department of, at Mississippi, Blair E. Batson, chairman, 189
Peer review, 342
Pennsylvania Hospital, 53
Pentagon, the, 116–19
Pepper, Claude, 39

Pepper, D., Sergeant Major, 80, 83
Pepper, O. H. Perry, 46, 56, 68–69, 71–72, 76, 107, 118, 123
Pepper, William, 33, 40
Perry, Theodore, 350
Perth Daily News, 324
Peru, mission to, 313–19
Peters, Jane, 207–8
Philadelphia Academy of Surgery, 147
Philadelphia College of Physicians Library, 54
Philadelphia General (Old Blockley) Hospital (PGH), 53, 54, 135
Philadelphia Inquirer, 33, 38
Philadelphia Music Appreciation Committee, successful distribution of low cost classical albums, 38
Phillips, Arthur, 48
Physiologic surgery, rise of, 120–23; some leaders in, 123
Pichlmayr, Rudolph, 311
Pinto, Lieutenant, 92
Plastic bags for blood storage, an early invention, 127
Pneumonia, lobar, 8
Pobol, Herr Doktor, 103
Political interference, in Mississippi education, 190
Poynor, Diggs, Captain, instructor in military tactics, University of Alabama, 1861–65, 7
Poynor, Dudley, 17
Poynor, Julia Ann. *See* Hardy, Julia Ann P.
Presbyterian church, 10
Presbyterian Hospital, 53
Professional practice audit, 342
"Prometheus Bound," Philadelphia Museum of Art, liver regeneration in, 38
Psoriasis, lack of cure, 62
Pulmonary surgery, development of, 160
Pump oxygenator, first human open-heart operation with (1952), 160; first at UMC, 233, 234

Quail hunting, bird dogs in, 15

Radiology, Department of, at Mississippi, Robert D. Sloan, Chairman, 188

Raju, Seshadri, 347, 350, 369
Ravdin, Elizabeth (Betty, "Sis"), 128
Ravdin, Isidor Schwaner, 125; birth, 124; education, 124; marriage, 124; positive relationship with basic scientists, 124–25; his gallbladder operation, 125–26; commander, 20th General Hospital in Assam, 126; Major General, 126; Chairman, Department of Surgery, University of Pennsylvania, 126; reorganization, Penn department of surgery after WW II, 126; his selection of Julian Johnson and Jonathan Rhoads, 126; etiquette of surgical consultations, 127; operation on President Eisenhower, 127; children, 128; atherosclerosis, complications of, 128; anti-Semitism, 129; as a public speaker, 129; respect for loyalty, 130; letter to James D. Hardy regarding Ravdin's memoirs, 130; death at seventy-eight, 131; "surgical conscience," 133; remarkable memory for patients' names, 134
Ravdin, Robert, 128
Ravdin, William, 128
Ravitch, Mark, 303
Reading, habit of, 13
Reagan, Nancy, 311–12
Reagan, Ronald, 311–12
Reconstruction, bitter memories of, 15
Red Cross, mobile refreshments unit at POE, 87
Reemtsma, Keith, 241, 271, 278, 334
Reilly, Frank, 34
Reisman, 87, 106
Renoir, 364
Research, importance of, achievements and future challenges, 365; requirements for successful pursuit of, 74; resident, value of, 217
Rhoads, Jonathan E., 32, 63, 124–26, 132; birth and achievements, 137, 138–39, 141, 144, 152, 153; career advice, 176, 309, 321, 334
Rice, James, 223
Richards, Dickinson W., 159
Richards, Victor, 334
Riegel, Cecilia, 124

Rimsky-Korsakov, 108
Rittenberg, David, 145–46
Roberts, Brooke, 151
Roberts, Dean, 196–97
Rodriguez, Jorğe A., 196, 236
Roffman, Larry, 80
Rommel, General, 82
Roosevelt, Franklin D., 16, 47, 90, 99
Rose, Edward, 65–66, 71
Rosenbach, Abraham, 306
Rosenthal, Otto, 124
Röska, Karl-Otto, 356
ROTC, required course, University of Alabama, 20
Royal College of Surgeons of Edinburgh, 321
Ruffin, Mary Ruth, 207–8
Rumble, Ruth, 68
Rundstedt, General, 86–90
Runyon, Damon, 141, 147–48, 168
Rushton, Fred, 369

Sabiston, David C., Jr., 311, 334
Saier, family of, Marseille, 108, 110
Sandblom, Philip, 326
Sanders, R. L., 176, 204
Sauer, Barry, 369
Schaefer, Sir Edward Sharpey, 124
Schenkin, Henry, 60
Schilling, John A., 334
Schwartz, Seymour I., 311
Schwegman, Cletus, 152
Scientific Foundations of Surgery, William Heinemann Medical Books, Ltd. (1981), 307
Scimeca, Officer, 110
Scott, Byron, 249
Scott, Captain, 87, 100
Scott, H. William, 309
Second opinion, requirements, 342
Sen, P. K., 147, 324
Senning, Ake, 311
Shannon, Walton, 202
Shelley, 94
Shires, G. Thomas, 309, 311, 334
Shumway, Norman E., 241, 261, 278–79, 285
Silver, James W., 234
Simmons, General, 117
Slaney, Geoffrey, 338

Sloan, Margaret, 127
Sloan, Robert D., 188
Smith, Ben, 85, 102–3
Smith, Betty, 149
Smith, George, 326
Smith, Robert R., 347
Smith, William, 62
Smithsonian Institution, 267, 276
Smithy, Horace G., 337
Smythe, Henry F., Jr., 36
Snavely, Robert, 188, 211, 225–26
Sobieski (ship), 94
Society of University Surgeons, 176
Southern Methodist University, 356
Spangler, Henry Lee, 33
Speranza, Vincenzo, 310, 311
Sprunt, Douglas, 169, 173
Stalin, Joseph, 63, 110–11, 330
Stark General Hospital, 79
Starr, Albert, 163
Starr, Isaac, 50, 73–76, 81, 118, 127
Starzl, Thomas E., 241, 252, 255, 279, 311
State Times, 234
Stewardship, professional, personal accountability for, 368
Stinchfield, Frank E., 309
Stofer, Raymond C., 261
Stokes, John, 48
Stokes, Joseph, 62, 66
Stokowski, Leopold, 38
Story, Mark T., 357
Streptokinase and streptodornase, 127
Student Promotions Committee, establishment of, 223, 224
Sulya, Louis, 184
Superspecialization, disadvantages of, in diagnosis and treatment, 71
Surgeon General's Library, 54
Surgeons become clinical physiologists, 123
Surgery and the Endocrine System, W. B. Saunders, 1952, 157
Surgery, by untrained physicians, 340
"Surgical conscience," 133
Surgical instruments and sutures, special requirements for delicate operations, 163
Surgical organization committee work, 320

Surgical practice, changes over past forty years, 362
Surgical residency training program, University of Mississippi Medical Center, establishment of, 211–12
Sutherland, Francis A., 334
Suzuki, Akio, 292
Swan, Henry, 334
Swift Creek Maneuver Area, 82, 86

Taussig, Helen, 159
Tavener, 110
Tchaikovsky, 32
Teaching assistant, biology and zoology, University of Alabama, 23
Tedder, 104
Teeter, John, 148, 168
Thevenet, André, *311*
Thomason, Douglas, 145
Thompson, Jesse E., 347, 349
"Thoracoplasty" surgeons, 160
Thorbeck, Raphael V., *311*
Thorn, George, 251
Thorpe, Edward, 41–42
Timmis, Hilary, 162, 252, 292
Tompkins, Souther, 61
Town-gown conflict, 190–93, 220–23
Tracy, G. Douglas, *311*
Transplantation: history of, 240–42; legal problems in, 250; American pioneers in, 241; autografts, 240; allografts, 240; Mendelian laws of genetic inheritance, 242; heterografts, 242; genetics in, 243, 245; allograft reaction in, 245; immunology in, 243, 245; tissue typing in, 243, 245; organ procurement and storage in, 246; ethical questions in, 246–50; immunosuppressive therapy in, 243, 245; "self vs. non-self" in, 245; xenograft, 245; of liver, 255, 256; of pancreas, 256, 257; of small bowel, 257–58; of parathyroid, 258; of adrenal, 258–59; utero-ovarian, 259–60; of heart, 260–61; auto-, of kidney, for ureteral injury, 252; of kidney, between identical twins, "permanently" successful, 252; of kidney, three vignettes, 253–55; of kidney, chimpanzee, in humans, 270–71; of lung, 264–68; of lung, first, in man, operative technique, 266; of lung, massive public interest in, 268; of heart, first, in man, a "dry run," 271; of heart, report of a case, 272–76; of heart, operative permit for (1964), 274; of heart, surgical team, 275; technique of, 276; of heart, *in situ*, 277; of heart, bitter criticism resulting from, 278; of heart, aftermath a searing experience, 280; immunological rejection a principal problem in, 288
Transplantation Society, Ethics Committee of, 250
Trede, Michael, 311
Trombone, in lieu of rifle, in ROTC, 20
Truman, Harry S., 113
Tuberculosis, rampant in liberated displaced persons, Germany, 98
Turner, Anne Cole Bass, 196
Turner, M. Don, 196, 203, 273, 369
Tuttle, Officer, 110
Twins, James and Julian, birth of, 5
Twiss, Maurine, 239, 277

Udy, Ruth, 99
Undergraduate Medical Association Day, 55
Underwood, J. D., 202
University of Pennsylvania Hospital army medical unit (20th General Hospital) in Assam, 63
University hospitals, obligation to set standards, 196
University of Alabama, 7, 8
University of Frankfurt (Germany), 356
University of Pennsylvania, School of Medicine, 31–57, 34
University of Tennessee, Memphis, 7, decision for, 154; negotiations with, 155
U.S. Army, service with, at the Pentagon, 116–19; in Europe, 78–117

Vaeth, George, 80
V-E Day, 104
Vallery-Radot, René, 22
Vanderbilt University, 356
Vane, John, 46
Van Gogh, 106

NO LONGER THE PROPERTY
OF THE
UNIVERSITY OF R. I. LIBRARY